TUMOR MICROENVIRONMENT AND MYELOMONOCYTIC CELLS

Edited by **Subhra K. Biswas**

Tumor Microenvironment and Myelomonocytic Cells
Edited by Subhra K. Biswas

Published by InTech
Janeza Trdine 9, 51000 Rijeka, Croatia

Publishing Process Manager Maja Jukic

Technical Editor Teodora Smiljanic

Cover Designer InTech Design Team

Additional hard copies can be obtained from orders@intechopen.com

Tumor Microenvironment and Myelomonocytic Cells, Edited by Subhra K. Biswas
p. cm.
ISBN 978-953-51-0439-1

For EU product safety concerns:
IN TECH d.o.o., Prolaz Marije Krucifikse Kozulić 3, 51000 Rijeka, Croatia,
info@intechopen.com or visit our website at intechopen.com.

Meet the editor

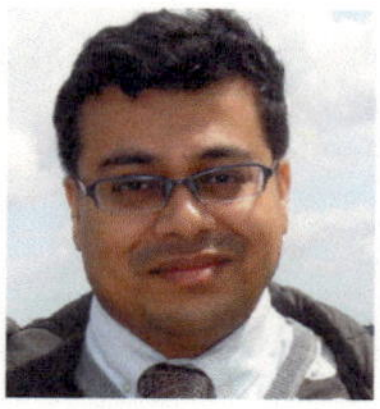

Dr. Biswas's research interests focus on investigating the role of monocytes and macrophages in different human diseases, in particular, cancer. Dr. Biswas completed his Ph.D in Biotechnology at Banaras Hindu University, India, following which he did his post-doctoral study at the Istituto di Ricerche Farmacologiche "Mario Negri" in Milan, Italy. He is a principal investigator at the Singapore Immunology Network (SIgN), Agency for Science, Technology & Research (A*STAR), Singapore. Dr. Biswas's major contribution in this field was the first molecular characterization of tumor associated macrophages. Dr. Biswas is a member of the American Association of Immunologists and European Macrophage and Dendritic Cell Society and an editorial board member of Scientific Reports, Cancer Microenvironment and Frontiers in Tumor Immunity.

Contents

Preface

Tumor microenvironment represents an extremely dynamic and diverse milieu consisting of different cell types (e.g. tumor cells, stromal cells), distinct physico-chemical stimuli (e.g. low oxygen or hypoxia) and a variety of humoral factors such as cytokines, chemokines and growth factors. The interplay of these different elements is crucial to tumor progression. Therefore, investigating the tumor microenvironment has a direct impact on the understanding of the mechanisms which regulate cancer progression.

Myelomonocytic cells have emerged as key players in the tumor microenvironment. In particular, tumor associated macrophages (TAMs) have served as the classical example of the tumor promoting actions of myelomonocytic cells. These cells constitute a major proportion of the inflammatory infiltrates associated with most solid tumors and a link between inflammation and cancer. One of the most direct evidence for the tumor promoting role of TAMs comes from studies which use transgenic approach to modulate TAM numbers in murine tumor models where TAM infiltration has been linked to tumor progression, angiogenesis and metastasis. Similarly, in many human cancers of the breast, cervix, bladder and prostrate, a high TAM density positively correlates with poor prognosis. More recently, other myelomonocytic cell types such as blood monocytes, Tie-2-Expressing Monocytes (TEMs), Myeloid-Derived Suppressor Cells (MDSCs), and Tumor Associated Neutrophils (TANs) have been shown to possess protumoral activity. Inspite of these evidences, several aspects of myelomonocytic cell repertoire in the tumor microenvironment remains to be understood. For example, the plasticity of these cells across different phases of cancer progression, the dialogue between these cells and other lymphocytic populations in the tumor tissues, and the possibility of re-programming the tumor microenvironment by strategies to modulate myelomonocytic cells *in vivo*.

The objective of this book is to present a comprehensive overview of the dynamic interaction between the tumor microenvironment and the myelomonocytic cells that leads to cancer progression. The focus is explaining how the tumor microenvironment polarizes the myelomonocytic cells to favor tumor growth and how these cells, in turn, contribute to the shaping and maintenance of the tumor microenvironment. Mechanisms regulating this process at the level of functional phenotypes, cytokine/chemokine circuits and molecular pathways have also been addressed. For the reader's ease, the book is divided into three broad sections: section 1 introduces some of the basic features of myelomonocytic cells and details the general functions and the diversity of these cells in the tumor microenvironment; Section 2 focusses on describing the tumor microenvironments of specific cancer types, such as brain cancer, liver cancer, oral cancer, lung cancer and melanoma and the role of myelomonocytic cells therein; Section 3 focusses on describing some new players (e.g. mesenchymal stem cells, microRNAs) and novel approaches (e.g. in vivo imaging) of studying the tumor microenvironments.

In the end, I would like to express my sincere gratitude to Profs Alberto Mantovani, Antonio Sica and Ajit Sodhi for mentoring me in the field of macrophage research. I am indebted to Saki, for her constant support and encouragement; to Prof. B. Lahiry for kindling my curiosity to look into the unknown. I am grateful to all my collaborators who have contributed to my research and the generous grant support from Biomedical Research Council (A*STAR). Finally, I would like to thank Maja and her colleagues at In Tech without whose help the production of this book would not have taken place.

Subhra K. Biswas, PhD
Principal Investigator
Singapore Immunology Network (SIgN),
Agency for Science, Technology & Research (A*STAR),
8A Biomedical Grove; #04 Immunos,
Singapore

Part 1

Myelomonocytic Cells – Phenotypic and Functional Diversity in Tumor Microenvironment

1

Cell Lineage Commitment and Tumor Microenvironment as Determinants for Tumor-Associated Myelomonocytic Cells Plasticity

Raffaella Bonecchi[1,2], Benedetta Savino[1], Matthieu Pesant[1] and Massimo Locati[1,2]
[1]*Istituto Clinico Humanitas IRCCS, Rozzano,*
[2]*Department of Translational Medicine, University of Milan, Milan, Italy*

1. Introduction

Myelomonocytic cells have long been recognized as key elements in tumor biology, with the potential to both elicit tumor and tissue destructive reactions and to promote tumor progression. Tumor-associated macrophages (TAM) from established tumors resemble alternative-activated macrophages associated with the resolution phase of inflammatory reactions and support tumor growth, angiogenesis, tissue remodeling, metastatization, and local immunosuppression. On the other hand, myeloid-derived suppressor cells are released from bone marrow pools in tumor-bearing animals and operate immunosuppressive activities in tumor-draining lymphoid organs, thus contributing to tumor escape from immune surveillance. The ambivalent role of myelomonocytic cells in tumor biology reflects their extraordinary plasticity. Tumor-derived signals in the local microenvironment have long been recognized for their ability to dictate macrophage-polarized activation. More recently, different monocyte subsets have been identified in both human and mouse, and cell lineage commitment is now emerging as a second element dictating cell functional polarization. We will here review current knowledge on the relative contribution of these two elements in the plasticity of myelomonocytic cells in the tumor setting.

2. Macrophage heterogeneity and polarization mechanisms

It is well established that tumors are environments of deregulated innate and adaptive immune responses. In this scenario, several evidences link tumor initiation and progression to chronic inflammation and recent findings have started dissecting the underlying cellular and molecular mechanisms. Macrophages represent one of the major myelomonocytic-derived cell types detectable within the tumor (Condeelis & Pollard 2006; Mantovani et al. 2008). It is now widely documented that tumor-associated macrophages (TAM) infiltration and biological activities within the tumor favor tumor growth/development (Pollard 2004; Lin et al. 2006; Mantovani et al. 2008), and consistently with this TAM infiltrate is usually associated with poor prognosis (Bingle et al. 2002; Lewis & Pollard 2006; Torroella-Kouri et al. 2009; Qian & Pollard 2010).

In contrast with classically activated macrophages (also known as M1 macrophages), in most tumors macrophages present an "alternative" activation state (Elgert et al. 1998). Originally based on *in vitro* studies inspired by the Th1/Th2 paradigma, macrophage activation can be schematically reconciled to two main phenotypes (Figure 1). Macrophages stimulated with the Th1 cytokine IFNγ and bacterial components such as LPS were named classically-activated macrophages or M1. They are characterized by a high production of IL-12 and IL-23, sustain the Th1 response by producing the chemokines CXCL9 and CXCL10, exhibit cytotoxic activity and high phagocytosis capacity, a high production or reactive oxygen intermediates (ROI), and display a good antigen presentation capability (Mantovani et al. 2002; Gordon 2003; Verreck et al. 2004; Gordon & Taylor 2005; Mantovani et al. 2005; Martinez et al. 2006). As a first line of defense against pathogens M1 play an important role in protection from viral and microbial infections. By their ability to produce high amounts a pro-inflammatory cytokines and mounting an immune response they also limit tumor growth/development. At the other extreme of the macrophage polarization spectrum are cells exposed to the Th2 prototypical cytokine IL-4, referred to as alternatively-activated macrophages or M2 macrophages (Stein et al. 1992). More recently, different forms of alternative activation polarization, collectively indicated as M2-like macrophages, have been reported as a consequence to activation by other stimuli, including the combination of immune complexes and TLR ligands, IL-10, TGFβ, and glucocorticoids (Mantovani et al. 2004). In general terms, hallmarks of M2 and M2-like cells are a high expression of negative

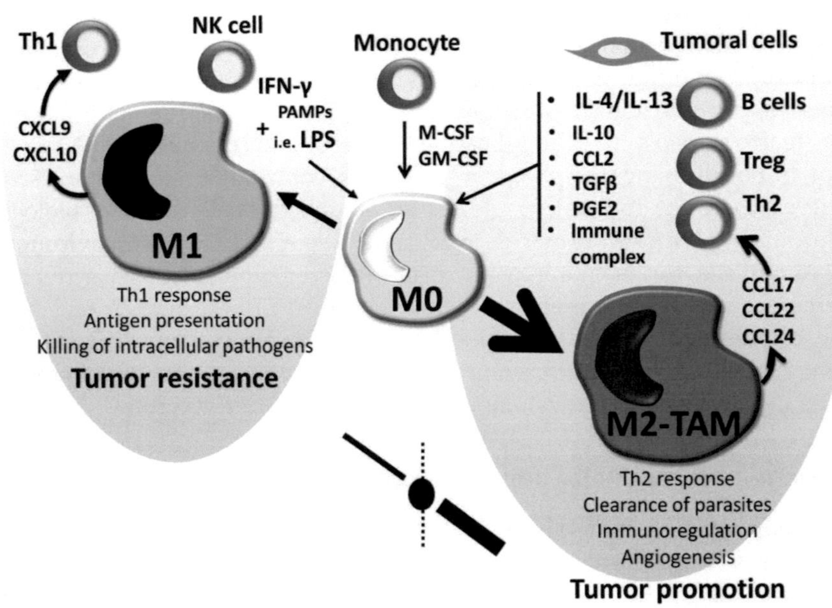

Macrophages differentiate from monocytes after M-CSF and/or GM-CSF stimulation. Subsequent polarization pathways include classical activation induced by IFNγ and LPS (M1 macrophages) and alternative activation triggered by IL-4/IL-13 (M2 macrophages). In the tumoral microenvironment, tumor-associated macrophages (TAMs) encounter diverse polarizing stimuli produced by tumoral cells, Th2 cells, Treg cells and B cells that skew their activation state to a phenotype resembling M2 macrophages, leading to tumor promotion/development.

Fig. 1. Macrophage polarization mechanisms and cancer: a dangerous imbalance.

regulators of the inflammatory response, including IL-10 and IL-1 receptor antagonist, and scavenger and galactose-type receptors (for example CD36 and the mannose receptor MRC1). M2 also produce abundant levels of the chemokines CCL17, CCL22 (Bonecchi et al. 1998) and CCL18 (Bonecchi et al. 2011) that in turn favor and sustain a Th2 response and tumor growth. Furthermore, M1 and M2 have distinct metabolic properties, as demonstrated by the dichotomic metabolic pathways of arginine (Munder et al. 1998; Hesse et al. 2001) and iron (Recalcati et al. 2010; Cairo et al. 2011). Major functions of M2 are their contribution in the clearance of parasites, wound healing and tissue remodeling, suppression of T-cell proliferation, pro-tumoral activity by virtue of their immunoregulatory and angiogenic abilities (Biswas & Mantovani 2010).

3. The tumor microenvironment: Macrophage polarity in Tumor-Associated Macrophages (TAM)

Several tumor-microenvironmental signals have been reported to instruct TAM polarization, including prostaglandin E2 (Rodriguez et al. 2005; Hagemann et al. 2006; Eruslanov et al. 2009; Eruslanov et al. 2010), migration-stimulating factor (MSF) (Solinas et al. 2010), and TGFβ (Flavell et al. 2010). Strong evidence also supports the relevance of M-CSF as a pro-tumoral factor attracting and triggering a M2-like polarization within the tumor. Indeed in human tumors, overproduction of M-CSF is associated with a poor clinical outcome in a wide range of cancers and several tumor types feature characteristics of an M-CSF-induced gene expression signature (Espinosa et al. 2009; Webster et al. 2010). This is consistent with transcriptional profiling analysis on *in vitro* differentiated macrophages, which have shown that M-CSF differentiated macrophages exhibit M2-like features, while GM-CSF differentiated macrophages exhibit M1-like features (Martinez et al. 2006; Fleetwood et al. 2007; Hamilton 2008). Accumulating experimental evidence from murine models of cancer further showed the pro-tumoral role of M-CSF. For example transplanted tumors' growth is impaired in M-CSF-deficient mice (Nowicki et al. 1996) and blockade of either M-CSF or is receptor leads to impaired tumor growth (Aharinejad et al. 2004; Kubota et al. 2009; Priceman et al. 2010). On the other hand, whereas no effect on tumor development was observed in the spontaneous mammary cancer model MMTV-PyMT in an M-CSF deficient background, the development of metastatic carcinoma was delayed (Lin et al. 2001). Angiogenesis is clearly a pro-tumoral feature as it provides the necessary "fuel" favoring tumor growth. In this context M-CSF has been shown to exert a pro-angiogenic effect in macrophages by inducing the production of VEGF (Curry et al. 2008).

A second pathway skewing TAM to the M2 phenotype is sustained by the Th2-derived cytokines IL-4 and IL-13. In the spontaneous mammary carcinoma model driven by PyMT both cytokines have been shown to be responsible for the M2 polarization of TAMs (DeNardo et al. 2009). In this model IL-4 derived from $CD4^+$ T cells and IL-13 derived from NKT cells instruct TAM an M2-like polarization leading to tumor development. Conversely, blockade of IL-4Rα led to a diminished M2-like gene expression profile and a switch to M1-associated gene expression, ultimately resulting in increased tumor surveillance. IL-4-induced M2 polarization of TAM has also been evidenced in a model of pancreatic cancer (Gocheva et al. 2010). IL-4 induced the activity of cathepsin in TAM, resulting in increased angiogenesis and tumor growth. The contribution of IL-13 to the M2 polarization of TAM has been demonstrated in the 4T1 mammary carcinoma model (Sinha et al. 2005). In this context, macrophages from CD1d-deficient mice (that lack NKT cells) show a M1 tumoricidal phenotype and metastasis resistance. IL-10 is also well known to induce an M2 phenotype. In tumor, IL-10 produced by Treg cells has been shown to dampen TAM capacity to mount a T cell mediated immune response (Kuang et al. 2009). B cells are also a source of tumoral IL-10. It has been demonstrated that IL-10 production by B-1 cells induced a M2 polarization of TAMs in a B16 melanoma model (Wong, S. C. et al. 2010). Besides the contribution of B cells-derived IL-10 in driving M2 polarization of TAM, new evidence support that B cells skew TAM to a M2 phenotype via production of T cell-dependent autoantibodies against an extracellular matrix component in a K14-HPV16 skin carcinogenesis model (de Visser et al. 2005; Andreu et al. 2010).

Finally, emerging evidence indicate that besides their major role in monocyte recruitment chemokines, CCL2 (MCP-1) in particular, may also be involved in macrophage polarization in the tumor burden (Roca et al. 2009). Indeed, human CD11b^{+} peripheral blood mononuclear cells induced to differentiate upon CCL2 stimulation upregulated M2 markers such as CD14 and CD206 (also known as Mannose Receptor 1). This M2 polarizing effect and thus pro-tumoral role of CCL2 is paralleled with the observation that many tumors overexpress CCL2 and these high levels have been associated with a bad outcome in cancer patients (Qian & Pollard 2010). It was furthermore recently reported in a murine breast-cancer model that CCL2 induced inflammatory monocytes infiltration in tumors (Qian et al. 2011). Moreover, tumor cells-derived CCL2 was shown to play a prominent role in metastasis development.

4. Cell lineage commitment: Monocyte subsets

Experimental evidence highlights that macrophage plasticity depends not only on the specific microenvironment encountered upon their extravasation from the circulation, but also on the existence of myelomonocytic subsets and lineage-committed TAM subpopulations that exploit diverse tumor-promoting activities (Coffelt et al. 2010b; Geissmann et al. 2010a; Geissmann et al. 2010b). On the basis of morphology and differential expression of antigenic markers, three types of blood monocytes (classical, intermediate, and nonclassical) have been described for both human and murine system (Ziegler-Heitbrock et al. 2010). In the mouse monocytes, which express CD115 (M-CSF receptor) and CD11b (Mac 1), are classified based on the expression level of Ly6C (one of the epitopes recognized by the anti-Gr-1 monoclonal antibody) in Ly6C^{high}CD43^{+} or classical monocytes, Ly6C^{high}CD43^{++} or intermediate monocytes and Ly6C^{low}CD43^{++}or nonclassical monocytes. These two subsets have been demonstrated to have different functions and migration patterns (Auffray et al. 2009), as classical monocytes are CX3CR1^{low}CCR2^{+}CD62L^{+} and are actively recruited to sites of inflammation whereas nonclassical monocytes were CX3CR1^{hi}CCR2^{-}CD62L^{-} and make homing to non-inflamed tissues. Recently, Geissman and colleagues demonstrated that the nonclassical monocyte subset constantly patrols the blood vessel wall and can be rapidly recruited to sites of inflammation before the arrival of classical monocytes (Auffray et al. 2007). The developmental relationship between the two monocyte subsets is still unclear. Experimental data suggest the possibility of a common precursor that gives rise to both classical and nonclassical monocytes. Adoptive transfer of classical monocytes demonstrated that this subset decreased the expression of Ly6C giving rise to nonclassical monocytes (Yrlid et al. 2006; Varol et al. 2007; Movahedi et al. 2010).

However, the generation of nonclassical monocytes has not been affected by antibody-mediated depletion or genetic defect in classical monocytes (Scatizzi et al. 2006; Feinberg et al. 2007; Mildner et al. 2007; Alder et al. 2008). Monocyte subsets were also identified in the human settings, with some consistency and some discrepancies as compared to the murine setting. Three human monocyte subsets were defined based on the expression levels of CD14 and CD16 (the FcγRIII molecule): classical monocytes ($CD14^{++}CD16^{-}$), intermediate monocytes ($CD14^{++}CD16^{+}$) and non-classical monocytes ($CD14^{+}CD16^{++}$). Gene expression profiles of these subsets indicates that they exhibit common gene expression patterns (at intermediate levels mirroring the CD14/CD16 levels) but also display unique features that potentially argue for distinct roles of these subsets in the immune process (Wong, K. L. et al. 2011; Zawada et al. 2011). Classical and non-classical monocytes have both pro-inflammatory activities for examples in response to LPS challenge but differ in the cytokine/chemokine repertoire they produce in response to LPS (Wong, K. L. et al. 2011). Moreover, non-classical monocytes show "patrolling" properties and appear to be very responsive to virus stimulation (Cros et al. 2010). So far, no specialized function has been assigned for intermediate monocytes but it is of note that their frequency is increased in cardiovascular diseases (Heine et al. 2008; Rogacev et al. 2011) and HIV (Ellery et al. 2007; Jaworowski et al. 2007). Tie2-expressing monocytes (TEM) were found in the nonclassical monocyte subset (De Palma et al. 2005). These monocytes play a non-redundant role in tumor neovascularization as their selective depletion resulted in reduced tumor angiogenesis in murine tumor models. TEM are selectively recruited to tumors by the Tie2 ligand angiopoietin-2 (ANG-2), which is expressed by tumor endothelium (Venneri et al. 2007; Coffelt et al. 2010a). Recent results indicate that Tie2 can be expressed also by classical and intermediate human monocytes (Zawada et al. 2011).

A discussed issue about monocyte heterogeneity is about identity and localization of their precursors. A compartmental reservoir of extramedullary monocytes has been identified in the subcapsular red pulp of the spleen (Swirski et al. 2009). These undifferentiated monocytes express Ly6C, rapidly amplified and are recruited to ischemic myocardium while their role in the tumor context is still unknown. Mobilization and proliferation of precursors in peripheral tissues has been studied as another mechanism to give rise to differentiated macrophages (Massberg et al. 2007). CCR2 ligands seem to play a central role for the mobilization of committed hematopoietic precursors to peripheral sites where they differentiate into M2 repair macrophages (Si et al. 2010). Hematopoietic precursors were found also in some tumor bearing-mice models (Kitamura et al. 2007; Deak et al. 2010) and probably they contribute to the mature macrophage pool. $CD34^{+}$ hematopoietic progenitors in presence of breast cancer cell culture medium differentiate in $CD11b^{+}$ myeloid cells that seem to be involved in the tumor angiogenesis and in the initiation of premetastatic niche. Proangiogenic $CD11b^{+}$ monocytes have been identified in the blood of tumor-bearing mice and cancer patients (Laurent et al. 2011).

At present our understanding of the relative role of monocyte subsets in tumor infiltration and biology is still largely incomplete. Classical monocytes represent one of the cellular components of a heterogeneous population of myeloid nature indicated as myeloid-derived suppressor cells (MDSC), which also includes immature monocytes and granulocytic cells (Sinha et al. 2007; Gabrilovich & Nagaraj 2009; Peranzoni et al. 2010). MDSC are functionally defined for their immunosuppressive functions, are expanded both at tumor site and in secondary lymphoid organs in tumor-bearing animals and in cancer patient blood samples, where their increase correlated with the clinical cancer stage (Diaz-Montero et al. 2009). Recently it has been demonstrated that classical monocytes preferentially infiltrate lung tumor metastasis, while nonclassical monocytes are mainly recruited to primary tumor site (Qian et al. 2011).

5. An integrated view

The different circulating monocyte subsets identified appear to be committed to distinct extravascular fates in the tumor microenvironment (Figure 2). Classical monocytes are thought to differentiate mainly toward M2-like macrophages (Sinha et al. 2007; Geissmann et al. 2010b), and several studies have showed that MDSC in the tumors differentiate into immunosuppressive TAM (Kusmartsev & Gabrilovich 2005; Movahedi et al. 2010) and tolerogenic dendritic cells (Liu et al. 2009; Augier et al. 2010). Conversely, in TS/A and 4T1 tumors classical monocytes have been shown to include the precursors of both M1-like TAM enriched in hypoxic regions of the tumor and M2-like macrophages (Movahedi et al. 2010). As TEM are concerned, it is interesting to note that ANG-2 induces an M2-like phenotype (Pucci et al. 2009). However, TEM depletion has no impact on TAM recruitment in murine tumor models (De Palma et al. 2005), suggesting that TEM likely represent a sub-population of monocytes distinct from TAM precursors. Finally, despite monocytes have long been considered the unique precursors of macrophages, local proliferation of tissue-resident macrophages has been demonstrated for many populations, as alveolar macrophages (Sawyer et al. 1982; Tarling et al. 1987; Landsman et al. 2007), splenic white-pulp and metallophilic macrophages (Wijffels et al. 1994), and liver Kupffer cells (Crofton et al. 1978),

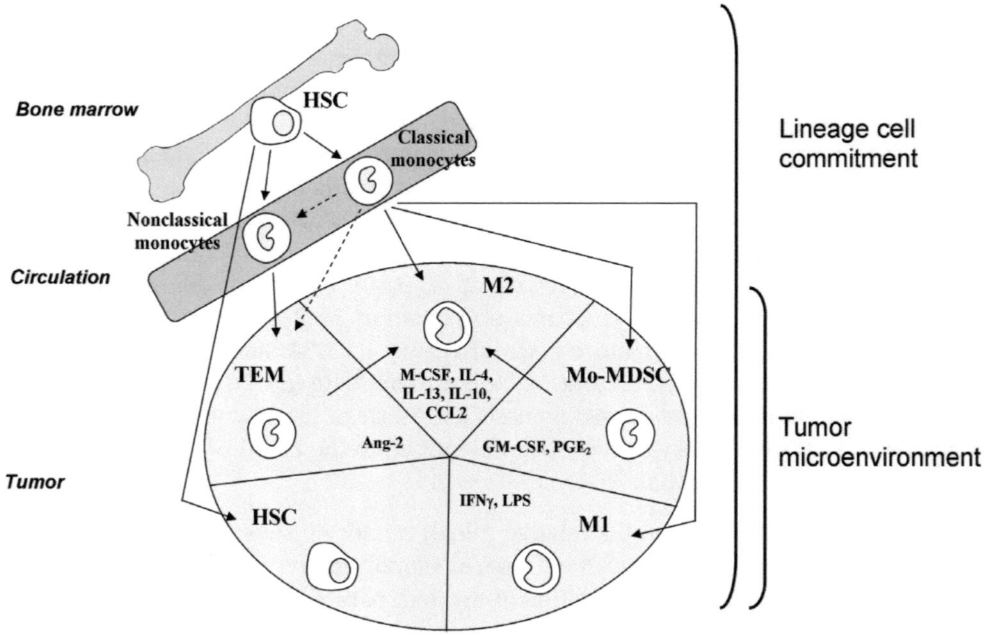

Fig. 2. Lineage commitment and tumor microenvironment in the generation of mononuclear phagocytes heterogeneity at the tumor site.

principally in homeostatic conditions. Of note, Allen and colleagues have also recently described IL-4-driven local proliferation of resident macrophages during helminth infections (Jenkins et al. 2011). In the context of cancer, it would thus be of great interest to address the potential effect of IL-4 on TAM proliferation to get a better insight in de novo recruitment of monocytes/macrophages versus local expansion of the existing pool of TAM.

The two main murine subsets, classical (Ly6C^{high}) and non-classical (Ly6C^{low}) monocytes, originate from hematopoietic precursors (HPC) in bone marrow and enter the tumor mass. Once in the tumor, exposure of monocytes and macrophages to different stimuli drive their polarization and function, resulting in the generation of the heterogeneous infiltrate. It remains unknown whether Ly6C^{low} nonclassical monocytes are generated through a Ly6C^{high} intermediate (dotted lines).

6. Conclusion

Macrophages are heterogeneous and plastic cells of the myelomonocytic lineage which adapt to the microenvironmental cues by changing their transcriptional program. Using cancer as a paradigm for macrophage polarization leads to the current view that various, if not all tumor-associated signals/factors/cytokines/chemokines/growth factors lead to a macrophage phenotype closely but at the same time different from the M2 type. Besides TAM, in tumors other monocyte/macrophages populations have been described, including MDSC, HPC and TEM, which display molecular and functional signatures resembling circulating monocytes subsets.

7. References

Aharinejad, S., P. Paulus, M. Sioud, M. Hofmann, K. Zins, R. Schafer, E. R. Stanley & D. Abraham (2004). "Colony-stimulating factor-1 blockade by antisense oligonucleotides and small interfering RNAs suppresses growth of human mammary tumor xenografts in mice." Cancer Res 64(15): 5378-84, ISSN 0008-5472

Alder, J. K., R. W. Georgantas, 3rd, R. L. Hildreth, I. M. Kaplan, S. Morisot, X. Yu, M. McDevitt & C. I. Civin (2008). "Kruppel-like factor 4 is essential for inflammatory monocyte differentiation in vivo." J Immunol 180(8): 5645-52, ISSN 0022-1767

Andreu, P., M. Johansson, N. I. Affara, F. Pucci, T. Tan, S. Junankar, L. Korets, J. Lam, D. Tawfik, D. G. DeNardo, L. Naldini, K. E. de Visser, M. De Palma & L. M. Coussens (2010). "FcRgamma activation regulates inflammation-associated squamous carcinogenesis." Cancer Cell 17(2): 121-34, ISSN 1878-3686

Auffray, C., D. Fogg, M. Garfa, G. Elain, O. Join-Lambert, S. Kayal, S. Sarnacki, A. Cumano, G. Lauvau & F. Geissmann (2007). "Monitoring of blood vessels and tissues by a population of monocytes with patrolling behavior." Science 317(5838): 666-70, ISSN 1095-9203

Auffray, C., M. H. Sieweke & F. Geissmann (2009). "Blood monocytes: development, heterogeneity, and relationship with dendritic cells." Annu Rev Immunol 27: 669-92, ISSN 0732-0582

Augier, S., T. Ciucci, C. Luci, G. F. Carle, C. Blin-Wakkach & A. Wakkach (2010). "Inflammatory blood monocytes contribute to tumor development and represent a privileged target to improve host immunosurveillance." J Immunol 185(12): 7165-73, ISSN 1550-6606

Bingle, L., N. J. Brown & C. E. Lewis (2002). "The role of tumour-associated macrophages in tumour progression: implications for new anticancer therapies." J Pathol 196(3): 254-65, ISSN 0022-3417

Biswas, S. K. & A. Mantovani (2010). "Macrophage plasticity and interaction with lymphocyte subsets: cancer as a paradigm." Nat Immunol 11(10): 889-96

Bonecchi, R., M. Locati & A. Mantovani (2011). "Chemokines and cancer: a fatal attraction." Cancer Cell 19(4): 434-5

Bonecchi, R., S. Sozzani, J. T. Stine, W. Luini, G. D'Amico, P. Allavena, D. Chantry & A. Mantovani (1998). "Divergent effects of interleukin-4 and interferon-gamma on macrophage-derived chemokine production: an amplification circuit of polarized T helper 2 responses." Blood 92(8): 2668-71

Cairo, G., S. Recalcati, A. Mantovani & M. Locati (2011). "Iron trafficking and metabolism in macrophages: contribution to the polarized phenotype." Trends Immunol 32(6): 241-7, ISSN 1471-4981

Coffelt, S. B., C. E. Lewis, L. Naldini, J. M. Brown, N. Ferrara & M. De Palma (2010a). "Elusive identities and overlapping phenotypes of proangiogenic myeloid cells in tumors." Am J Pathol 176(4): 1564-76, ISSN 1525-2191

Coffelt, S. B., A. O. Tal, A. Scholz, M. De Palma, S. Patel, C. Urbich, S. K. Biswas, C. Murdoch, K. H. Plate, Y. Reiss & C. E. Lewis (2010b). "Angiopoietin-2 regulates gene expression in TIE2-expressing monocytes and augments their inherent proangiogenic functions." Cancer Res 70(13): 5270-80, ISSN 1538-7445

Condeelis, J. & J. W. Pollard (2006). "Macrophages: obligate partners for tumor cell migration, invasion, and metastasis." Cell 124(2): 263-6, ISSN 0092-8674

Crofton, R. W., M. M. Diesselhoff-den Dulk & R. van Furth (1978). "The origin, kinetics, and characteristics of the Kupffer cells in the normal steady state." J Exp Med 148(1): 1-17, ISSN 0022-1007

Cros, J., N. Cagnard, K. Woollard, N. Patey, S. Y. Zhang, B. Senechal, A. Puel, S. K. Biswas, D. Moshous, C. Picard, J. P. Jais, D. D'Cruz, J. L. Casanova, C. Trouillet & F. Geissmann (2010). "Human CD14dim monocytes patrol and sense nucleic acids and viruses via TLR7 and TLR8 receptors." Immunity 33(3): 375-86, ISSN 1097-4180

Curry, J. M., T. D. Eubank, R. D. Roberts, Y. Wang, N. Pore, A. Maity & C. B. Marsh (2008). "M-CSF signals through the MAPK/ERK pathway via Sp1 to induce VEGF production and induces angiogenesis in vivo." PLoS One 3(10): e3405, ISSN 1932-6203

De Palma, M., M. A. Venneri, R. Galli, L. Sergi Sergi, L. S. Politi, M. Sampaolesi & L. Naldini (2005). "Tie2 identifies a hematopoietic lineage of proangiogenic monocytes required for tumor vessel formation and a mesenchymal population of pericyte progenitors." Cancer Cell 8(3): 211-26, ISSN 1535-6108

de Visser, K. E., L. V. Korets & L. M. Coussens (2005). "De novo carcinogenesis promoted by chronic inflammation is B lymphocyte dependent." Cancer Cell 7(5): 411-23,

Deak, E., S. Gottig, B. Ruster, V. Paunescu, E. Seifried, J. Gille & R. Henschler (2010). "Bone marrow derived cells in the tumour microenvironment contain cells with primitive haematopoietic phenotype." J Cell Mol Med 14(7): 1946-52, ISSN 1582-4934

DeNardo, D. G., J. B. Barreto, P. Andreu, L. Vasquez, D. Tawfik, N. Kolhatkar & L. M. Coussens (2009). "CD4(+) T cells regulate pulmonary metastasis of mammary carcinomas by enhancing protumor properties of macrophages." Cancer Cell 16(2): 91-102, ISSN 1878-3686

Diaz-Montero, C. M., M. L. Salem, M. I. Nishimura, E. Garrett-Mayer, D. J. Cole & A. J. Montero (2009). "Increased circulating myeloid-derived suppressor cells correlate with clinical cancer stage, metastatic tumor burden, and doxorubicin-cyclophosphamide chemotherapy." Cancer Immunol Immunother 58(1): 49-59, ISSN 1432-0851

Elgert, K. D., D. G. Alleva & D. W. Mullins (1998). "Tumor-induced immune dysfunction: the macrophage connection." J Leukoc Biol 64(3): 275-90, ISSN 0741-5400

Ellery, P. J., E. Tippett, Y. L. Chiu, G. Paukovics, P. U. Cameron, A. Solomon, S. R. Lewin, P. R. Gorry, A. Jaworowski, W. C. Greene, S. Sonza & S. M. Crowe (2007). "The CD16+ monocyte subset is more permissive to infection and preferentially harbors HIV-1 in vivo." J Immunol 178(10): 6581-9, ISSN 0022-1767

Eruslanov, E., I. Daurkin, J. Ortiz, J. Vieweg & S. Kusmartsev (2010). "Pivotal Advance: Tumor-mediated induction of myeloid-derived suppressor cells and M2-polarized macrophages by altering intracellular PGE catabolism in myeloid cells." J Leukoc Biol 88(5): 839-48, ISSN 1938-3673

Eruslanov, E., S. Kaliberov, I. Daurkin, L. Kaliberova, D. Buchsbaum, J. Vieweg & S. Kusmartsev (2009). "Altered expression of 15-hydroxyprostaglandin dehydrogenase in tumor-infiltrated CD11b myeloid cells: a mechanism for immune evasion in cancer." J Immunol 182(12): 7548-57, ISSN 1550-6606

Espinosa, I., A. H. Beck, C. H. Lee, S. Zhu, K. D. Montgomery, R. J. Marinelli, K. N. Ganjoo, T. O. Nielsen, C. B. Gilks, R. B. West & M. van de Rijn (2009). "Coordinate expression of colony-stimulating factor-1 and colony-stimulating factor-1-related proteins is associated with poor prognosis in gynecological and nongynecological leiomyosarcoma." Am J Pathol 174(6): 2347-56, ISSN 1525-2191

Feinberg, M. W., A. K. Wara, Z. Cao, M. A. Lebedeva, F. Rosenbauer, H. Iwasaki, H. Hirai, J. P. Katz, R. L. Haspel, S. Gray, K. Akashi, J. Segre, K. H. Kaestner, D. G. Tenen & M. K. Jain (2007). "The Kruppel-like factor KLF4 is a critical regulator of monocyte differentiation." EMBO J 26(18): 4138-48, ISSN 0261-4189

Flavell, R. A., S. Sanjabi, S. H. Wrzesinski & P. Licona-Limon (2010). "The polarization of immune cells in the tumour environment by TGFbeta." Nat Rev Immunol 10(8): 554-67, ISSN 1474-1741

Fleetwood, A. J., T. Lawrence, J. A. Hamilton & A. D. Cook (2007). "Granulocyte-macrophage colony-stimulating factor (CSF) and macrophage CSF-dependent macrophage phenotypes display differences in cytokine profiles and transcription factor activities: implications for CSF blockade in inflammation." J Immunol 178(8): 5245-52, ISSN 0022-1767

Gabrilovich, D. I. & S. Nagaraj (2009). "Myeloid-derived suppressor cells as regulators of the immune system." Nat Rev Immunol 9(3): 162-74, ISSN 1474-1741

Geissmann, F., S. Gordon, D. A. Hume, A. M. Mowat & G. J. Randolph (2010a). "Unravelling mononuclear phagocyte heterogeneity." Nat Rev Immunol 10(6): 453-60, ISSN 1474-1741

Geissmann, F., M. G. Manz, S. Jung, M. H. Sieweke, M. Merad & K. Ley (2010b). "Development of monocytes, macrophages, and dendritic cells." Science 327(5966): 656-61, ISSN 1095-9203

Gocheva, V., H. W. Wang, B. B. Gadea, T. Shree, K. E. Hunter, A. L. Garfall, T. Berman & J. A. Joyce (2010). "IL-4 induces cathepsin protease activity in tumor-associated macrophages to promote cancer growth and invasion." Genes Dev 24(3): 241-55, ISSN 1549-5477

Gordon, S. (2003). "Alternative activation of macrophages." Nat Rev Immunol 3(1): 23-35, ISSN 1474-1733

Gordon, S. & P. R. Taylor (2005). "Monocyte and macrophage heterogeneity." Nat Rev Immunol 5(12): 953-64, ISSN 1474-1733

Hagemann, T., J. Wilson, F. Burke, H. Kulbe, N. F. Li, A. Pluddemann, K. Charles, S. Gordon & F. R. Balkwill (2006). "Ovarian cancer cells polarize macrophages toward a tumor-associated phenotype." J Immunol 176(8): 5023-32, ISSN 0022-1767

Hamilton, J. A. (2008). "Colony-stimulating factors in inflammation and autoimmunity." Nat Rev Immunol 8(7): 533-44, ISSN 1474-1741

Heine, G. H., C. Ulrich, E. Seibert, S. Seiler, J. Marell, B. Reichart, M. Krause, A. Schlitt, H. Kohler & M. Girndt (2008). "CD14(++)CD16+ monocytes but not total monocyte numbers predict cardiovascular events in dialysis patients." Kidney Int 73(5): 622-9, ISSN 1523-1755

Hesse, M., M. Modolell, A. C. La Flamme, M. Schito, J. M. Fuentes, A. W. Cheever, E. J. Pearce & T. A. Wynn (2001). "Differential regulation of nitric oxide synthase-2 and arginase-1 by type 1/type 2 cytokines in vivo: granulomatous pathology is shaped by the pattern of L-arginine metabolism." J Immunol 167(11): 6533-44, ISSN 0022-1767

Jaworowski, A., D. D. Kamwendo, P. Ellery, S. Sonza, V. Mwapasa, E. Tadesse, M. E. Molyneux, S. J. Rogerson, S. R. Meshnick & S. M. Crowe (2007). "CD16+ monocyte subset preferentially harbors HIV-1 and is expanded in pregnant Malawian women with Plasmodium falciparum malaria and HIV-1 infection." J Infect Dis 196(1): 38-42, 0022-1899 (Print)

0022-1899 (Linking)

Jenkins, S. J., D. Ruckerl, P. C. Cook, L. H. Jones, F. D. Finkelman, N. van Rooijen, A. S. MacDonald & J. E. Allen (2011). "Local macrophage proliferation, rather than recruitment from the blood, is a signature of TH2 inflammation." Science 332(6035): 1284-8, ISSN

Kitamura, T., K. Kometani, H. Hashida, A. Matsunaga, H. Miyoshi, H. Hosogi, M. Aoki, M. Oshima, M. Hattori, A. Takabayashi, N. Minato & M. M. Taketo (2007). "SMAD4-deficient intestinal tumors recruit CCR1+ myeloid cells that promote invasion." Nat Genet 39(4): 467-75, ISSN 1061-4036

Kuang, D. M., Q. Zhao, C. Peng, J. Xu, J. P. Zhang, C. Wu & L. Zheng (2009). "Activated monocytes in peritumoral stroma of hepatocellular carcinoma foster immune privilege and disease progression through PD-L1." J Exp Med 206(6): 1327-37,

Kubota, Y., K. Takubo, T. Shimizu, H. Ohno, K. Kishi, M. Shibuya, H. Saya & T. Suda (2009). "M-CSF inhibition selectively targets pathological angiogenesis and lymphangiogenesis." J Exp Med 206(5): 1089-102, ISSN 1540-9538

Kusmartsev, S. & D. I. Gabrilovich (2005). "STAT1 signaling regulates tumor-associated macrophage-mediated T cell deletion." J Immunol 174(8): 4880-91, ISSN 0022-1767

Landsman, L., C. Varol & S. Jung (2007). "Distinct differentiation potential of blood monocyte subsets in the lung." J Immunol 178(4): 2000-7, ISSN 0022-1767

Laurent, J., E. F. Hull, C. Touvrey, F. Kuonen, Q. Lan, G. Lorusso, M. A. Doucey, L. Ciarloni, N. Imaizumi, G. C. Alghisi, E. Fagiani, K. Zaman, R. Stupp, M. Shibuya, J. F. Delaloye, G. Christofori & C. Ruegg (2011). "Proangiogenic factor PlGF programs CD11b(+) myelomonocytes in breast cancer during differentiation of their hematopoietic progenitors." Cancer Res 71(11): 3781-91, ISSN 1538-7445

Lewis, C. E. & J. W. Pollard (2006). "Distinct role of macrophages in different tumor microenvironments." Cancer Res 66(2): 605-12, ISSN 0008-5472

Lin, E. Y., J. F. Li, L. Gnatovskiy, Y. Deng, L. Zhu, D. A. Grzesik, H. Qian, X. N. Xue & J. W. Pollard (2006). "Macrophages regulate the angiogenic switch in a mouse model of breast cancer." Cancer Res 66(23): 11238-46, ISSN 0008-5472

Lin, E. Y., A. V. Nguyen, R. G. Russell & J. W. Pollard (2001). "Colony-stimulating factor 1 promotes progression of mammary tumors to malignancy." J Exp Med 193(6): 727-40, ISSN 0022-1007

Liu, Q., C. Zhang, A. Sun, Y. Zheng, L. Wang & X. Cao (2009). "Tumor-educated CD11bhighIalow regulatory dendritic cells suppress T cell response through arginase I." J Immunol 182(10): 6207-16, ISSN 1550-6606

Mantovani, A., P. Allavena, A. Sica & F. Balkwill (2008). "Cancer-related inflammation." Nature 454(7203): 436-44, ISSN 1476-4687

Mantovani, A., A. Sica & M. Locati (2005). "Macrophage polarization comes of age." Immunity 23(4): 344-6, ISSN 1074-7613

Mantovani, A., A. Sica, S. Sozzani, P. Allavena, A. Vecchi & M. Locati (2004). "The chemokine system in diverse forms of macrophage activation and polarization." Trends Immunol 25(12): 677-86, ISSN 1471-4906

Mantovani, A., S. Sozzani, M. Locati, P. Allavena & A. Sica (2002). "Macrophage polarization: tumor-associated macrophages as a paradigm for polarized M2 mononuclear phagocytes." Trends Immunol 23(11): 549-55, ISSN 1471-4906

Martinez, F. O., S. Gordon, M. Locati & A. Mantovani (2006). "Transcriptional profiling of the human monocyte-to-macrophage differentiation and polarization: new molecules and patterns of gene expression." J Immunol 177(10): 7303-11, ISSN 0022-1767

Massberg, S., P. Schaerli, I. Knezevic-Maramica, M. Kollnberger, N. Tubo, E. A. Moseman, I. V. Huff, T. Junt, A. J. Wagers, I. B. Mazo & U. H. von Andrian (2007). "Immunosurveillance by hematopoietic progenitor cells trafficking through blood, lymph, and peripheral tissues." Cell 131(5): 994-1008, ISSN 0092-8674

Mildner, A., H. Schmidt, M. Nitsche, D. Merkler, U. K. Hanisch, M. Mack, M. Heikenwalder, W. Bruck, J. Priller & M. Prinz (2007). "Microglia in the adult brain arise from Ly-6ChiCCR2+ monocytes only under defined host conditions." Nat Neurosci 10(12): 1544-53, ISSN 1097-6256

Movahedi, K., D. Laoui, C. Gysemans, M. Baeten, G. Stange, J. Van den Bossche, M. Mack, D. Pipeleers, P. In't Veld, P. De Baetselier & J. A. Van Ginderachter (2010). "Different tumor microenvironments contain functionally distinct subsets of macrophages derived from Ly6C(high) monocytes." Cancer Res 70(14): 5728-39, ISSN 1538-7445

Munder, M., K. Eichmann & M. Modolell (1998). "Alternative metabolic states in murine macrophages reflected by the nitric oxide synthase/arginase balance: competitive regulation by CD4+ T cells correlates with Th1/Th2 phenotype." J Immunol 160(11): 5347-54, ISSN 0022-1767

Nowicki, A., J. Szenajch, G. Ostrowska, A. Wojtowicz, K. Wojtowicz, A. A. Kruszewski, M. Maruszynski, S. L. Aukerman & W. Wiktor-Jedrzejczak (1996). "Impaired tumor growth in colony-stimulating factor 1 (CSF-1)-deficient, macrophage-deficient op/op mouse: evidence for a role of CSF-1-dependent macrophages in formation of tumor stroma." Int J Cancer 65(1): 112-9,

Peranzoni, E., S. Zilio, I. Marigo, L. Dolcetti, P. Zanovello, S. Mandruzzato & V. Bronte (2010). "Myeloid-derived suppressor cell heterogeneity and subset definition." Curr Opin Immunol 22(2): 238-44, ISSN 1879-0372

Pollard, J. W. (2004). "Tumour-educated macrophages promote tumour progression and metastasis." Nat Rev Cancer 4(1): 71-8, ISSN 1474-175X

Priceman, S. J., J. L. Sung, Z. Shaposhnik, J. B. Burton, A. X. Torres-Collado, D. L. Moughon, M. Johnson, A. J. Lusis, D. A. Cohen, M. L. Iruela-Arispe & L. Wu (2010). "Targeting distinct tumor-infiltrating myeloid cells by inhibiting CSF-1 receptor: combating tumor evasion of antiangiogenic therapy." Blood 115(7): 1461-71, ISSN 1528-0020

Pucci, F., M. A. Venneri, D. Biziato, A. Nonis, D. Moi, A. Sica, C. Di Serio, L. Naldini & M. De Palma (2009). "A distinguishing gene signature shared by tumor-infiltrating Tie2-expressing monocytes, blood "resident" monocytes, and embryonic macrophages suggests common functions and developmental relationships." Blood 114(4): 901-14, ISSN 1528-0020

Qian, B. Z., J. Li, H. Zhang, T. Kitamura, J. Zhang, L. R. Campion, E. A. Kaiser, L. A. Snyder & J. W. Pollard (2011). "CCL2 recruits inflammatory monocytes to facilitate breast-tumour metastasis." Nature 475(7355): 222-5, ISSN 1476-4687

Qian, B. Z. & J. W. Pollard (2010). "Macrophage diversity enhances tumor progression and metastasis." Cell 141(1): 39-51, ISSN 1097-4172

Recalcati, S., M. Locati, A. Marini, P. Santambrogio, F. Zaninotto, M. De Pizzol, L. Zammataro, D. Girelli & G. Cairo (2010). "Differential regulation of iron homeostasis during human macrophage polarized activation." Eur J Immunol 40(3): 824-35, ISSN 1521-4141

Roca, H., Z. S. Varsos, S. Sud, M. J. Craig, C. Ying & K. J. Pienta (2009). "CCL2 and interleukin-6 promote survival of human CD11b+ peripheral blood mononuclear cells and induce M2-type macrophage polarization." J Biol Chem 284(49): 34342-54, ISSN 1083-351X

Rodriguez, P. C., C. P. Hernandez, D. Quiceno, S. M. Dubinett, J. Zabaleta, J. B. Ochoa, J. Gilbert & A. C. Ochoa (2005). "Arginase I in myeloid suppressor cells is induced by COX-2 in lung carcinoma." J Exp Med 202(7): 931-9, ISSN 0022-1007

Rogacev, K. S., S. Seiler, A. M. Zawada, B. Reichart, E. Herath, D. Roth, C. Ulrich, D. Fliser & G. H. Heine (2011). "CD14++CD16+ monocytes and cardiovascular outcome in patients with chronic kidney disease." Eur Heart J 32(1): 84-92, ISSN 1522-9645

Sawyer, R. T., P. H. Strausbauch & A. Volkman (1982). "Resident macrophage proliferation in mice depleted of blood monocytes by strontium-89." Lab Invest 46(2): 165-70, ISSN 0023-6837

Scatizzi, J. C., J. Hutcheson, E. Bickel, J. M. Woods, K. Klosowska, T. L. Moore, G. K. Haines, 3rd & H. Perlman (2006). "p21Cip1 is required for the development of monocytes and their response to serum transfer-induced arthritis." Am J Pathol 168(5): 1531-41, ISSN 0002-9440

Si, Y., C. L. Tsou, K. Croft & I. F. Charo (2010). "CCR2 mediates hematopoietic stem and progenitor cell trafficking to sites of inflammation in mice." J Clin Invest 120(4): 1192-203, ISSN 1558-8238

Sinha, P., V. K. Clements, A. M. Fulton & S. Ostrand-Rosenberg (2007). "Prostaglandin E2 promotes tumor progression by inducing myeloid-derived suppressor cells." Cancer Res 67(9): 4507-13, ISSN 0008-5472

Sinha, P., V. K. Clements & S. Ostrand-Rosenberg (2005). "Interleukin-13-regulated M2 macrophages in combination with myeloid suppressor cells block immune surveillance against metastasis." Cancer Res 65(24): 11743-51, ISSN 0008-5472

Solinas, G., S. Schiarea, M. Liguori, M. Fabbri, S. Pesce, L. Zammataro, F. Pasqualini, M. Nebuloni, C. Chiabrando, A. Mantovani & P. Allavena (2010). "Tumor-conditioned macrophages secrete migration-stimulating factor: a new marker for M2-polarization, influencing tumor cell motility." J Immunol 185(1): 642-52, ISSN 1550-6606

Stein, M., S. Keshav, N. Harris & S. Gordon (1992). "Interleukin 4 potently enhances murine macrophage mannose receptor activity: a marker of alternative immunologic macrophage activation." J Exp Med 176(1): 287-92, ISSN 0022-1007

Swirski, F. K., M. Nahrendorf, M. Etzrodt, M. Wildgruber, V. Cortez-Retamozo, P. Panizzi, J. L. Figueiredo, R. H. Kohler, A. Chudnovskiy, P. Waterman, E. Aikawa, T. R. Mempel, P. Libby, R. Weissleder & M. J. Pittet (2009). "Identification of splenic reservoir monocytes and their deployment to inflammatory sites." Science 325(5940): 612-6, ISSN 1095-9203

Tarling, J. D., H. S. Lin & S. Hsu (1987). "Self-renewal of pulmonary alveolar macrophages: evidence from radiation chimera studies." J Leukoc Biol 42(5): 443-6, ISSN 0741-5400

Torroella-Kouri, M., R. Silvera, D. Rodriguez, R. Caso, A. Shatry, S. Opiela, D. Ilkovitch, R. A. Schwendener, V. Iragavarapu-Charyulu, Y. Cardentey, N. Strbo & D. M. Lopez (2009). "Identification of a subpopulation of macrophages in mammary tumor-bearing mice that are neither M1 nor M2 and are less differentiated." Cancer Res 69(11): 4800-9, ISSN 1538-7445

Varol, C., L. Landsman, D. K. Fogg, L. Greenshtein, B. Gildor, R. Margalit, V. Kalchenko, F. Geissmann & S. Jung (2007). "Monocytes give rise to mucosal, but not splenic, conventional dendritic cells." J Exp Med 204(1): 171-80, ISSN 0022-1007

Venneri, M. A., M. De Palma, M. Ponzoni, F. Pucci, C. Scielzo, E. Zonari, R. Mazzieri, C. Doglioni & L. Naldini (2007). "Identification of proangiogenic TIE2-expressing monocytes (TEMs) in human peripheral blood and cancer." Blood 109(12): 5276-85, ISSN 0006-4971

Verreck, F. A., T. de Boer, D. M. Langenberg, M. A. Hoeve, M. Kramer, E. Vaisberg, R. Kastelein, A. Kolk, R. de Waal-Malefyt & T. H. Ottenhoff (2004). "Human IL-23-

producing type 1 macrophages promote but IL-10-producing type 2 macrophages subvert immunity to (myco)bacteria." Proc Natl Acad Sci U S A 101(13): 4560-5, ISSN 0027-8424

Webster, J. A., A. H. Beck, M. Sharma, I. Espinosa, B. Weigelt, M. Schreuder, K. D. Montgomery, K. C. Jensen, M. van de Rijn & R. West (2010). "Variations in stromal signatures in breast and colorectal cancer metastases." J Pathol 222(2): 158-65, ISSN 1096-9896

Wijffels, J. F., Z. de Rover, R. H. Beelen, G. Kraal & N. van Rooijen (1994). "Macrophage subpopulations in the mouse spleen renewed by local proliferation." Immunobiology 191(1): 52-64, ISSN 0171-2985

Wong, K. L., J. J. Tai, W. C. Wong, H. Han, X. Sem, W. H. Yeap, P. Kourilsky & S. C. Wong (2011). "Gene expression profiling reveals the defining features of the classical, intermediate, and nonclassical human monocyte subsets." Blood 118(5): e16-31, ISSN 1528-0020

Wong, S. C., A. L. Puaux, M. Chittezhath, I. Shalova, T. S. Kajiji, X. Wang, J. P. Abastado, K. P. Lam & S. K. Biswas (2010). "Macrophage polarization to a unique phenotype driven by B cells." Eur J Immunol 40(8): 2296-307, ISSN 1521-4141

Yrlid, U., C. D. Jenkins & G. G. MacPherson (2006). "Relationships between distinct blood monocyte subsets and migrating intestinal lymph dendritic cells in vivo under steady-state conditions." J Immunol 176(7): 4155-62, ISSN 0022-1767

Zawada, A. M., K. S. Rogacev, B. Rotter, P. Winter, R. R. Marell, D. Fliser & G. H. Heine (2011). "SuperSAGE evidence for CD14++CD16+ monocytes as a third monocyte subset." Blood 118(12): e50-61, ISSN 1528-0020

Ziegler-Heitbrock, L., P. Ancuta, S. Crowe, M. Dalod, V. Grau, D. N. Hart, P. J. Leenen, Y. J. Liu, G. MacPherson, G. J. Randolph, J. Scherberich, J. Schmitz, K. Shortman, S. Sozzani, H. Strobl, M. Zembala, J. M. Austyn & M. B. Lutz (2010). "Nomenclature of monocytes and dendritic cells in blood." Blood 116(16): e74-80, ISSN 1528-0020

2

Functions of Diverse Myeloid Cells in the Tumor Micro-Environment

A. Sica[1,2*], C. Porta[2], E. Riboldi[2], M. Erreni[1] and P. Allavena[1*]
[1]*Dpt Immunology and Inflammation, IRCCS Humanitas Clinical Institute, Rozzano, Milan,*
[2]*DiSCAFF, University of Piemonte Orientale A. Avogadro, Novara, Italy*

1. Introduction

Myeloid cells are abundant in solid tumors and early infiltrate neoplastic lesions since the first stages of tumourigenesis, usually preceding other leukocytes (e.g. lymphocytes). (Clark et al., 2007) In the last decades there has been growing evidence that infiltrating T lymphocytes (CD3+ CD8+CD45RO+) are associated with favourable prognosis in human colorectal cancer (Laghi et al., 2009; Pages et al., 2005) melanoma, ovarian and breast cancer (Clemente et al., 1996; Mahmoud et al., 2011; Vesely et al., 2011; Zhang et al., 2003) In marked contrast, cells of the innate immunity, like myeloid cells, are most frequently associated with poor clinical outcomes. A number of studies have demonstrated that tumor-associated myeloid cells (TAMCs) have the ability to support tumor cell proliferation and invasion, activate the neo-angiogenic switch, and suppress anti-tumor immune responses. (DeNardo et al., 2009; Mantovani et al., 2004a; Martinez et al., 2009; Pollard, 2004; Qian and Pollard, 2010; Talmadge et al., 2007) Thus, in a simplified scheme, adaptive immunity is usually protective and limit tumour progression, while innate immunity favours disease development. However, research in recent years have added a further level of complexity, as components of the adaptive immunity (e.g. IL-4-producing CD4 T cells and antibody-producing B cells) have been shown to activate innate immune cells in a pro-tumour manner. (DeNardo et al., 2009; Wang and Joyce, 2010) Therefore, the dynamic interplay between tumor-infiltrating cells of the innate and adaptive immunity is of paramount importance for the outcome of tumour progression or regression.

Tumor-associated myeloid cells (TAMCs) include at least four different myeloid populations **(Figure 1)**: 1) tumor-associated macrophages (TAMs), considered crucial orchestrators of cancer-related inflammation (Mantovani et al., 2008), promoting angiogenesis, immunosuppression, tissue remodelling and metastasis (Sica, 2010); 2) the angiogenic monocytes expressing the tunica internal endothelial kinase 2 (Tie2), the angiopoietin receptor, playing a key role in tumor angiogenesis (De Palma et al., 2005); 3) the Ly6G and Ly6C subsets of an heterogeneous population of immature myeloid cells, called myeloid-derived suppressor cells (MDSCs) for their ability to suppress T cells

* Corresponding Authors

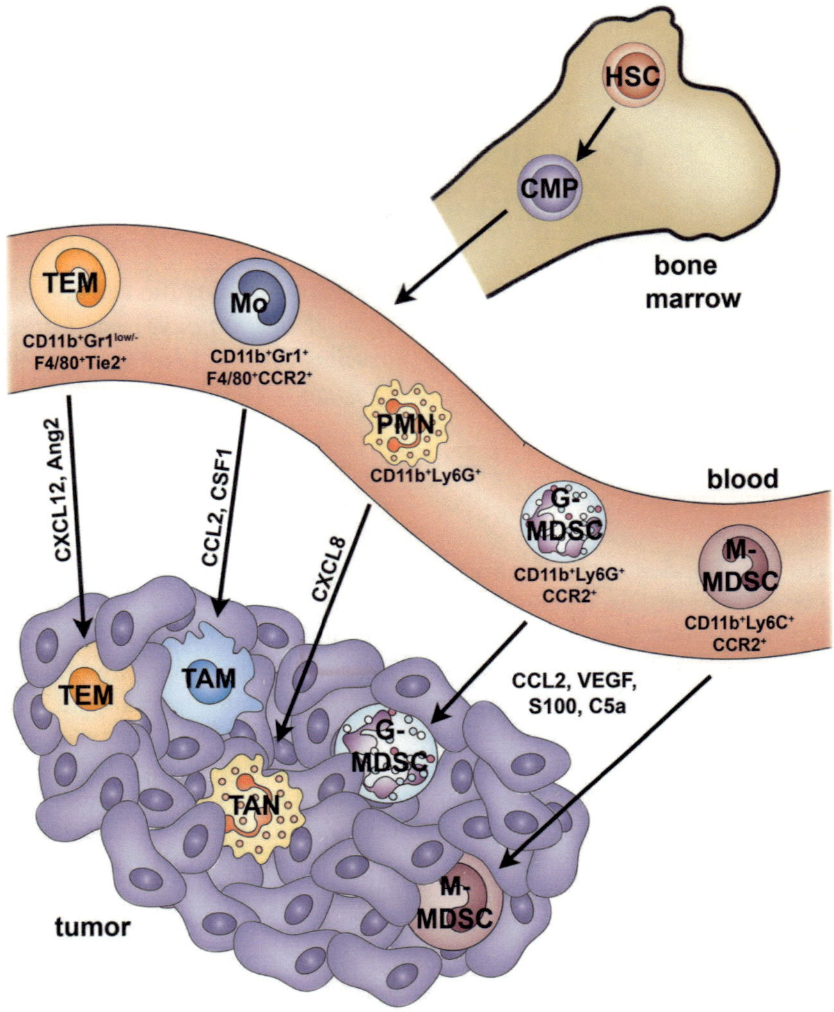

Fig. 1. **Pathways of differentiation and accumulation of TAMCs.** In the bone marrow hematopoietic stem cell (HSC) differentiate into common myeloid progenitors (CMPs), which can subsequently differentiate into different subsets of circulating myeloid cells: monocytes (Mo), Tie2-expressing monocytes (TEM), neutrophils (PMN), and granulocytic and monocytic myeloid-suppressor cells (G-MDSC and M-MDSC). Tumors secrete factors which sustain myelopoiesis, and promote both the recruitment and pro-tumor differentiation of circulating myeloid cells. TAMs are recruited into the tumor site by chemotactic factors (eg. CCL2, CSF-1) and represent the prominent phagocytes population orchestrating cancer-related inflammation. TEMs derive from circulating Tie2+ monocytes and are recruited in tumors by hypoxia-inducible chemoattractants, such as Ang2 and CXCL12. Tumor-associated neutrophils (TANs) stem from circulating neutrophils and are recruited in tumors by chemokines (e.g. CXCL8). TANs participate in tumor promotion by the expression of crucial pro-angiogenic factors. During tumour progression an heterogeneous population of myeloid cells (G-MDSC and M-MDSC) accumulate in blood and lymphoid organs. MDSCs may be recruited by selected chemoattractants (CCL2, S-100, VEGF, C5a) into the tumor microenvironment, where they contribute to suppression of the adaptive immunity.

functions, which accumulate mainly in blood and lymphoid organs during tumor progression, but may also be recruited to the tumor site (Sica and Bronte, 2007); 4) tumor-associated neutrophils (TANs) that, despite their short half-life, have been recently proven to participate in tumor promotion by the expression of crucial pro-angiogenic factors (Fridlender et al., 2009).

TAMCs originate in the bone marrow where hematopoietic stem cells (HSCs) differentiate into common myeloid precursors (CMPs), which subsequently give rise to different subsets of circulating cells: immature myeloid cells (IMCs) that can be further subdivided in a granulocytic ($CD11b^+/Ly6G^+$) and a monocytic ($CD11b^+/Ly6C^+$) subpopulation, monocytes ($CD11b^+/Gr1^+/F4/80^+/CCR2^+$), Tie2-expressing monocytes ($CD11b^+/Gr1^{low/-}/Tie2^+$) and neutrophils ($CD11b^+Ly6G^+$) (Mantovani et al., 2009). Tumors secrete factors which sustain myelopoiesis, promote the recruitment of circulating cells into the tumor mass, and orientate their functional differentiation to their own advantage (Mantovani et al., 2009; Sica and Bronte, 2007). In addition, Dendritic cells (DCs) also belong to the family of myeloid cells stemming from CMPs. Cells with dendritic characteristics are scarcely present in neoplastic tissues (Murdoch et al., 2008). Tumor-associated DCs generally show an immature phenotype and are poor inducers of effective responses to tumor antigens. The properties of these cells have been extensively reviewed elsewhere (Ma et al., 2011; Palucka et al., 2010) and are not discussed here.

2. Pro-tumour functions of tumor-associated myeloid cells

2.1 Tumor-associated macrophages

TAMs derive from circulating monocytes which are recruited at tumor sites by a number of diverse chemoattractants secreted by tumour and stromal cells. For instance the chemokine CCL2 was discovered as a tumour-derived factor inducing chemotaxis in monocytes.(Bottazzi et al., 1983; Zachariae et al., 1990) Other chemokines these include : CCL3, CCL4, CCL5, CXCL12 (Balkwill, 2004; Konishi et al., 1996; Schioppa et al., 2003). Non-chemokine chemotactic factors are also important, for instance: urokinase plasminogen activator (uPa) (Zhang et al., 2011), M-CSF, TGFβ; fibroblast growth factor, FGF; vascular endothelial growth factor, VEGF) (Joyce and Pollard, 2009; Lin et al., 2002; Sica and Bronte, 2007) and antimicrobial peptides (β-defensin-3, BD-3) (Jin et al., 2010). Many of these molecules correlate with TAMs infiltration in different types of tumor, while other (eg. uPa, BD-3) are specifically associated with certain types of cancer, prostate and gastric cancer respectively (Jin et al., 2010; Zhang et al., 2011).

Once in tumours, monocytes differentiate to macrophages, primarily because of the presence of M-CSF produced by tumour cells, and polarize to tumour-educated macrophages by exposure to the local milieu rich in immune-suppressive mediators such as IL-10, TGFβ and VEGF.

Macrophages are versatile cells that are capable of displaying different functional activities, some of which are antagonistic: they can be immuno-stimulatory or immune suppressive, and either promote or restrain inflammation. (Auffray et al., 2009; Gordon and Taylor, 2005; Hamilton, 2008; Mantovani et al., 2004b; Martinez et al., 2009) Macrophage heterogeneity has been simplified in the macrophage polarization concept where the two extreme phenotypes, the M1 and M2 macrophages, have distinct features. (Allavena et al., 2008; Goerdt and

Orfanos, 1999; Gordon and Taylor, 2005; Mantovani et al., 1992; Pollard, 2009; Stein et al., 1992) M1 or classically-activated macrophages are stimulated by bacterial products and Th1 cytokines (e.g. IFNγ); they are potent effectors that produce inflammatory and immuno-stimulating cytokines to elicit the adaptive immune response, secrete reactive oxygen species (ROS) and nitrogen intermediates and may have cytotoxic activity to transformed cells. M2 or alternatively activated macrophages differentiate in micro-environments rich in Th2 cytokines (e.g. IL-4, IL-13); they have high scavenging activity, produce several growth factors that activate the process of tissue repair and suppress adaptive immune responses. (Gordon and Martinez, 2010; Mantovani et al., 2005; Qian and Pollard, 2010)

While this M1 vs M2 dual subsets simplification offers a mechanistic model of the functional polarization of macrophages, tissue microenvironments are likely to elicit simultaneous activation of different signalling pathways with opposite influence on macrophage functions, contributing to the extensive heterogeneity in patterns of gene expression seen in macrophages (Gratchev et al., 2008; Murray and Wynn, 2011; Ravasi et al., 2002; Riches, 1995; Stout et al., 2005; Tannenbaum et al., 1988). This in vivo functional skewing of myeloid populations is an emerging paradigm of tumor-mediated immunosuppression, where myeloid cell plasticity plays as a double-edged sword (Mantovani and Sica, 2010; Sica and Bronte, 2007). In early phases, high production of M1 inflammatory mediators (e.g. tumor necrosis factor, TNF; reactive oxygen species, ROS) appears to support neoplastic transformation (Sica and Bronte, 2007), whereas in established cancers the expression of M2-like phenotypes with immunosuppressive, pro-angiogenic and tissue remodelling activities promotes immune escape, tumor growth and malignancy (Dinapoli et al., 1996; Mantovani and Sica, 2010; Movahedi et al., 2010; Pollard, 2004; Saccani et al., 2006; Sica and Bronte, 2007; Sica et al., 2008; Sica et al., 2000).

In molecular profiling studies, murine TAMs from fibrosarcoma showed several features of M2 macrophages: arginase-I, YM1, FIZZ1, MGL2, VEGF, osteopontin and MMPs, as well as an immunosuppressive phenotype : high IL-10, TGFβ and low IL-12, RNI and MHC II, which correlate functionally to reduced cytotoxicity and antigen-presenting capacity. (Biswas et al., 2006; Hagemann et al., 2009; Ojalvo et al., 2010) Similar findings were found in human TAMs from ovarian cancer patients.(Allavena et al., 2010) We compared the expression of upregulated genes in human TAMs with the profiling of in vitro-polarized M1 and M2 macrophages. Several genes (e.g. osteopontin, fibronectin, scavenger and mannose receptors) were similarly upregulated in TAMs and in M2 macrophages. By the Principal Component Analysis, the global profiling of TAMs fell much closer to that of M2-polarized macrophages. (Solinas et al., 2010)

However, TAMs heterogeneity is starting to emerge, likely depending on the tumour type and micro-environmental cues. (Lewis and Pollard, 2006; Movahedi et al., 2010) Notably, murine TAMs showed also the expression of typical M1 factors such as IFN-inducible chemokines (CCL5, CXCL9, CXCL10, CXCL16). (Biswas et al., 2006; Stout and Suttles, 2005)

TAMs influence fundamental aspects of tumour biology, as shown in **figure 2**. Among the well documented pro-tumour functions of TAMs is the production of trophic and activating factors for tumour and stromal cells (e.g.EGF, FGF, VEGF, PDGF, TGFβ). These growth factors directly promote the proliferation of tumour cells and increase the resistance to apoptotic stimuli (Ingman et al., 2006; Kalluri and Zeisberg, 2006; Mantovani et al., 2008; Moussai et al., 2011) The cytokine IL-6, released by TAMs, is important to sustain the

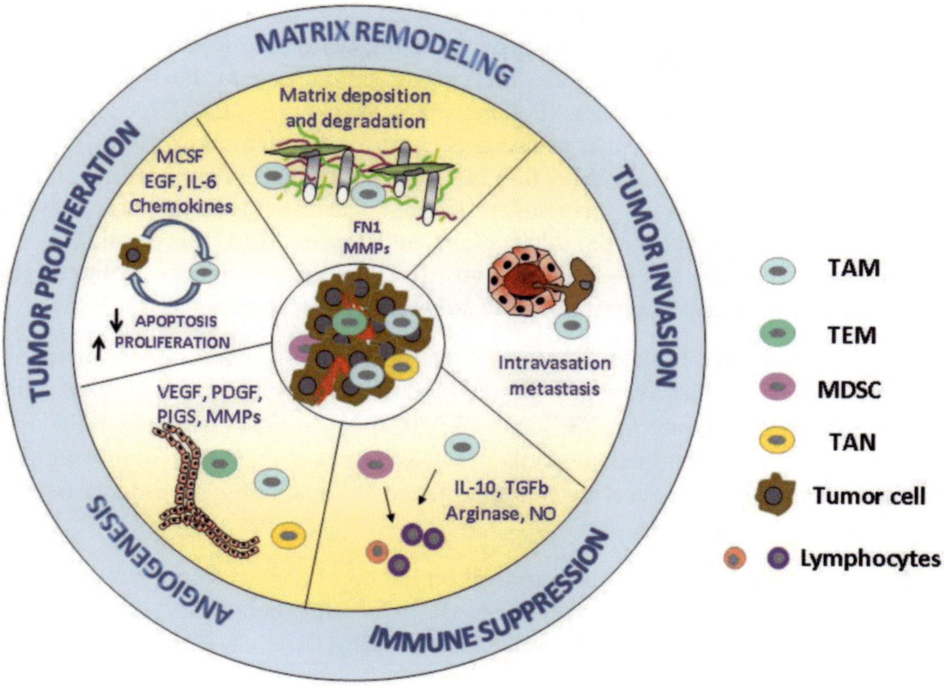

Fig. 2. **Pro-tumour functions of Tumour-Associated Myeloid Cells (TAMCs)**. Different types of TAMCs promote the progression of tumors. TAMs rescue neoplastic cells from apoptotic stimuli and stimulate their proliferation, by producing several growth factors and cytokines (e.g.EGF, IL-6). TAMs, TEMs and TAN activate angiogenesis, via VEGF, MMPs and other angiogenic factors. TAMs have an intense proteolityic activity and degrade the extra-cellular matrix, but also produce matrix proteins, such fibronectin (FN1). TAMs favour tumour cell intravasation and dissemination to distant sites. TAMs and MDSC induce immune suppression by producing suppressive mediators such as IL-10 and TGFβ, arginase 1 and nitric oxide (NO).

survival and proliferation of malignant cells in tumours of epithelial and hematopoietic origin. (Bollrath et al., 2009; Fukuda et al., 2011; Grivennikov et al., 2009; Lesina et al., ; Ribatti and Vacca, 2009) TAMs are also a major source of proteolytic enzymes that degrade the ECM, thus favouring the release of matrix-bound growth factors. (Joyce and Pollard, 2009; Mantovani et al., 2008)

TAMs a key effectors of the "angiogenic switch" where the balance between pro- and anti-angiogenic factors, commonly present in tissues, tilts towards a pro-angiogenic outcome. (Baeriswyl and Christofori, 2009; Du et al., 2008; Murdoch et al., 2008; Zumsteg et al., 2009) In hypoxic conditions the transcription factor HIF-1alpha induces in TAMs the production of VEGF and of the angiogenic chemokine CXCL8. (Lewis et al., 2000)

TAMs are probably the most active contributors to the incessant matrix remodelling present within tumours, as they produce several MMPs and other proteolytic enzymes. (Mason and Joyce, 2011) Tumour cells exploit the ECM degradation mediated by TAMs to invade locally, penetrate into vessels and disseminate to give distant metastasis. (Wyckoff et al.,

2007) TAMs aiding cancer cell invasion have been directly visualized in experimental tumours in vivo by multiphoton microscopy: by using fluorescently labelled cells Wyckoff and colleagues showed that tumour cell intravasation occurs next to perivascular macrophages in mammary tumours. (Pollard, 2008; Wyckoff et al., 2007) Further, it has been recently shown that cathepsin protease activity, by IL-4-stimulated TAMs, promotes tumour invasion.(Gocheva et al., 2010) IL-4 is produced by tumour-infiltrating CD4 T cells and there is mounting evidence of its relevance in the polarization of macrophages with pro-tumour functions. (DeNardo et al., 2009; Wang and Joyce, 2010) The chemokine CCL18 produced by TAMs has been recently shown to play a critical role in promoting breast cancer invasiveness by activating tumour cell adherence to ECM. (Chen et al., 2011)

We recently found that human TAMs and in vitro tumour-conditioned macrophages express high levels of the Migration Stimulation Factor (MSF), (Solinas et al., 2010) a truncated isoform of Fibronectin. (Schor et al., 2003) Macrophage-secreted MSF displays potent chemotactic activity to tumour cells in vitro,(Solinas et al., 2010) confirming that the pro-invasive phenotype of cancer cells is modulated by macrophage products released in the tumour-micro-environment.

Further support to the concept of a reciprocal interaction between tumour cells and TAMs was provided by a recent paper where SNAIL-expressing keratinocytes became locally invasive after macrophage recruitment elicited by M-CSF. (Du et al., 2010)

In line with the above experimental evidence, high numbers of infiltrating TAMs have been significantly associated with advanced tumours and poor patient prognosis, in the majority of human tumours.(Bingle et al., 2002; Mantovani et al., 2008; Pollard, 2004; Qian and Pollard, 2010) There are, however, notable exceptions to this pro-tumour phenotype, probably dictated by their functional polarization. One such exception is human colorectal cancer, where some studies reported that TAMs density is associated with better prognosis.(Forssell et al., 2007; Ohno et al., 2003; Sconocchia et al., 2011) The localization of TAMs within colorectal cancers appears of primary importance: the number of peritumoural macrophages with high expression of costimulatory molecules (CD80 and CD86), but not of those within the cancer stroma, was associated with improved disease-free survival.(Ohtani et al., 1997; Sugita et al., 2002)

Specific TAMs subsets identified by surface markers may have predictive values: in lung adenocarcinoma, the number of TAMs CD204+ (scavenger receptor) showed a strong association with poor outcome while the total CD68+ population did not. (Ohtaki et al., 2010)

Macrophage-related gene signatures have been identified in human tumours such as ovarian and breast cancer, soft tissue sarcoma and follicular B lymphoma; (Beck et al., 2009; Finak et al., 2008; Ghassabeh et al., 2006; Lenz et al., 2008) in classic Hodgkin's lymphoma, tumours with increased number of CD68+ TAMs were significantly associated with shortened progression-free survival. (Steidl et al., 2010)

Recent addition to the molecular repertoire of TAMs includes semaphorin 4D (Sema4D) (Sierra et al., 2008) and growth arrest-specific 6 (Gas6) (Loges et al., 2010), which are respectively involved in promoting tumor angiogenesis and cancer cell proliferation.

2.2 Tie2-expressing onocytes/macrophages (TEMs)

Tie2-expressing monocytes/macrophages (TEMs) are a small subset of myeloid cells characterized by the expression of the angiopoietin receptor Tie2 and powerful pro-angiogenic activity (De Palma and Naldini, 2009; De Palma et al., 2005; Murdoch et al., 2007; Venneri et al., 2007). They derive from circulating Tie2-expressing monocytes which are recruited in tumors by hypoxia-induced endothelial-derived chemotactic factors, such as Ang-2 and CXCL12 (Coffelt et al., 2011; Murdoch et al., 2007; Venneri et al., 2007; Welford et al., 2011b) The CXCL12-CXCR4 axis is a well known circuit driving accumulation of TAMs in hypoxic areas of solid tumors (Schioppa et al., 2003). In addition, it has been demonstrated that pharmacological inhibition of CXCR4 is associated with a significant reduction of TEM recruitment into mammary tumors (Welford et al., 2011b). Both ablation and adoptive transfer studies have demonstrated that TEMs are crucial promoters of tumor angiogenesis (De Palma et al., 2005; De Palma et al., 2003; Venneri et al., 2007). In two models of mammary tumours and orthotopic human gliomas, Ganciclovir-driven ablation of Tie2$^+$ monocytes induced a significant reduction of both tumour mass and vasculature, demonstrating their importance in tumour angiogenesis and growth (De Palma et al., 2005; De Palma et al., 2003; Venneri et al., 2007). In line, adoptive transfer studies demonstrated that subcutaneous co-injection of tumor cells with TEMs increases tumor vascularization (De Palma et al., 2005).

Strikingly, gene expression analysis highlighted that TEMs are highly related to TAMs, but express a more pronounced M2-skewed gene signature, with higher expression of M2 genes, including arginase 1 (Arg1), scavenger receptors (CD163; Mannose receptor 1, Mrc1; Macrophage scavenger receptor 2, Msr2; stabilin-1) and lower levels of pro-inflammatory molecules (IL-1β; prostaglandin endoperoxide synthase 2/cyclooxygenase 2, PTGS2/COX2; IL-12; TNF; inducible nitric oxide synthase, iNOS; CCL5; CXCL10; CXCL11) (Pucci et al., 2009). These results suggested that Tie2$^+$ monocytes could be a distinct lineage of myeloid cells, committed to execute physiologic pro-angiogenic and tissue-remodeling programs, which can be co-opted by tumors (Andreu et al., 2010). Noteworthy, human Tie2$^+$ circulating monocytes express high levels of pro-angiogenic genes (e.g. VEGF-A; Matrix metallopeptidase 9, MMP9; COX2; wingless-related MMTV integration site 5A, WNT5A) and are powerful inducers of endothelial cells activation (Coffelt et al., 2010). In agreement, sub-cutaneous tumors growing in Ang-2-overexpressing mice showed increased number of TEMs associated with enhanced microvessels density (Coffelt et al., 2010). Tie2 engagement by Ang-2 in both mouse and human TEMs not only elicits a chemotactic response but also enhances their pro-tumoral activities (Coffelt et al., 2010). It was also recently demonstrated that Ang-2 levels in 4T1 mammary tumors correlates with both TEM-derived IL-10 and Treg infiltration, resulting in suppression of T cells proliferation (Coffelt et al., 2011). In contrast, Ang-2 inhibited the expression of M1 cytokines (IL-12 and TNFα) in TEMs exposed to hypoxia (Murdoch et al., 2007).

2.3 Myeloid-Derived Suppressor Cells (MDSCs)

MDSCs represent an heterogenous population of cells whose common characteristics are an immature state and the ability to suppress T-cell responses both *in vitro* and *in vivo* (Gabrilovich and Nagaraj, 2009; Ostrand-Rosenberg and Sinha, 2009).

MDSC recruitment and expansion are regulated by several cytokines, chemokines and transcription factors (Sica and Bronte, 2007). It has been demonstrated that among chemokine receptors, CCR2 plays a pivotal role in the recruitment and turnover of MDSC to the tumour site (Sawanobori et al., 2008). Furthermore, the C5a complement component, which interacts with a G protein-coupled receptor, has been shown to play a role in MDSC recruitment and activation in a cervix cancer model (Markiewski et al., 2008). Some factors which are found in the tumour microenvironment, such as pro-inflammatory S-100 proteins, are also crucial for MDSC recruitment. Sinha and co-workers demonstrated that MDSCs can produce S-100 proteins by themselves, providing evidence for an autocrine loop that promotes MDSC recruitment (Cheng et al., 2008; Sinha et al., 2008).

MDSCs possess several mechanisms for immune suppression: 1) depletion of arginine, mediated by Arg1 and iNOS; 2) production of ROS; 3) post-translational modifications of T cell receptor (TCR) mediated by peroxynitrite generation; 4) depletion of cysteine; 5) production of TGFβ; 6) induction of Tregs (Bronte et al., 2005; Huang et al., 2006; Movahedi et al., 2008; Nagaraj et al., 2007; Srivastava et al., 2010; Terabe et al., 2003; Yang et al., 2006; Youn et al., 2008). In healthy individuals, IMCs differentiate in mature granulocytes, macrophages or dendritic cells, whereas in pathological conditions they expand into MDSCs. MDSCs have been observed in cancer, chronic infectious diseases, and autoimmunity. In tumor-bearing mice, MDSCs accumulate within primary and metastatic tumors, in the bone marrow, spleen and peripheral blood. In cancer patients, MDSCs have been identified in the blood.

Recent studies have contributed to partially clarify the biology of MDSCs. In mice, two major subsets were identified on the basis of their morphology and the expression of Ly6 family glycoproteins: monocytic MDSCs (M-MDSCs) and granulocytic MDSCs (G-MDSCs). M-MDSCs are $CD11b^+$ $Ly6G^-$ $Ly6C^{high}$ cells with monocyte-like morphology, while G-MDSCs are $CD11b^+$ $Ly6G^+$ $Ly6C^{low}$ with granulocyte-like morphology (Ostrand-Rosenberg and Sinha, 2009). Cells with similar phenotype, precursors of myeloid cells, are present in physiological conditions, but they are devoid of immunosuppressive activity. These cells, therefore, should not be named MDSCs (Youn and Gabrilovich, 2010). Other markers of MDSC subsets are: IL-4Rα (CD124), F4/80, CD80, and CSF-1R (CD115) (Sica and Bronte, 2007). The characterization of MDSCs deeply suffers from the lack of specific markers. However, recent characterizations have identified human MDSCs as $CD34^+$ $CD33^+$ $CD11b^+$ $HLA\text{-}DR^-$ cells (Ostrand-Rosenberg and Sinha, 2009). The ability to differentiate into mature DCs and macrophages *in vitro* has been shown to be restricted to M-MDSCs (Youn et al., 2008). M-MDSC-mediated immune suppression does not require cell-cell contact, but utilizes up-regulation of iNOS and Arg1, as well as production of immunosuppressive cytokines (Gabrilovich and Nagaraj, 2009). On the contrary, G-MDSCs suppress antigen-specific responses using mechanisms, including the release of ROS, that require prolonged cell-cell contact between MDSC and T cell (Gabrilovich and Nagaraj, 2009). The C5a subunit of the complement system appears a key regulator of MDSC functions, by modulating their migration and ROS production (Markiewski et al., 2008).

Several factors produced by tumors have been implicated in the differentiation of MDSCs, including granulocyte monocytes-colony stimulating factor (GM-CSF), macrophage-monocytes-colony stimulating factor (M-CSF), IL-6, IL-1β, VEGF and PGE2 (Gabrilovich and Nagaraj, 2009; Marigo et al., 2010). The transcription factor CCAT/enhancer binding protein β (C/EBPβ) proved to be the key player in the process of MDSC development (Marigo et al., 2010). It has been proposed that two signals are needed for the expansion and function of MDSCs: one factor (e.g. GM-CSF) prevents the differentiation in mature myeloid cells, and a second signal, provided by pro-inflammatory molecules such as IFNγ, activate MDSCs (Condamine and Gabrilovich, 2011).

A remarkable relation exists between MDSCs and TAMs. MDSCs are able to skew TAMs differentiation toward a tumor-promoting type-2 phenotype (Sinha et al., 2007). The cross-talk between MDSCs and macrophages requires cell-cell contact, then MDSCs release IL-10 to reduce IL-12 production by macrophages. MDSCs from an IL-1β enriched tumor microenvironment produce more IL-10 and are more potent down-regulators of macrophage-released IL-12 (Bunt et al., 2009). Circulating MDSCs can differentiate into $Gr1^-$ $F4/80^+$ TAMs in the tumor site (Kusmartsev and Gabrilovich, 2005) and this conversion is driven by tumor hypoxia (Corzo et al., 2010).

Because of their tumor-promoting activities, MDSCs are associated with type-2 immune responses, however accumulating evidence shows that MDSCs have characteristics of both M1 and M2 macrophages (Sica and Bronte, 2007). As an example, MDSCs express both Arg1 and iNOS, where these enzyme are differentially expressed by M1 (iNOS) and M2 (Arg1) macrophages. A recent study, investigating the molecular mechanisms behind MDSC differentiation, demonstrated an essential role of paired-immunoglobulin receptors (PIRs) in the differentiation of M1 or M2 MDSCs (Ma et al., 2011). The balance between PIR-A and PIR-B modulates MDSC polarization. In support of this, growth of Lewis lung carcinoma was significantly retarded in PIR-B-deficient mice (*Lilrb3-/-*) and PIR-B-deficient M-MDSCs expressed high levels of the M1 molecules iNOS.

MDSCs contribute to tumor growth also by non-immune mechanisms, including the promotion of angiogenesis. MDSCs isolated from murine tumors express high levels of metalloproteases, including MMP9 (Murdoch et al., 2008). MMP9 increases the bioavailability of VEGF sequestered in the extracellular matrix. Further in the tumor microenvironment and in proangiogenic culture conditions, MDSCs acquire endothelial markers such as CD31 and VEGF receptor 2 (VEGFR2) and the ability to directly incorporate into tumor endothelium (Yang et al., 2004). In agreement, tumor refractoriness to anti-VEGF therapy was shown to be mediated by $CD11b^+GR1^+$ myeloid cells (Shojaei et al., 2007a; Shojaei et al., 2007b).

2.4 Tumor-Associated Neutrophils (TANs)

Tumor-associated neutrophils (TANs) have received little interest by immunologists, also based on their short life span. However, new evidence contradicts this view, in that cytokines like IL-1 or microenvironment conditions such as hypoxia can prolong PMN survival (Sica et al., 2011). TANs are present in various tumors, including kidney, breast, colon, and lung (Houghton, 2010), and are recruited by locally secreted chemotactic factors. As an example, several carcinoma cells produce CXCL8, a prototypic chemoattractant for neutrophils (Bellocq et al., 1998). Furthermore, tumor-derived TGFβ promotes neutrophils migration both directly and indirectly, by regulating the expression of adhesion molecules in the endothelium (Flavell et al., 2010).

Neutrophils are able to produce various cytokines and chemokines that can influence not only immune and antimicrobial responses, but other processes such as hematopoiesis, wound healing, and angiogenesis (Cassatella et al., 2009; Mantovani, 2009; Piccard et al., 2011; Zhang et al., 2009). Despite little attention has been paid to TANs, clinical evidence indicates that their presence is a negative prognostic indicator. A correlation between TANs infiltrate and poor outcome has been described in renal cell carcinoma, bronchoalveolar cell carcinoma, and breast cancer (Jensen et al., 2009; Yang et al., 2005). In agreement, preclinical studies experimenting PMN depletion confirmed the detrimental nature of TANs (Pekarek et al., 1995; Tazawa et al., 2003).

Neutrophils contribute to tumor growth by promoting angiogenesis, cell proliferation, and metastasis (Houghton, 2010). Similarly to macrophages, a recent report described the functional plasticity of neutrophils (Fridlender et al., 2009). The authors investigated the effects of SM16, a TGFβ receptor kinase antagonist in murine lung cancer and mesothelioma models using syngeneic tumor xenografts and the orthotopic LSL-K-ras tumor model. Depletion of neutrophils by a specific anti-Ly6G antibody resulted in a significantly reduced effect of SM16, suggesting that neutrophils participate to the antitumor activity of TGFβ blockade, most likely by the production of oxygen radicals. Also, depletion of neutrophils affected the activation of $CD8^+$ CTLs. Fridlender and colleagues propose a new paradigm in which resident TANs acquire a protumor phenotype, largely driven by TGFβ, to become "N2 neutrophils". If TGFβ is blocked, neutrophils acquire an antitumor phenotype to become "N1 neutrophils" (Fridlender et al., 2009).

It was suggested that N1- and N2-type neutrophils are cells with a different degree of activation (i.e. fully activated or weakly activated neutrophils, respectively) rather than two alternatively activated cell subtypes (Gregory and Houghton, 2011). It is also object of debate the existence of two distinct populations, namely N2-polarized TANs and granulocytic MDSCs, that seem to overlap for many characteristics. In the absence of specific markers, it cannot be determined if N2 neutrophils within the tumors are granulocytic MDSCs recruited from the spleen or whether they are blood-derived neutrophils converted to an N2 phenotype by the tumor microenvironment. In support to the existence of N2-polarized TANs, Fridlender et al. emphasize that TGFβ-blockade does not alter blood neutrophils, splenic myeloid cells ($CD11b^+$), or splenic MDSCs, selectively acting on the intratumor activation of neutrophils. Also, TANs characterized in Fridlender's study have clear features of mature neutrophils, while MDSCs mostly exhibit an immature morphology (Mantovani, 2009).

3. Therapeutic approaches targeting TAMCs

The frequent association of TAMCs with poor prognosis makes these cells reasonable targets of biological anti-cancer therapies. Further, in the last few years there has been increasing evidence that TAMCs are strongly implicated in the failure of conventional chemotherapy and anti-angiogenic therapy.(Ferrara, 2010; Welford et al., 2011a) Accumulation of myeloid CD11b+Gr1+ cells (including TAMs, MDSC and immature cells) in tumours renders them refractory to angiogenic blockade by VEGF antibodies. (Shojaei and Ferrara, 2008) This effect was traced to a VEGF-independent pathway driven by the G-CSF-induced protein Bv8. (Shojaei et al., 2007b) Further, pharmacological inhibition of TEMs in tumour-bearing mice markedly increased the efficacy of therapeutic treatment with a vascular-disrupting agent.

3.1 TAMs and TEMs

Elimination of TAMs at tumor sites, or inhibition of their survival could result in improved prognosis. Earlier and more recent studies of macrophage depletion in experimental settings have been successful to limit tumour growth and metastatic spread (Aharinejad et al., 2009; Lin et al., 2001; Mantovani et al., 1992), and to achieve better therapeutic responses (De Palma et al., 2007; Ferrara, 2010; Gabrilovich and Nagaraj, 2009; Marigo et al., 2008; Welford et al., 2011a)

A number of studies have shown that the bisphosphonate clodronate encapsulated in liposomes is an efficient reagent for the depletion of macrophages in vivo. Clodronate-depletion of TAMs in tumour-bearing mice resulted in reduced angiogenesis and decreased tumour growth and metastatization.(Brown and Holen, 2009; Zeisberger et al., 2006) Moreover, the combination of clodronate with sorafenib, an available inhibitor of tyrosine protein kinases (e.g,VEGFR and PDGFR), significantly increased the efficacy of sorafenib alone in a xenograft model of hepatocellular carcinoma. In clinical practice, bisphosphonates are employed to treat osteoporosis; current applications in cancer therapy include their use to treat skeletal metastases in Multiple Myeloma, prostate and breast cancer. Treatment with zoledronic acid was associated with a significant reduction of skeletal-related events and, possibly, direct apoptotic effects in tumour cells. (Martin et al., 2010; Morgan et al., ; Zhang et al., 2010)

Our group reported that the anti-tumour agent of marine origin, Trabectedin (Yondelis), was unexpectedly found to be highly cytotoxic to mononuclear phagocytes, including TAMs. This cytotoxic effect is remarkably selective, as neutrophils and lymphocytes were not affected. (Allavena et al., 2005; D'Incalci and Galmarini, 2010)

A second approach is to inhibit the recruitment of circulating monocytes in tumour tissues.

The M-CSF receptor (M-CSFR) is exclusively expressed by monocytes-macrophages. In patients with advanced tumours, clinical studies are under way to check the feasibility and possibly clinical efficacy of inhibitors to the CSF-1R. Among the many chemokines expressed in the tumour micro-environment, CCL2 (or Monocyte Chemotactic Protein-1) occupies a prominent role and has been selected for therapeutic purposes. Pre-clinical studies have shown that anti-CCL2 antibodies or antagonists to its receptor CCR2, given in combination with chemotherapy, were able to induce tumour regression and yielded to improved survival in prostate mouse cancer models (Li et al., 2009; Loberg et al., 2007; Popivanova et al., 2009)

In the opposite direction, another approach is to exploit the tumor-homing ability of TAMCs: after all, they are at the right place at the right time. Indeed, delivery of cytokines and cytotoxic proteins to tumors by means of gene modified cells represents a promising strategy to treat cancer. It was recently shown that TEMs could be used to deliver interferon-alpha (IFNα), a potent cytokine with angiostatic and antiproliferative activity (De Palma et al., 2008), thanks to the preferential homing of TEMs to the tumors (De Palma and Naldini, 2009).

A fourth and more recent approach is to 're-educate' TAMs to exert anti-tumour responses protective for the host, ideally by using factors able to revert TAMs into M1-macrophages, with potential anti-tumour activity. It is becoming accepted that macrophages are flexible and able to switch from one polarization state to the other. (Pelegrin and Surprenant, 2009)

This was achieved in experimental mouse tumours, by injecting the TLR9 agonist CpG-oligodeoxynucleotide (CpG-ODN), coupled with anti-IL-10 receptor.(Guiducci et al., 2005) or the chemokine CCL16 (Cappello et al., 2004). CpG-ODN synergized also with an agonist anti-CD40 mAb to revert TAMs displaying anti-tumour activity. (Buhtoiarov et al., 2011) A remarkable anti-tumour effect of re-directed macrophages has been recently reported in human pancreatic cancer with the use of agonist anti-CD40 mAb. (Beatty et al., 2011) Still in the same direction, a recent report showed that the plasma protein histidine-rich glycoprotein (HRG) known for its inhibitory effects on angiogenesis (Juarez et al., 2002; Olsson et al., 2004) is able to skew TAMs polarization into M1-like phenotype by down-regulation of the placental growth factor (PlGF), a member of the VEGF family. In mice, HRG promoted anti-tumour immune responses and normalization of the vessel network. (Rolny et al., 2011)

Direct activation with IFNγ, a prototypical M1-polarizing cytokine, has been shown to re-educate TAMs (Duluc et al., 2009) and there is evidence for antitumor activity of this molecule in minimal residual disease (Mantovani and Sica, 2010). Inhibition of STAT3 activity, required for IL-10 biological functions and gene transcription, restored production of pro-inflammatory mediators (IL-12 and TNF-α) by infiltrating leukocytes and promoted tumour inhibition (Kortylewski et al., 2005). Recent results suggest that SHIP1 functions in vivo to repress M2 macrophage skewing. Consistent with this, Ship1−/− mice display enhanced tumor implant growth (Rauh et al., 2005). In agreement, inhibition of the M2 polarizing p50 NF-κB activity resulted in restoration of M1 inflammation and tumor inhibition in different cancer mouse models (fibrosarcoma, melanoma)(Saccani A. et al Cancer Res 2006) (Porta et al., 2009)

3.2 MDSC

The translational potential of MDSC research is dual. The immunosuppressive activity of MDSCs could be exploited to inhibit immune responses in autoimmune diseases and organ transplantation. Conversely, elimination of MDSCs could be essential in cancer patients undergoing active (vaccination) or passive (adoptive transfer of *ex-vivo* expanded anti-tumor T cells) immunotherapy. A possible approach to contrast MDSC pro-tumoral activities consists in the promotion of MDSC differentiation into mature cells devoid of suppressive activity. Vitamin A represents an interesting candidate to restore immunosurveillance. In fact, Vitamin A metabolites stimulate the differentiation of myeloid progenitor cells into DCs and macrophages and reduce MDSC accumulation (Gabrilovich et al., 2001; Kusmartsev et al., 2003). A clinical trial testing the effects of all-*trans*-retinoic acid (ATRA) in patients with metastatic renal cell carcinoma showed the efficacy of this compound in reducing MDSCs in peripheral blood. The decrease in MDSC number correlated with improved-antigen-specific T cell responses (Mirza et al., 2006). It has been reported that some chemotherapeutic drugs, such as gemcitabine, are able to eliminate MDSCs, without affecting T cells, B cells, NK cells, and macrophages (Ko et al., 2007; Suzuki et al., 2005). Another strategy is aimed to inhibit MDSC suppressive function. Compounds under investigation for this ability belong to COX2 inhibitors, phosphodiesterase 5 (PDE5) inhibitors, and NO-releasing non-steroidal anti-inflammatory drugs (NSAIDs) (Gabrilovich and Nagaraj, 2009). Preclinical evidence supports the use of IL-1 antagonists in treating human metastatic disease. Blocking IL-1 activity, mainly IL-1β, reduces both metastasis and tumor growth (Dinarello, 2010). Recently, it was shown that the effect is also mediated by the decrease of MDSC accumulation and suppressive activity (Ostrand-Rosenberg and Sinha, 2009). It has also been reported that $CD11b^+$ $Gr1^+$ cells enhance tumor refractoriness to anti-VEGF antibody (bevacizumab) treatment (Shojaei et al., 2007a). In this situation, MDSCs release the pro-angiogenic protein Bv8 that surrogates VEGF in the stimulation of tumor angiogenesis (Shojaei et al., 2007b). Because Bv8 is also important in MDSC mobilization and homing to the tumor site, this is an interesting candidate for cancer therapy.

3.3 TANs

TAN depletion represents a potential therapeutic approach for cancer cure (Tazzyman et al., 2009). However, since oncologic patients are already immunocompromized individuals, a complete ablation of neutrophils is not desirable. Alternatively, given that activated neutrophils can kill tumor cells through the release of toxic substances, it would be of interest to modulate TAN phenotype, with a switch from N2- towards N1-polarization. Nevertheless, this plan would lead to the generation of highly cytotoxic cells and could result in excessive tissue damage, potentially lethal. A more manageable therapeutic strategy can target neutrophils recruitment to tumors. Inhibition of CXCR2-mediated PMN chemotaxis with a specific antibody or a CXCR2 antagonist has been successfully tested in pre-clinical experimentation (Gregory and Houghton, 2011). The description of the pivotal role of TGFβ in the promotion of a protumor phenotype of TAN suggests that therapies contrasting this cytokine could contribute to re-educate neutrophils in the tumor microenvironment (Flavell et al., 2010). Interestingly, a recent study showed that the CCL2-driven accumulation of TAMs limits the influx of neutrophils in solid tumors by a yet unidentified mechanism. If TAMs accumulation is suppressed, neutrophils are recruited to the tumor providing a secondary source of MMP-9. Therefore, in the absence of TAMs, TANs provide alternative paracrine support for tumor angiogenesis and progression (Pahler et al., 2008). Hence, the elimination of TAMs alone may be insufficient to eradicate myeloid cell support to tumor growth .

4. Conclusions

Recent results indicate that tumour development promotes expansion and functional skewing of different myeloid cell populations, leading to accumulation of protumoral TAMC populations, which include TAMs, TEMs, MDSCs and TANs. These myeloid cell populations display distinct specialized functions, as well as overlapping activities (eg. angiogenesis). It is becoming evident that TAMCs appear to constitute a robust pro-tumour system and the functional elimination of a single myeloid population may be insufficient to eradicate their support to tumor growth. New strategies able to target different myeloid cell populations, simultaneously, are therefore desirable.

New evidence indicates that pathways promoting polarized functions of either macrophages (eg. M1 vs M2) or neutrophils (N1 vs N2) may share common constituents. (Mantovani, 2009) Understanding of this convergent pathways may offer common target/s and strategies to therapeutically affect the pro-tumoral networks established by TAMCs.

5. References

Aharinejad, S., Sioud, M., Lucas, T. and Abraham, D. (2009) Targeting stromal-cancer cell interactions with siRNAs. *Methods Mol Biol*, 487, 243-266.

Allavena, P., Chieppa, M., Bianchi, G., Solinas, G., Fabbri, M., Laskarin, G. and Mantovani, A. (2010) Engagement of the mannose receptor by tumoral mucins activates an immune suppressive phenotype in human tumor-associated macrophages. *Clin Dev Immunol*, 2010, 547179.

Allavena, P., Sica, A., Garlanda, C. and Mantovani, A. (2008) The Yin-Yang of tumor-associated macrophages in neoplastic progression and immune surveillance. *Immunol Rev*, 222, 155-161.

Allavena, P., Signorelli, M., Chieppa, M., Erba, E., Bianchi, G., Marchesi, F., Olimpio, C.O., Bonardi, C., Garbi, A., Lissoni, A., de Braud, F., Jimeno, J. and D'Incalci, M. (2005) Anti-inflammatory properties of the novel antitumor agent yondelis (trabectedin): inhibition of macrophage differentiation and cytokine production. *Cancer Res*, 65, 2964-2971.

Andreu, P., Johansson, M., Affara, N.I., Pucci, F., Tan, T., Junankar, S., Korets, L., Lam, J., Tawfik, D., DeNardo, D.G., Naldini, L., de Visser, K.E., De Palma, M. and Coussens, L.M. (2010) FcRgamma activation regulates inflammation-associated squamous carcinogenesis. *Cancer Cell*, 17, 121-134.

Auffray, C., Sieweke, M.H. and Geissmann, F. (2009) Blood monocytes: development, heterogeneity, and relationship with dendritic cells. *Annu Rev Immunol*, 27, 669-692.

Baeriswyl, V. and Christofori, G. (2009) The angiogenic switch in carcinogenesis. *Semin Cancer Biol*, 19, 329-337.

Balkwill, F. (2004) Cancer and the chemokine network. *Nat Rev Cancer*, 4, 540-550.

Beatty, G.L., Chiorean, E.G., Fishman, M.P., Saboury, B., Teitelbaum, U.R., Sun, W., Huhn, R.D., Song, W., Li, D., Sharp, L.L., Torigian, D.A., O'Dwyer, P.J. and Vonderheide, R.H. (2011) CD40 agonists alter tumor stroma and show efficacy against pancreatic carcinoma in mice and humans. *Science*, 331, 1612-1616.

Beck, A.H., Espinosa, I., Edris, B., Li, R., Montgomery, K., Zhu, S., Varma, S., Marinelli, R.J., van de Rijn, M. and West, R.B. (2009) The macrophage colony-stimulating factor 1 response signature in breast carcinoma. *Clin Cancer Res*, 15, 778-787.

Bellocq, A., Antoine, M., Flahault, A., Philippe, C., Crestani, B., Bernaudin, J.F., Mayaud, C., Milleron, B., Baud, L. and Cadranel, J. (1998) Neutrophil alveolitis in bronchioloalveolar carcinoma: induction by tumor-derived interleukin-8 and relation to clinical outcome. *Am J Pathol*, 152, 83-92.

Bingle, L., Brown, N.J. and Lewis, C.E. (2002) The role of tumour-associated macrophages in tumour progression: implications for new anticancer therapies. *J Pathol*, 196, 254-265.

Biswas, S.K., Gangi, L., Paul, S., Schioppa, T., Saccani, A., Sironi, M., Bottazzi, B., Doni, A., Vincenzo, B., Pasqualini, F., Vago, L., Nebuloni, M., Mantovani, A. and Sica, A. (2006) A distinct and unique transcriptional program expressed by tumor-associated macrophages (defective NF-kappaB and enhanced IRF-3/STAT1 activation). *Blood*, 107, 2112-2122.

Bollrath, J., Phesse, T.J., von Burstin, V.A., Putoczki, T., Bennecke, M., Bateman, T., Nebelsiek, T., Lundgren-May, T., Canli, O., Schwitalla, S., Matthews, V., Schmid, R.M., Kirchner, T., Arkan, M.C., Ernst, M. and Greten, F.R. (2009) gp130-mediated

Stat3 activation in enterocytes regulates cell survival and cell-cycle progression during colitis-associated tumorigenesis. *Cancer Cell*, 15, 91-102.

Bottazzi, B., Polentarutti, N., Acero, R., Balsari, A., Boraschi, D., Ghezzi, P., Salmona, M. and Mantovani, A. (1983) Regulation of the macrophage content of neoplasms by chemoattractants. *Science*, 220, 210-212.

Bronte, V., Kasic, T., Gri, G., Gallana, K., Borsellino, G., Marigo, I., Battistini, L., Iafrate, M., Prayer-Galetti, T., Pagano, F. and Viola, A. (2005) Boosting antitumor responses of T lymphocytes infiltrating human prostate cancers. *J Exp Med*, 201, 1257-1268.

Brown, H.K. and Holen, I. (2009) Anti-tumour effects of bisphosphonates--what have we learned from in vivo models? *Curr Cancer Drug Targets*, 9, 807-823.

Buhtoiarov, I.N., Sondel, P.M., Wigginton, J.M., Buhtoiarova, T.N., Yanke, E.M., Mahvi, D.A. and Rakhmilevich, A.L. (2011) Anti-tumour synergy of cytotoxic chemotherapy and anti-CD40 plus CpG-ODN immunotherapy through repolarization of tumour-associated macrophages. *Immunology*, 132, 226-239.

Bunt, S.K., Clements, V.K., Hanson, E.M., Sinha, P. and Ostrand-Rosenberg, S. (2009) Inflammation enhances myeloid-derived suppressor cell cross-talk by signaling through Toll-like receptor 4. *J Leukoc Biol*, 85, 996-1004.

Cappello, P., Caorsi, C., Bosticardo, M., De Angelis, S., Novelli, F., Forni, G. and Giovarelli, M. (2004) CCL16/LEC powerfully triggers effector and antigen-presenting functions of macrophages and enhances T cell cytotoxicity. *J Leukoc Biol*, 75, 135-142.

Cassatella, M.A., Locati, M. and Mantovani, A. (2009) Never underestimate the power of a neutrophil. *Immunity*, 31, 698-700.

Chen, J., Yao, Y., Gong, C., Yu, F., Su, S., Chen, J., Liu, B., Deng, H., Wang, F., Lin, L., Yao, H., Su, F., Anderson, K.S., Liu, Q., Ewen, M.E., Yao, X. and Song, E. (2011) CCL18 from tumor-associated macrophages promotes breast cancer metastasis via PITPNM3. *Cancer Cell*, 19, 541-555.

Cheng, P., Corzo, C.A., Luetteke, N., Yu, B., Nagaraj, S., Bui, M.M., Ortiz, M., Nacken, W., Sorg, C., Vogl, T., Roth, J. and Gabrilovich, D.I. (2008) Inhibition of dendritic cell differentiation and accumulation of myeloid-derived suppressor cells in cancer is regulated by S100A9 protein. *J Exp Med*, 205, 2235-2249.

Clark, C.E., Hingorani, S.R., Mick, R., Combs, C., Tuveson, D.A. and Vonderheide, R.H. (2007) Dynamics of the immune reaction to pancreatic cancer from inception to invasion. *Cancer Res*, 67, 9518-9527.

Clemente, C.G., Mihm, M.C., Jr., Bufalino, R., Zurrida, S., Collini, P. and Cascinelli, N. (1996) Prognostic value of tumor infiltrating lymphocytes in the vertical growth phase of primary cutaneous melanoma. *Cancer*, 77, 1303-1310.

Coffelt, S.B., Chen, Y.Y., Muthana, M., Welford, A.F., Tal, A.O., Scholz, A., Plate, K.H., Reiss, Y., Murdoch, C., De Palma, M. and Lewis, C.E. (2011) Angiopoietin 2 Stimulates TIE2-Expressing Monocytes To Suppress T Cell Activation and To Promote Regulatory T Cell Expansion. *J Immunol*, 186, 4183-4190.

Coffelt, S.B., Tal, A.O., Scholz, A., De Palma, M., Patel, S., Urbich, C., Biswas, S.K., Murdoch, C., Plate, K.H., Reiss, Y. and Lewis, C.E. (2010) Angiopoietin-2 regulates gene expression in TIE2-expressing monocytes and augments their inherent proangiogenic functions. *Cancer Res*, 70, 5270-5280.

Condamine, T. and Gabrilovich, D.I. (2011) Molecular mechanisms regulating myeloid-derived suppressor cell differentiation and function. *Trends Immunol*, 32, 19-25.

Corzo, C.A., Condamine, T., Lu, L., Cotter, M.J., Youn, J.I., Cheng, P., Cho, H.I., Celis, E., Quiceno, D.G., Padhya, T., McCaffrey, T.V., McCaffrey, J.C. and Gabrilovich, D.I. (2010) HIF-1alpha regulates function and differentiation of myeloid-derived suppressor cells in the tumor microenvironment. *J Exp Med*, 207, 2439-2453.

D'Incalci, M. and Galmarini, C.M. (2010) A review of trabectedin (ET-743): a unique mechanism of action. *Mol Cancer Ther*, 9, 2157-2163.

De Palma, M., Mazzieri, R., Politi, L.S., Pucci, F., Zonari, E., Sitia, G., Mazzoleni, S., Moi, D., Venneri, M.A., Indraccolo, S., Falini, A., Guidotti, L.G., Galli, R. and Naldini, L. (2008) Tumor-targeted interferon-alpha delivery by Tie2-expressing monocytes inhibits tumor growth and metastasis. *Cancer Cell*, 14, 299-311.

De Palma, M., Murdoch, C., Venneri, M.A., Naldini, L. and Lewis, C.E. (2007) Tie2-expressing monocytes: regulation of tumor angiogenesis and therapeutic implications. *Trends Immunol*, 28, 519-524.

De Palma, M. and Naldini, L. (2009) Tie2-expressing monocytes (TEMs): novel targets and vehicles of anticancer therapy? *Biochim Biophys Acta*, 1796, 5-10.

De Palma, M., Venneri, M.A., Galli, R., Sergi Sergi, L., Politi, L.S., Sampaolesi, M. and Naldini, L. (2005) Tie2 identifies a hematopoietic lineage of proangiogenic monocytes required for tumor vessel formation and a mesenchymal population of pericyte progenitors. *Cancer Cell*, 8, 211-226.

De Palma, M., Venneri, M.A., Roca, C. and Naldini, L. (2003) Targeting exogenous genes to tumor angiogenesis by transplantation of genetically modified hematopoietic stem cells. *Nat Med*, 9, 789-795.

DeNardo, D.G., Barreto, J.B., Andreu, P., Vasquez, L., Tawfik, D., Kolhatkar, N. and Coussens, L.M. (2009) CD4(+) T cells regulate pulmonary metastasis of mammary carcinomas by enhancing protumor properties of macrophages. *Cancer Cell*, 16, 91-102.

Dinapoli, M.R., Calderon, C.L. and Lopez, D.M. (1996) The altered tumoricidal capacity of macrophages isolated from tumor-bearing mice is related to reduce expression of the inducible nitric oxide synthase gene. *J Exp Med*, 183, 1323-1329.

Dinarello, C.A. (2010) Why not treat human cancer with interleukin-1 blockade? *Cancer Metastasis Rev*, 29, 317-329.

Du, F., Nakamura, Y., Tan, T.L., Lee, P., Lee, R., Yu, B. and Jamora, C. (2010) Expression of snail in epidermal keratinocytes promotes cutaneous inflammation and hyperplasia conducive to tumor formation. *Cancer Res*, 70, 10080-10089.

Du, R., Lu, K.V., Petritsch, C., Liu, P., Ganss, R., Passegue, E., Song, H., Vandenberg, S., Johnson, R.S., Werb, Z. and Bergers, G. (2008) HIF1alpha induces the recruitment of bone marrow-derived vascular modulatory cells to regulate tumor angiogenesis and invasion. *Cancer Cell*, 13, 206-220.

Duluc, D., Corvaisier, M., Blanchard, S., Catala, L., Descamps, P., Gamelin, E., Ponsoda, S., Delneste, Y., Hebbar, M. and Jeannin, P. (2009) Interferon-gamma reverses the immunosuppressive and protumoral properties and prevents the generation of human tumor-associated macrophages. *Int J Cancer*, 125, 367-373.

Ferrara, N. (2010) Role of myeloid cells in vascular endothelial growth factor-independent tumor angiogenesis. *Curr Opin Hematol*, 17, 219-224.

Finak, G., Bertos, N., Pepin, F., Sadekova, S., Souleimanova, M., Zhao, H., Chen, H., Omeroglu, G., Meterissian, S., Omeroglu, A., Hallett, M. and Park, M. (2008) Stromal gene expression predicts clinical outcome in breast cancer. *Nat Med*, 14, 518-527.

Flavell, R.A., Sanjabi, S., Wrzesinski, S.H. and Licona-Limon, P. (2010) The polarization of immune cells in the tumour environment by TGFbeta. *Nat Rev Immunol*, 10, 554-567.

Forssell, J., Oberg, A., Henriksson, M.L., Stenling, R., Jung, A. and Palmqvist, R. (2007) High macrophage infiltration along the tumor front correlates with improved survival in colon cancer. *Clin Cancer Res*, 13, 1472-1479.

Fridlender, Z.G., Sun, J., Kim, S., Kapoor, V., Cheng, G., Ling, L., Worthen, G.S. and Albelda, S.M. (2009) Polarization of tumor-associated neutrophil phenotype by TGF-beta: "N1" versus "N2" TAN. *Cancer Cell*, 16, 183-194.

Fukuda, A., Wang, S.C., Morris, J.P.t., Folias, A.E., Liou, A., Kim, G.E., Akira, S., Boucher, K.M., Firpo, M.A., Mulvihill, S.J. and Hebrok, M. (2011) Stat3 and MMP7 contribute to pancreatic ductal adenocarcinoma initiation and progression. *Cancer Cell*, 19, 441-455.

Gabrilovich, D.I. and Nagaraj, S. (2009) Myeloid-derived suppressor cells as regulators of the immune system. *Nat Rev Immunol*, 9, 162-174.

Gabrilovich, D.I., Velders, M.P., Sotomayor, E.M. and Kast, W.M. (2001) Mechanism of immune dysfunction in cancer mediated by immature Gr-1+ myeloid cells. *J Immunol*, 166, 5398-5406.

Ghassabeh, G.H., De Baetselier, P., Brys, L., Noel, W., Van Ginderachter, J.A., Meerschaut, S., Beschin, A., Brombacher, F. and Raes, G. (2006) Identification of a common gene signature for type II cytokine-associated myeloid cells elicited in vivo in different pathologic conditions. *Blood*, 108, 575-583.

Gocheva, V., Wang, H.W., Gadea, B.B., Shree, T., Hunter, K.E., Garfall, A.L., Berman, T. and Joyce, J.A. (2010) IL-4 induces cathepsin protease activity in tumor-associated macrophages to promote cancer growth and invasion. *Genes Dev*, 24, 241-255.

Goerdt, S. and Orfanos, C.E. (1999) Other functions, other genes: alternative activation of antigen-presenting cells. *Immunity*, 10, 137-142.

Gordon, S. and Martinez, F.O. (2010) Alternative activation of macrophages: mechanism and functions. *Immunity*, 32, 593-604.

Gordon, S. and Taylor, P.R. (2005) Monocyte and macrophage heterogeneity. *Nat Rev Immunol*, 5, 953-964.

Gratchev, A., Kzhyshkowska, J., Kannookadan, S., Ochsenreiter, M., Popova, A., Yu, X., Mamidi, S., Stonehouse-Usselmann, E., Muller-Molinet, I., Gooi, L. and Goerdt, S. (2008) Activation of a TGF-beta-specific multistep gene expression program in mature macrophages requires glucocorticoid-mediated surface expression of TGF-beta receptor II. *J Immunol*, 180, 6553-6565.

Gregory, A.D. and Houghton, A.M. (2011) Tumor-Associated Neutrophils: New Targets for Cancer Therapy. *Cancer Res*.

Grivennikov, S., Karin, E., Terzic, J., Mucida, D., Yu, G.Y., Vallabhapurapu, S., Scheller, J., Rose-John, S., Cheroutre, H., Eckmann, L. and Karin, M. (2009) IL-6 and Stat3 are required for survival of intestinal epithelial cells and development of colitis-associated cancer. *Cancer Cell*, 15, 103-113.

Guiducci, C., Vicari, A.P., Sangaletti, S., Trinchieri, G. and Colombo, M.P. (2005) Redirecting in vivo elicited tumor infiltrating macrophages and dendritic cells towards tumor rejection. *Cancer Res*, 65, 3437-3446.

Hagemann, T., Biswas, S.K., Lawrence, T., Sica, A. and Lewis, C.E. (2009) Regulation of macrophage function in tumors: the multifaceted role of NF-kappaB. *Blood*, 113, 3139-3146.

Hamilton, J.A. (2008) Colony-stimulating factors in inflammation and autoimmunity. *Nat Rev Immunol*, 8, 533-544.

Houghton, A.M. (2010) The paradox of tumor-associated neutrophils: fueling tumor growth with cytotoxic substances. *Cell Cycle*, 9, 1732-1737.

Huang, B., Pan, P.Y., Li, Q., Sato, A.I., Levy, D.E., Bromberg, J., Divino, C.M. and Chen, S.H. (2006) Gr-1+CD115+ immature myeloid suppressor cells mediate the development of tumor-induced T regulatory cells and T-cell anergy in tumor-bearing host. *Cancer Res*, 66, 1123-1131.

Ingman, W.V., Wyckoff, J., Gouon-Evans, V., Condeelis, J. and Pollard, J.W. (2006) Macrophages promote collagen fibrillogenesis around terminal end buds of the developing mammary gland. *Dev Dyn*, 235, 3222-3229.

Jensen, H.K., Donskov, F., Marcussen, N., Nordsmark, M., Lundbeck, F. and von der Maase, H. (2009) Presence of intratumoral neutrophils is an independent prognostic factor in localized renal cell carcinoma. *J Clin Oncol*, 27, 4709-4717.

Jin, G., Kawsar, H.I., Hirsch, S.A., Zeng, C., Jia, X., Feng, Z., Ghosh, S.K., Zheng, Q.Y., Zhou, A., McIntyre, T.M. and Weinberg, A. (2010) An Antimicrobial Peptide Regulates Tumor-Associated Macrophage Trafficking via the Chemokine Receptor CCR2, a Model for Tumorigenesis. *PLoS ONE*, 5, e10993.

Joyce, J.A. and Pollard, J.W. (2009) Microenvironmental regulation of metastasis. *Nat Rev Cancer*, 9, 239-252.

Juarez, J.C., Guan, X., Shipulina, N.V., Plunkett, M.L., Parry, G.C., Shaw, D.E., Zhang, J.C., Rabbani, S.A., McCrae, K.R., Mazar, A.P., Morgan, W.T. and Donate, F. (2002) Histidine-proline-rich glycoprotein has potent antiangiogenic activity mediated through the histidine-proline-rich domain. *Cancer Res*, 62, 5344-5350.

Kalluri, R. and Zeisberg, M. (2006) Fibroblasts in cancer. *Nat Rev Cancer*, 6, 392-401.

Ko, H.J., Kim, Y.J., Kim, Y.S., Chang, W.S., Ko, S.Y., Chang, S.Y., Sakaguchi, S. and Kang, C.Y. (2007) A combination of chemoimmunotherapies can efficiently break self-tolerance and induce antitumor immunity in a tolerogenic murine tumor model. *Cancer Res*, 67, 7477-7486.

Konishi, T., Okabe, H., Katoh, H., Fujiyama, Y. and Mori, A. (1996) Macrophage inflammatory protein-1 alpha expression in non-neoplastic and neoplastic lung tissue. *Virchows Arch*, 428, 107-111.

Kortylewski, M., Kujawski, M., Wang, T., Wei, S., Zhang, S., Pilon-Thomas, S., Niu, G., Kay, H., Mule, J., Kerr, W.G., Jove, R., Pardoll, D. and Yu, H. (2005) Inhibiting Stat3 signaling in the hematopoietic system elicits multicomponent antitumor immunity. *Nat Med*, 11, 1314-1321.

Kusmartsev, S., Cheng, F., Yu, B., Nefedova, Y., Sotomayor, E., Lush, R. and Gabrilovich, D. (2003) All-trans-retinoic acid eliminates immature myeloid cells from tumor-bearing mice and improves the effect of vaccination. *Cancer Res*, 63, 4441-4449.

Kusmartsev, S. and Gabrilovich, D.I. (2005) STAT1 signaling regulates tumor-associated macrophage-mediated T cell deletion. *J Immunol*, 174, 4880-4891.

Laghi, L., Bianchi, P., Miranda, E., Balladore, E., Pacetti, V., Grizzi, F., Allavena, P., Torri, V., Repici, A., Santoro, A., Mantovani, A., Roncalli, M. and Malesci, A. (2009) CD3+ cells at the invasive margin of deeply invading (pT3-T4) colorectal cancer and risk of post-surgical metastasis: a longitudinal study. *Lancet Oncol*, 10, 877-884.

Lenz, G., Wright, G., Dave, S.S., Xiao, W., Powell, J., Zhao, H., Xu, W., Tan, B., Goldschmidt, N., Iqbal, J., Vose, J., Bast, M., Fu, K., Weisenburger, D.D., Greiner, T.C., Armitage, J.O., Kyle, A., May, L., Gascoyne, R.D., Connors, J.M., Troen, G., Holte, H., Kvaloy, S., Dierickx, D., Verhoef, G., Delabie, J., Smeland, E.B., Jares, P., Martinez, A., Lopez-Guillermo, A., Montserrat, E., Campo, E., Braziel, R.M., Miller, T.P., Rimsza, L.M., Cook, J.R., Pohlman, B., Sweetenham, J., Tubbs, R.R., Fisher, R.I., Hartmann, E., Rosenwald, A., Ott, G., Muller-Hermelink, H.K., Wrench, D., Lister, T.A., Jaffe, E.S., Wilson, W.H., Chan, W.C. and Staudt, L.M. (2008) Stromal gene signatures in large-B-cell lymphomas. *N Engl J Med*, 359, 2313-2323.

Lesina, M., Kurkowski, M.U., Ludes, K., Rose-John, S., Treiber, M., Kloppel, G., Yoshimura, A., Reindl, W., Sipos, B., Akira, S., Schmid, R.M. and Algul, H. Stat3/Socs3 activation by IL-6 transsignaling promotes progression of pancreatic intraepithelial neoplasia and development of pancreatic cancer. *Cancer Cell*, 19, 456-469.

Lewis, C.E. and Pollard, J.W. (2006) Distinct role of macrophages in different tumor microenvironments. *Cancer Res*, 66, 605-612.

Lewis, J.S., Landers, R.J., Underwood, J.C., Harris, A.L. and Lewis, C.E. (2000) Expression of vascular endothelial growth factor by macrophages is up-regulated in poorly vascularized areas of breast carcinomas. *J Pathol*, 192, 150-158.

Li, X., Loberg, R., Liao, J., Ying, C., Snyder, L.A., Pienta, K.J. and McCauley, L.K. (2009) A destructive cascade mediated by CCL2 facilitates prostate cancer growth in bone. *Cancer Res*, 69, 1685-1692.

Lin, E.Y., Gouon-Evans, V., Nguyen, A.V. and Pollard, J.W. (2002) The macrophage growth factor CSF-1 in mammary gland development and tumor progression. *J Mammary Gland Biol Neoplasia*, 7, 147-162.

Lin, E.Y., Nguyen, A.V., Russell, R.G. and Pollard, J.W. (2001) Colony-stimulating factor 1 promotes progression of mammary tumors to malignancy. *J Exp Med*, 193, 727-740.

Loberg, R.D., Ying, C., Craig, M., Day, L.L., Sargent, E., Neeley, C., Wojno, K., Snyder, L.A., Yan, L. and Pienta, K.J. (2007) Targeting CCL2 with systemic delivery of neutralizing antibodies induces prostate cancer tumor regression in vivo. *Cancer Res*, 67, 9417-9424.

Loges, S., Schmidt, T., Tjwa, M., van Geyte, K., Lievens, D., Lutgens, E., Vanhoutte, D., Borgel, D., Plaisance, S., Hoylaerts, M., Luttun, A., Dewerchin, M., Jonckx, B. and Carmeliet, P. (2010) Malignant cells fuel tumor growth by educating infiltrating leukocytes to produce the mitogen Gas6. *Blood*, 115, 2264-2273.

Ma, G., Pan, P.Y., Eisenstein, S., Divino, C.M., Lowell, C.A., Takai, T. and Chen, S.H. (2011) Paired Immunoglobin-like Receptor-B Regulates the Suppressive Function and Fate of Myeloid-Derived Suppressor Cells. *Immunity*, 34, 385-395.

Mahmoud, S.M., Paish, E.C., Powe, D.G., Macmillan, R.D., Grainge, M.J., Lee, A.H., Ellis, I.O. and Green, A.R. (2011) Tumor-infiltrating CD8+ lymphocytes predict clinical outcome in breast cancer. *J Clin Oncol*, 29, 1949-1955.

Mantovani, A. (2009) The yin-yang of tumor-associated neutrophils. *Cancer Cell*, 16, 173-174.

Mantovani, A., Allavena, P. and Sica, A. (2004a) Tumour-associated macrophages as a prototypic type II polarised phagocyte population: role in tumour progression. *Eur J Cancer*, 40, 1660-1667.

Mantovani, A., Allavena, P., Sica, A. and Balkwill, F. (2008) Cancer-related inflammation. *Nature*, 454, 436-444.

Mantovani, A., Bottazzi, B., Colotta, F., Sozzani, S. and Ruco, L. (1992) The origin and function of tumor-associated macrophages. *Immunol Today*, 13, 265-270.

Mantovani, A. and Sica, A. (2010) Macrophages, innate immunity and cancer: balance, tolerance, and diversity. *Curr Opin Immunol*, 22, 231-237.

Mantovani, A., Sica, A., Allavena, P., Garlanda, C. and Locati, M. (2009) Tumor-associated macrophages and the related myeloid-derived suppressor cells as a paradigm of the diversity of macrophage activation. *Hum Immunol*, 70, 325-330.

Mantovani, A., Sica, A. and Locati, M. (2005) Macrophage polarization comes of age. *Immunity*, 23, 344-346.

Mantovani, A., Sica, A., Sozzani, S., Allavena, P., Vecchi, A. and Locati, M. (2004b) The chemokine system in diverse forms of macrophage activation and polarization. *Trends Immunol*, 25, 677-686.

Marigo, I., Bosio, E., Solito, S., Mesa, C., Fernandez, A., Dolcetti, L., Ugel, S., Sonda, N., Bicciato, S., Falisi, E., Calabrese, F., Basso, G., Zanovello, P., Cozzi, E., Mandruzzato, S. and Bronte, V. (2010) Tumor-induced tolerance and immune suppression depend on the C/EBPbeta transcription factor. *Immunity*, 32, 790-802.

Marigo, I., Dolcetti, L., Serafini, P., Zanovello, P. and Bronte, V. (2008) Tumor-induced tolerance and immune suppression by myeloid derived suppressor cells. *Immunol Rev*, 222, 162-179.

Markiewski, M.M., DeAngelis, R.A., Benencia, F., Ricklin-Lichtsteiner, S.K., Koutoulaki, A., Gerard, C., Coukos, G. and Lambris, J.D. (2008) Modulation of the antitumor immune response by complement. *Nat Immunol*, 9, 1225-1235.

Martin, C.K., Werbeck, J.L., Thudi, N.K., Lanigan, L.G., Wolfe, T.D., Toribio, R.E. and Rosol, T.J. (2010) Zoledronic acid reduces bone loss and tumor growth in an orthotopic xenograft model of osteolytic oral squamous cell carcinoma. *Cancer Res*, 70, 8607-8616.

Martinez, F.O., Helming, L. and Gordon, S. (2009) Alternative activation of macrophages: an immunologic functional perspective. *Annu Rev Immunol*, 27, 451-483.

Mason, S.D. and Joyce, J.A. (2011) Proteolytic networks in cancer. *Trends Cell Biol*, 21, 228-237.

Mirza, N., Fishman, M., Fricke, I., Dunn, M., Neuger, A.M., Frost, T.J., Lush, R.M., Antonia, S. and Gabrilovich, D.I. (2006) All-trans-retinoic acid improves differentiation of myeloid cells and immune response in cancer patients. *Cancer Res*, 66, 9299-9307.

Morgan, G.J., Davies, F.E., Gregory, W.M., Cocks, K., Bell, S.E., Szubert, A.J., Navarro-Coy, N., Drayson, M.T., Owen, R.G., Feyler, S., Ashcroft, A.J., Ross, F., Byrne, J., Roddie, H., Rudin, C., Cook, G., Jackson, G.H. and Child, J.A. (2010) First-line treatment with zoledronic acid as compared with clodronic acid in multiple myeloma (MRC Myeloma IX): a randomised controlled trial. *Lancet*, 376, 1989-1999.

Moussai, D., Mitsui, H., Pettersen, J.S., Pierson, K.C., Shah, K.R., Suarez-Farinas, M., Cardinale, I.R., Bluth, M.J., Krueger, J.G. and Carucci, J.A. (2011) The human cutaneous squamous cell carcinoma microenvironment is characterized by increased lymphatic density and enhanced expression of macrophage-derived VEGF-C. *J Invest Dermatol*, 131, 229-236.

Movahedi, K., Guilliams, M., Van den Bossche, J., Van den Bergh, R., Gysemans, C., Beschin, A., De Baetselier, P. and Van Ginderachter, J.A. (2008) Identification of discrete tumor-induced myeloid-derived suppressor cell subpopulations with distinct T cell-suppressive activity. *Blood*, 111, 4233-4244.

Movahedi, K., Laoui, D., Gysemans, C., Baeten, M., Stange, G., Van den Bossche, J., Mack, M., Pipeleers, D., In't Veld, P., De Baetselier, P. and Van Ginderachter, J.A. (2010) Different tumor microenvironments contain functionally distinct subsets of macrophages derived from Ly6C(high) monocytes. *Cancer Res*, 70, 5728-5739.

Murdoch, C., Muthana, M., Coffelt, S.B. and Lewis, C.E. (2008) The role of myeloid cells in the promotion of tumour angiogenesis. *Nat Rev Cancer*, 8, 618-631.

Murdoch, C., Tazzyman, S., Webster, S. and Lewis, C.E. (2007) Expression of Tie-2 by human monocytes and their responses to angiopoietin-2. *J Immunol*, 178, 7405-7411.

Murray, P.J. and Wynn, T.A. (2011) Obstacles and opportunities for understanding macrophage polarization. *J Leukoc Biol*, 89, 557-563.

Nagaraj, S., Gupta, K., Pisarev, V., Kinarsky, L., Sherman, S., Kang, L., Herber, D.L., Schneck, J. and Gabrilovich, D.I. (2007) Altered recognition of antigen is a mechanism of CD8+ T cell tolerance in cancer. *Nat Med*, 13, 828-835.

Ohno, S., Inagawa, H., Dhar, D.K., Fujii, T., Ueda, S., Tachibana, M., Suzuki, N., Inoue, M., Soma, G. and Nagasue, N. (2003) The degree of macrophage infiltration into the cancer cell nest is a significant predictor of survival in gastric cancer patients. *Anticancer Res*, 23, 5015-5022.

Ohtaki, Y., Ishii, G., Nagai, K., Ashimine, S., Kuwata, T., Hishida, T., Nishimura, M., Yoshida, J., Takeyoshi, I. and Ochiai, A. (2010) Stromal macrophage expressing CD204 is associated with tumor aggressiveness in lung adenocarcinoma. *J Thorac Oncol*, 5, 1507-1515.

Ohtani, H., Naito, Y., Saito, K. and Nagura, H. (1997) Expression of costimulatory molecules B7-1 and B7-2 by macrophages along invasive margin of colon cancer: a possible antitumor immunity? *Lab Invest*, 77, 231-241.

Ojalvo, L.S., Whittaker, C.A., Condeelis, J.S. and Pollard, J.W. (2010) Gene expression analysis of macrophages that facilitate tumor invasion supports a role for Wnt-signaling in mediating their activity in primary mammary tumors. *J Immunol*, 184, 702-712.

Olsson, A.K., Larsson, H., Dixelius, J., Johansson, I., Lee, C., Oellig, C., Bjork, I. and Claesson-Welsh, L. (2004) A fragment of histidine-rich glycoprotein is a potent inhibitor of tumor vascularization. *Cancer Res*, 64, 599-605.

Ostrand-Rosenberg, S. and Sinha, P. (2009) Myeloid-derived suppressor cells: linking inflammation and cancer. *J Immunol*, 182, 4499-4506.

Pages, F., Berger, A., Camus, M., Sanchez-Cabo, F., Costes, A., Molidor, R., Mlecnik, B., Kirilovsky, A., Nilsson, M., Damotte, D., Meatchi, T., Bruneval, P., Cugnenc, P.H., Trajanoski, Z., Fridman, W.H. and Galon, J. (2005) Effector memory T cells, early metastasis, and survival in colorectal cancer. *N Engl J Med*, 353, 2654-2666.

Pahler, J.C., Tazzyman, S., Erez, N., Chen, Y.Y., Murdoch, C., Nozawa, H., Lewis, C.E. and Hanahan, D. (2008) Plasticity in tumor-promoting inflammation: impairment of macrophage recruitment evokes a compensatory neutrophil response. *Neoplasia*, 10, 329-340.

Palucka, K., Ueno, H., Zurawski, G., Fay, J. and Banchereau, J. (2010) Building on dendritic cell subsets to improve cancer vaccines. *Curr Opin Immunol*, 22, 258-263.

Pekarek, L.A., Starr, B.A., Toledano, A.Y. and Schreiber, H. (1995) Inhibition of tumor growth by elimination of granulocytes. *J Exp Med*, 181, 435-440.

Pelegrin, P. and Surprenant, A. (2009) Dynamics of macrophage polarization reveal new mechanism to inhibit IL-1beta release through pyrophosphates. *Embo J*, 28, 2114-2127.

Piccard, H., Muschel, R.J. and Opdenakker, G. (2011) On the dual roles and polarized phenotypes of neutrophils in tumor development and progression. *Crit Rev Oncol Hematol*.

Pollard, J.W. (2004) Tumour-educated macrophages promote tumour progression and metastasis. *Nat Rev Cancer*, 4, 71-78.

Pollard, J.W. (2008) Macrophages define the invasive microenvironment in breast cancer. *J Leukoc Biol*, 84, 623-630.

Pollard, J.W. (2009) Trophic macrophages in development and disease. *Nat Rev Immunol*, 9, 259-270.

Popivanova, B.K., Kostadinova, F.I., Furuichi, K., Shamekh, M.M., Kondo, T., Wada, T., Egashira, K. and Mukaida, N. (2009) Blockade of a chemokine, CCL2, reduces chronic colitis-associated carcinogenesis in mice. *Cancer Res*, 69, 7884-7892.

Porta, C., Rimoldi, M., Raes, G., Brys, L., Ghezzi, P., Di Liberto, D., Dieli, F., Ghisletti, S., Natoli, G., De Baetselier, P., Mantovani, A. and Sica, A. (2009) Tolerance and M2 (alternative) macrophage polarization are related processes orchestrated by p50 nuclear factor kappaB. *Proc Natl Acad Sci U S A*, 106, 14978-14983.

Pucci, F., Venneri, M.A., Biziato, D., Nonis, A., Moi, D., Sica, A., Di Serio, C., Naldini, L. and De Palma, M. (2009) A distinguishing gene signature shared by tumor-infiltrating Tie2-expressing monocytes, blood "resident" monocytes, and embryonic macrophages suggests common functions and developmental relationships. *Blood*, 114, 901-914.

Qian, B.Z. and Pollard, J.W. (2010) Macrophage diversity enhances tumor progression and metastasis. *Cell*, 141, 39-51.

Rauh, M.J., Ho, V., Pereira, C., Sham, A., Sly, L.M., Lam, V., Huxham, L., Minchinton, A.I., Mui, A. and Krystal, G. (2005) SHIP represses the generation of alternatively activated macrophages. *Immunity*, 23, 361-374.

Ravasi, T., Wells, C., Forest, A., Underhill, D.M., Wainwright, B.J., Aderem, A., Grimmond, S. and Hume, D.A. (2002) Generation of diversity in the innate immune system: macrophage heterogeneity arises from gene-autonomous transcriptional probability of individual inducible genes. *J Immunol*, 168, 44-50.

Ribatti, D. and Vacca, A. (2009) The role of monocytes-macrophages in vasculogenesis in multiple myeloma. *Leukemia*, 23, 1535-1536.

Riches, D.W. (1995) Signalling heterogeneity as a contributing factor in macrophage functional diversity. *Semin Cell Biol*, 6, 377-384.

Rolny, C., Mazzone, M., Tugues, S., Laoui, D., Johansson, I., Coulon, C., Squadrito, M.L., Segura, I., Li, X., Knevels, E., Costa, S., Vinckier, S., Dresselaer, T., Akerud, P., De Mol, M., Salomaki, H., Phillipson, M., Wyns, S., Larsson, E., Buysschaert, I., Botling,

J., Himmelreich, U., Van Ginderachter, J.A., De Palma, M., Dewerchin, M., Claesson-Welsh, L. and Carmeliet, P. (2011) HRG inhibits tumor growth and metastasis by inducing macrophage polarization and vessel normalization through downregulation of PlGF. *Cancer Cell*, 19, 31-44.

Saccani, A., Schioppa, T., Porta, C., Biswas, S.K., Nebuloni, M., Vago, L., Bottazzi, B., Colombo, M.P., Mantovani, A. and Sica, A. (2006) p50 nuclear factor-kappaB overexpression in tumor-associated macrophages inhibits M1 inflammatory responses and antitumor resistance. *Cancer Res*, 66, 11432-11440.

Sawanobori, Y., Ueha, S., Kurachi, M., Shimaoka, T., Talmadge, J.E., Abe, J., Shono, Y., Kitabatake, M., Kakimi, K., Mukaida, N. and Matsushima, K. (2008) Chemokine-mediated rapid turnover of myeloid-derived suppressor cells in tumor-bearing mice. *Blood*, 111, 5457-5466.

Schioppa, T., Uranchimeg, B., Saccani, A., Biswas, S.K., Doni, A., Rapisarda, A., Bernasconi, S., Saccani, S., Nebuloni, M., Vago, L., Mantovani, A., Melillo, G. and Sica, A. (2003) Regulation of the chemokine receptor CXCR4 by hypoxia. *J Exp Med*, 198, 1391-1402.

Schor, S.L., Ellis, I.R., Jones, S.J., Baillie, R., Seneviratne, K., Clausen, J., Motegi, K., Vojtesek, B., Kankova, K., Furrie, E., Sales, M.J., Schor, A.M. and Kay, R.A. (2003) Migration-stimulating factor: a genetically truncated onco-fetal fibronectin isoform expressed by carcinoma and tumor-associated stromal cells. *Cancer Res*, 63, 8827-8836.

Sconocchia, G., Zlobec, I., Lugli, A., Calabrese, D., Iezzi, G., Karamitopoulou, E., Patsouris, E.S., Peros, G., Horcic, M., Tornillo, L., Zuber, M., Droeser, R., Muraro, M.G., Mengus, C., Oertli, D., Ferrone, S., Terracciano, L. and Spagnoli, G.C. (2011) Tumor infiltration by FcgammaRIII (CD16)+ myeloid cells is associated with improved survival in patients with colorectal carcinoma. *Int J Cancer*, 128, 2663-2672.

Shojaei, F. and Ferrara, N. (2008) Refractoriness to antivascular endothelial growth factor treatment: role of myeloid cells. *Cancer Res*, 68, 5501-5504.

Shojaei, F., Wu, X., Malik, A.K., Zhong, C., Baldwin, M.E., Schanz, S., Fuh, G., Gerber, H.P. and Ferrara, N. (2007a) Tumor refractoriness to anti-VEGF treatment is mediated by CD11b+Gr1+ myeloid cells. *Nat Biotechnol*, 25, 911-920.

Shojaei, F., Wu, X., Zhong, C., Yu, L., Liang, X.H., Yao, J., Blanchard, D., Bais, C., Peale, F.V., van Bruggen, N., Ho, C., Ross, J., Tan, M., Carano, R.A., Meng, Y.G. and Ferrara, N. (2007b) Bv8 regulates myeloid-cell-dependent tumour angiogenesis. *Nature*, 450, 825-831.

Sica, A. (2010) Role of tumour-associated macrophages in cancerrelated inflammation. *Exp Oncol*, 32, 153-158.

Sica, A. and Bronte, V. (2007) Altered macrophage differentiation and immune dysfunction in tumor development. *J Clin Invest*, 117, 1155-1166.

Sica, A., Larghi, P., Mancino, A., Rubino, L., Porta, C., Totaro, M.G., Rimoldi, M., Biswas, S.K., Allavena, P. and Mantovani, A. (2008) Macrophage polarization in tumour progression. *Semin Cancer Biol*, 18, 349-355.

Sica, A., Melillo, G. and Varesio, L. (2011) Hypoxia: a double-edged sword of immunity. *J Mol Med*.

Sica, A., Saccani, A., Bottazzi, B., Polentarutti, N., Vecchi, A., van Damme, J. and Mantovani, A. (2000) Autocrine production of IL-10 mediates defective IL-12 production and NF-kappa B activation in tumor-associated macrophages. *J Immunol*, 164, 762-767.

Sierra, J.R., Corso, S., Caione, L., Cepero, V., Conrotto, P., Cignetti, A., Piacibello, W., Kumanogoh, A., Kikutani, H., Comoglio, P.M., Tamagnone, L. and Giordano, S. (2008) Tumor angiogenesis and progression are enhanced by Sema4D produced by tumor-associated macrophages. *J Exp Med*, 205, 1673-1685.

Sinha, P., Clements, V.K., Bunt, S.K., Albelda, S.M. and Ostrand-Rosenberg, S. (2007) Cross-talk between myeloid-derived suppressor cells and macrophages subverts tumor immunity toward a type 2 response. *J Immunol*, 179, 977-983.

Sinha, P., Okoro, C., Foell, D., Freeze, H.H., Ostrand-Rosenberg, S. and Srikrishna, G. (2008) Proinflammatory S100 proteins regulate the accumulation of myeloid-derived suppressor cells. *J Immunol*, 181, 4666-4675.

Solinas, G., Schiarea, S., Liguori, M., Fabbri, M., Pesce, S., Zammataro, L., Pasqualini, F., Nebuloni, M., Chiabrando, C., Mantovani, A. and Allavena, P. (2010) Tumor-conditioned macrophages secrete migration-stimulating factor: a new marker for M2-polarization, influencing tumor cell motility. *J Immunol*, 185, 642-652.

Srivastava, M.K., Sinha, P., Clements, V.K., Rodriguez, P. and Ostrand-Rosenberg, S. (2010) Myeloid-derived suppressor cells inhibit T-cell activation by depleting cystine and cysteine. *Cancer Res*, 70, 68-77.

Steidl, C., Lee, T., Shah, S.P., Farinha, P., Han, G., Nayar, T., Delaney, A., Jones, S.J., Iqbal, J., Weisenburger, D.D., Bast, M.A., Rosenwald, A., Muller-Hermelink, H.K., Rimsza, L.M., Campo, E., Delabie, J., Braziel, R.M., Cook, J.R., Tubbs, R.R., Jaffe, E.S., Lenz, G., Connors, J.M., Staudt, L.M., Chan, W.C. and Gascoyne, R.D. (2010) Tumor-associated macrophages and survival in classic Hodgkin's lymphoma. *N Engl J Med*, 362, 875-885.

Stein, M., Keshav, S., Harris, N. and Gordon, S. (1992) Interleukin 4 potently enhances murine macrophage mannose receptor activity: a marker of alternative immunologic macrophage activation. *J Exp Med*, 176, 287-292.

Stout, R.D., Jiang, C., Matta, B., Tietzel, I., Watkins, S.K. and Suttles, J. (2005) Macrophages sequentially change their functional phenotype in response to changes in microenvironmental influences. *J Immunol*, 175, 342-349.

Stout, R.D. and Suttles, J. (2005) Immunosenescence and macrophage functional plasticity: dysregulation of macrophage function by age-associated microenvironmental changes. *Immunol Rev*, 205, 60-71.

Sugita, J., Ohtani, H., Mizoi, T., Saito, K., Shiiba, K., Sasaki, I., Matsuno, S., Yagita, H., Miyazawa, M. and Nagura, H. (2002) Close association between Fas ligand (FasL; CD95L)-positive tumor-associated macrophages and apoptotic cancer cells along invasive margin of colorectal carcinoma: a proposal on tumor-host interactions. *Jpn J Cancer Res*, 93, 320-328.

Suzuki, E., Kapoor, V., Jassar, A.S., Kaiser, L.R. and Albelda, S.M. (2005) Gemcitabine selectively eliminates splenic Gr-1+/CD11b+ myeloid suppressor cells in tumor-bearing animals and enhances antitumor immune activity. *Clin Cancer Res*, 11, 6713-6721.

Talmadge, J.E., Donkor, M. and Scholar, E. (2007) Inflammatory cell infiltration of tumors: Jekyll or Hyde. *Cancer Metastasis Rev*, 26, 373-400.

Tannenbaum, C.S., Koerner, T.J., Jansen, M.M. and Hamilton, T.A. (1988) Characterization of lipopolysaccharide-induced macrophage gene expression. *J Immunol*, 140, 3640-3645.

Tazawa, H., Okada, F., Kobayashi, T., Tada, M., Mori, Y., Une, Y., Sendo, F., Kobayashi, M. and Hosokawa, M. (2003) Infiltration of neutrophils is required for acquisition of metastatic phenotype of benign murine fibrosarcoma cells: implication of inflammation-associated carcinogenesis and tumor progression. *Am J Pathol*, 163, 2221-2232.

Tazzyman, S., Lewis, C.E. and Murdoch, C. (2009) Neutrophils: key mediators of tumour angiogenesis. *Int J Exp Pathol*, 90, 222-231.

Terabe, M., Matsui, S., Park, J.M., Mamura, M., Noben-Trauth, N., Donaldson, D.D., Chen, W., Wahl, S.M., Ledbetter, S., Pratt, B., Letterio, J.J., Paul, W.E. and Berzofsky, J.A. (2003) Transforming growth factor-beta production and myeloid cells are an effector mechanism through which CD1d-restricted T cells block cytotoxic T lymphocyte-mediated tumor immunosurveillance: abrogation prevents tumor recurrence. *J Exp Med*, 198, 1741-1752.

Venneri, M.A., De Palma, M., Ponzoni, M., Pucci, F., Scielzo, C., Zonari, E., Mazzieri, R., Doglioni, C. and Naldini, L. (2007) Identification of proangiogenic TIE2-expressing monocytes (TEMs) in human peripheral blood and cancer. *Blood*, 109, 5276-5285.

Vesely, M.D., Kershaw, M.H., Schreiber, R.D. and Smyth, M.J. (2011) Natural innate and adaptive immunity to cancer. *Annu Rev Immunol*, 29, 235-271.

Wang, H.W. and Joyce, J.A. (2010) Alternative activation of tumor-associated macrophages by IL-4: priming for protumoral functions. *Cell Cycle*, 9, 4824-4835.

Welford, A.F., Biziato, D., Coffelt, S.B., Nucera, S., Fisher, M., Pucci, F., Di Serio, C., Naldini, L., De Palma, M., Tozer, G.M. and Lewis, C.E. (2011a) TIE2-expressing macrophages limit the therapeutic efficacy of the vascular-disrupting agent combretastatin A4 phosphate in mice. *J Clin Invest*, 121, 1969-1973.

Welford, A.F., Biziato, D., Coffelt, S.B., Nucera, S., Fisher, M., Pucci, F., Serio, C.D., Naldini, L., Palma, M.D., Tozer, G.M. and Lewis, C.E. (2011b) TIE2-expressing macrophages limit the therapeutic efficacy of the vascular-disrupting agent combretastatin A4 phosphate in mice. *The Journal of Clinical Investigation*, 0, 0-0.

Wyckoff, J.B., Wang, Y., Lin, E.Y., Li, J.F., Goswami, S., Stanley, E.R., Segall, J.E., Pollard, J.W. and Condeelis, J. (2007) Direct visualization of macrophage-assisted tumor cell intravasation in mammary tumors. *Cancer Res*, 67, 2649-2656.

Yang, L., DeBusk, L.M., Fukuda, K., Fingleton, B., Green-Jarvis, B., Shyr, Y., Matrisian, L.M., Carbone, D.P. and Lin, P.C. (2004) Expansion of myeloid immune suppressor Gr+CD11b+ cells in tumor-bearing host directly promotes tumor angiogenesis. *Cancer Cell*, 6, 409-421.

Yang, P., Bamlet, W.R., Sun, Z., Ebbert, J.O., Aubry, M.C., Krowka, M.J., Taylor, W.R., Marks, R.S., Deschamps, C., Swensen, S.J., Wieben, E.D., Cunningham, J.M., Melton, L.J. and de Andrade, M. (2005) Alpha1-antitrypsin and neutrophil elastase imbalance and lung cancer risk. *Chest*, 128, 445-452.

Yang, R., Cai, Z., Zhang, Y., Yutzy, W.H.t., Roby, K.F. and Roden, R.B. (2006) CD80 in immune suppression by mouse ovarian carcinoma-associated Gr-1+CD11b+ myeloid cells. *Cancer Res*, 66, 6807-6815.

Youn, J.I. and Gabrilovich, D.I. (2010) The biology of myeloid-derived suppressor cells: the blessing and the curse of morphological and functional heterogeneity. *Eur J Immunol*, 40, 2969-2975.

Youn, J.I., Nagaraj, S., Collazo, M. and Gabrilovich, D.I. (2008) Subsets of myeloid-derived suppressor cells in tumor-bearing mice. *J Immunol*, 181, 5791-5802.

Zachariae, C.O., Anderson, A.O., Thompson, H.L., Appella, E., Mantovani, A., Oppenheim, J.J. and Matsushima, K. (1990) Properties of monocyte chemotactic and activating factor (MCAF) purified from a human fibrosarcoma cell line. *J Exp Med*, 171, 2177-2182.

Zeisberger, S.M., Odermatt, B., Marty, C., Zehnder-Fjallman, A.H., Ballmer-Hofer, K. and Schwendener, R.A. (2006) Clodronate-liposome-mediated depletion of tumour-associated macrophages: a new and highly effective antiangiogenic therapy approach. *Br J Cancer*, 95, 272-281.

Zhang, J., Sud, S., Mizutani, K., Gyetko, M.R. and Pienta, K.J. (2011) Activation of urokinase plasminogen activator and its receptor axis is essential for macrophage infiltration in a prostate cancer mouse model. *Neoplasia*, 13, 23-30.

Zhang, L., Conejo-Garcia, J.R., Katsaros, D., Gimotty, P.A., Massobrio, M., Regnani, G., Makrigiannakis, A., Gray, H., Schlienger, K., Liebman, M.N., Rubin, S.C. and Coukos, G. (2003) Intratumoral T cells, recurrence, and survival in epithelial ovarian cancer. *N Engl J Med*, 348, 203-213.

Zhang, W., Zhu, X.D., Sun, H.C., Xiong, Y.Q., Zhuang, P.Y., Xu, H.X., Kong, L.Q., Wang, L., Wu, W.Z. and Tang, Z.Y. (2010) Depletion of tumor-associated macrophages enhances the effect of sorafenib in metastatic liver cancer models by antimetastatic and antiangiogenic effects. *Clin Cancer Res*, 16, 3420-3430.

Zhang, X., Majlessi, L., Deriaud, E., Leclerc, C. and Lo-Man, R. (2009) Coactivation of Syk kinase and MyD88 adaptor protein pathways by bacteria promotes regulatory properties of neutrophils. *Immunity*, 31, 761-771.

Zumsteg, A., Baeriswyl, V., Imaizumi, N., Schwendener, R., Ruegg, C. and Christofori, G. (2009) Myeloid cells contribute to tumor lymphangiogenesis. *PLoS One*, 4, e7067.

3

Monocyte Subsets and Their Role in Tumor Progression

Andrea I. Doseff* and Arti Parihar

Department of Internal Medicine, Division of Pulmonary, Allergy, Critical Care and Sleep, Department of Molecular Genetics, The Heart and Lung Research Institute, The Ohio State University, Columbus, OH, USA

1. Introduction

Monocytes are essential components of the innate immune system responsible for phagocytosis of pathogens, dead cells, and anti-tumor activities. These cells are involved in a remarkably diverse array of homeostatic processes ranging from host defense to tissue turnover and are emerging as key players in the pathophysiology of several diseases including atherosclerosis, arthritis, obesity, autoimmunity, and cancer. These mononuclear blood cells respond to "self" and "non-self" stimulatory signals by mediating immune responses, controlling inflammatory cytokines, and accumulating at sites of "danger". Thus, monocytes play a critical role in the protection against invaders. In the case of invader "tumors", monocyte accumulation has been shown to promote neoangiogenesis and tumor progression. This paradoxical role of monocytes in normal and tumor development may result in the polarized expression of either pro- or anti-tumor functions. Recognition of diverse monocyte subsets helps explain the plethora of functions attributed to monocytes in acute and chronic inflammatory diseases. Microenvironmental signals, to which monocytes are exposed, play a key role in the setting of their phenotype selectively tuning their functions. In the tumor microenvironment, recruitment of selected monocyte subsets and the inhibition of the apoptotic program promote increase numbers of macrophages in the tumor. A complex network of differentiation factors and inflammatory stimuli determine monocyte life span by blocking the apoptotic pathway and activating a myriad of survival pathways. The present chapter will discuss molecular changes that dictate the fate and behavior of monocyte subsets contributing to tumor biology. In addition, we will discuss the antagonistic and synergistic interplay of transcriptional and posttranscriptional regulatory networks that contribute to the specification of monocytic cell fate and their contribution in tumor progression. The recognition of these molecular networks will furnish strategies to decrease monocytic cell recruitment, survival at the tumor sites, and facilitate monocytic "re-education" programs reestablishing their normal anti-tumor function helping to define novel therapeutic strategy against cancer and other inflammatory diseases.

* Corresponding Author

2. Monocyte subsets: Molecular and functional heterogeneity

Heterogeneous populations of monocytes originate from common myeloid precursor cells and are responsible for controlling inflammation, tissue repair, stimulating angiogenesis, tumor progression, and growth. These populations are dynamic, capable to adapt their identity, fate, and immunological function in response to environmental cues. Monocytes help to neutralize self or non-self danger signals through innate mechanisms. In this defensive reaction, the blood and lymphatic vascular system are essential partners. In addition, recruitment of monocytic cells leads to new blood vessel formation or angiogenesis, a central feature of tumor growth. Monocytes act as defenders, secreting cytokines and in turn modulate other cells of the innate and adaptive immune system trying to combat the tumor. Interestingly, cues from the tumor microenvironment promote changes in monocytic cells fate and immune function leading to changes in myelogenous populations that ensure tumor growth and metastasis, in a co-adaptation process yet not well understood.

The tumor microenvironment is a complex milieu composed of cellular and noncellular (matrix) components. Myeloid cells, among others monocytes/macrophages, constitute about 50% of the infiltrating cells (Pollard, 2004). The origins and identities of tumor infiltrating myeloid cells have been recently uncovered as technical advances helped identify these heterogeneous subsets.

Circulating human and mouse monocytes are broadly classified on the basis of surface receptor markers and biological responses into three subtypes. Based on the recently approved nomenclature by the Nomenclature Committee of the International Union of Immunological Societies (Ziegler-Heitbrock et al., 2010) human monocyte subtypes are categorized into "classical" expressing high levels of CD14 and lacking CD16 expression ($CD14^{++}CD16^{-}$ or $CD16^{-}$) constituting ~90% of the population and the remaining 10% expressing CD14 and CD16 or FcγIII receptor ($CD14^{+}CD16^{+}$). The latest group is further subdivided based on the level of CD14 and CD16 expression into "intermediate" ($CD14^{++}CD16^{+}$ or $CD16^{+}$) and "non-classical" ($CD14^{+}CD16^{++}$ or $CD16^{++}$) (Parihar et al., 2010; Ziegler-Heitbrock et al., 2010) (Fig. 1). The mouse circulating monocyte counterparts are classified into three types based on the expression of the surface glycoprotein Ly6C and the transmembrane sialoglycoprotein CD43. These are "classical: $Ly6C^{++}CD43^{+}$, "intermediate": $Ly6C^{++}CD43^{++}$ and "non-classical": $Ly6C^{+}CD43^{++}$ monocytes (Ziegler-Heitbrock et al., 2010). Ly6C is part of the epitope of granulocyte differentiation antigen-1 (Gr-1), also recognized by Gr-1 antibodies (Hanninen et al., 1997). Hence, $Ly6C^{++}$ ($Ly6C^{high}$) monocytes are $Gr\text{-}1^{+}$ and $Ly6C^{+}$ ($Ly6C^{low}$) are $Gr\text{-}1^{-}$ (Geissmann et al., 2010). Classical mouse monocytes ($Ly6C^{high}$ $CD43^{+}$) express $CCR2^{+}$ and $CD62L^{+}$ and low levels of the chemokine receptor CX_3CR1^{low}, whereas non-classical ($LY6C^{low}CD43^{++}$) are CX_3CR1^{high} but $CCR2^{-}CD62L^{-}$ (Auffray et al., 2009). Recently, closer association has been shown between the human classical, intermediate, and mouse $Ly6C^{high}$, irrespective of CD16 expression while the $Ly6C^{low}$ correspond to non-classical $CD14^{low}CD16^{++}$ monocytes (Cros et al., 2010) (Fig. 1).

Several types of myeloid cells are important components of the tumor stroma contributing to diverse tumor-promoting activities including Tumor-Infiltrating Monocytes (TIM) and Tumor-Associated Macrophages (TAM) (Hanahan & Weinberg, 2011) (Fig. 1). Circulating

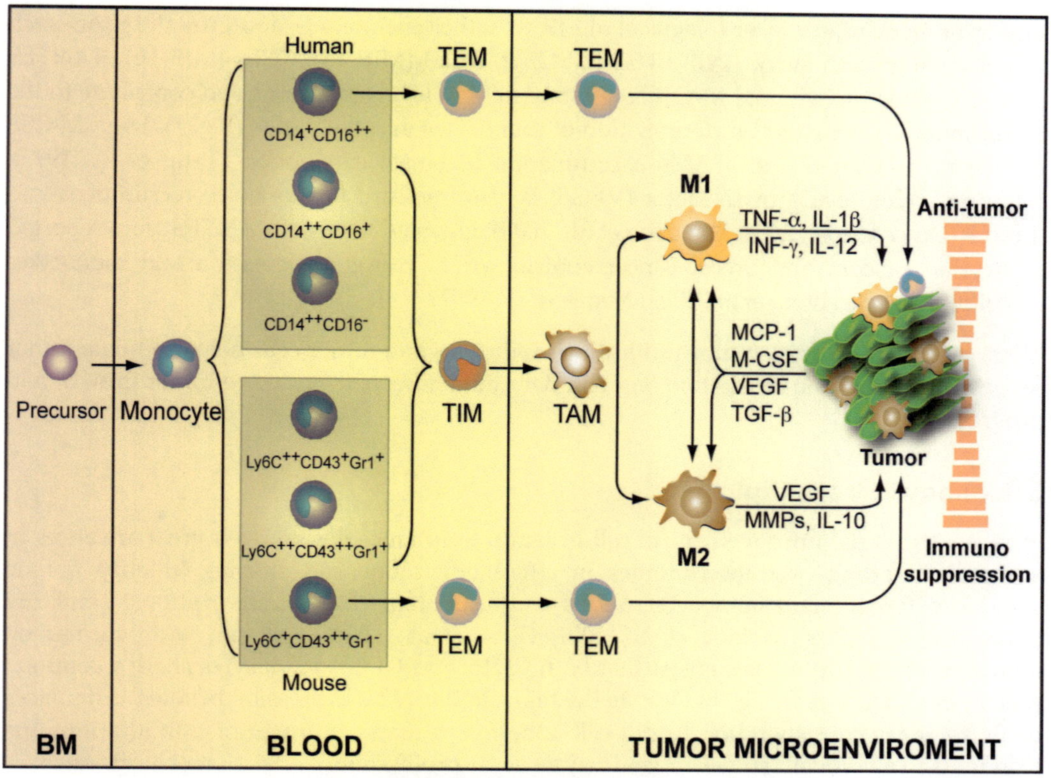

Fig. 1. Role of monocytes and macrophages in tumor progression. Heterogeneous monocyte populations arising from a common precursor have been described. Different monocyte subsets contribute to the infiltration of myelogenous cells such as TIM, TEM, and TAM into the tumor, which in paracrine and autocrine manner contribute to angiogenesis, tumor progression, and growth. Plastic behavior of TAMs from M1 to M2 as well as other infiltrated monocytes is characterized by distinct cytokine and chemokine profiles promoting an anti-tumoral or immunosuppressive environment respectively co-adapting to the tumor microenvironment.

monocytes expressing Tie-2 [angiopoietin-2 (Ang-2)] named TEM, comprised within $CD14^{+}CD16^{++}$ human monocytes and mice $Ly6C^{+}$ ($Ly6C^{low}$) are recruited to the tumor where they have been shown to be essential for angiogenesis (Venneri et al., 2007). In a mammary adenocarcinoma tumor model the majority of tumor infiltrating monocytes differentiating into TAM were $Ly6C^{++}$ (Movahedi et al., 2010). The tumor environment not only attracts myeloid cells but also modulates their fate resulting in a shift in hematopoiesis leading to an increase in myeloid cell accumulation in bone marrow, blood, spleen, and at the tumor site (Almand et al., 2001; Bronte et al., 2000; Mantovani et al., 2008).

Monocyte recruitment to the tumor site is greatly influenced by several factors. Among others, the prototype CC chemokine MCP-1 (monocyte chemoattractant protein-1; also known as CCL2) secreted by malignant cells increases monocyte infiltration (Gu et al., 1999). Significantly higher levels of MCP-1 have been reported in patients with primary ovarian cancer and melanoma (Negus et al., 1995) and MCP-1 down-regulation decreased monocyte migration in ovarian cancer (Negus et al., 1998). Other chemokines and growth factors such as placental growth factor (PGF), TGF-β, PGE-2, CCL3 (MIP-1α), CCL4 (MIP-1β), RANTES (also known as CCL-5), and M-CSF, are found at high levels in tumors and contribute to the recruitment, survival, and differentiation of monocytes into the tumor (Fig. 1). High M-CSF expression is related with TAMs accumulation in breast carcinomas (Tang et al., 1992). Vascular endothelial growth factor (VEGF) is also involved in monocyte recruitment into tumors (Dineen et al., 2008; Murdoch et al., 2008). Elevated levels of RANTES were reported in ovarian cancer and breast cancer contributed to cancer progression and monocytes recruitment (Azenshtein et al., 2002; Negus et al., 1997).

Thus, secreted factors by tumor-infiltrating monocytes and tumor cells help modulate tumor growth and monocyte infiltration and fate determination contributing to tumor growth and progression.

3. Monocytic transcriptomes

In recent years the improvement in cell isolation techniques has allowed great advances in the understanding of transcriptomes in circulating monocytes helping identify unique signatures for different monocyte subsets and share remarkably transcriptional similarity (Ancuta et al., 2009; Mobley et al., 2007; Zhao et al., 2009). Genome wide studies on monocytes transcriptomes suggest that both $CD16^-$ and $CD16^+$ monocytes share a common precursor (Ancuta et al., 2009). Despite the high similarity on expression profiles, differences relate to genes corresponding to cell-cell adhesion, trafficking, inflammation and immune responses, cell cycle, signal trasnduction and proliferation. Strict statistical analysis indicated as few as ~ 60 differentially expressed genes between monocyte subsets (Ancuta et al., 2009).

Classical monocytes ($CD14^+CD16^-$) have higher expression of genes involved in adhesion such as CCR2, CD62L and CD11b. In addition, the genes related to inflammation, angiogenesis and wound healing are also highly expressed in classical monocytes, revealing its implication in tissue repair (Wong et al., 2011). These classical monocytes also express higher level of CD14 and the cytokine IL-8 (Mobley et al., 2007). In these monocytes all phagocytosis enhancing proteins were highly expressed including levels of CD93, the receptor for complement component C1q1 (C1q1R), a component of a larger receptor complex for C1q complement factor and mannose-binding lectin (MBL2) (Ancuta et al., 2009). Furthermore, classical monocytes also showed high level expression of proinflammatory molecules such as S100A12, S100A9, S1008, and were among the top 50 most highly expressed genes (Wong et al., 2011).

$CD16^+$ subsets possess a more differentiated profile with increased expression of macrophage and dendritic cell-like genes, probably indicating a more advanced stage of differentiation of these cells (Ancuta et al., 2009). These cells express high levels of genes involved in antigen processing, antimicrobial activity and host defense. High expression of genes encoding defensins, lysosomal proteases including cathepsins and elastase have been found (Mobley et al., 2007). Intermediate monocytes ($CD14^{++}$ $CD16^+$) showed enrichment for genes under major histocompatibility complex (MHC) class II processing and presenting, these genes mainly includes CD47, HLA-DO and CD40. MARCO (macrophage receptor with collagenous structure) is also one of the highly expressed gene in the intermediate subset of monocytes (Wong et al., 2011). CD16+ monocytes express higher levels of TNF-α and chemokine receptor CX3CR1, CX3CR2 and colony-stimulating factor 1 receptor (CSF1R), the receptor for macrophage colony-stimulating factor (M-CSF) than classical CD16- monocytes (Ancuta et al., 2009; Wong et al., 2011; Zhao et al., 2009). Proteomic analysis also showed small differences with only 235 proteins differentially expressed between the monocyte subsets (Martinez, 2009). In addition to CD16, higher expression of the hematopoietic cell kinase (HCK) and the tyrosine protein kinase (LYN) were observed (Zhao et al., 2009). Interestingly the nonclassical monocytes (CD16++) showed the gene enrichment in the category of cytoskeleton rearrangement and phagocytosis. Genes related to phagocytosis such as LYN, HCK, ITAM of FCRs, C1QA, C1QB and also SLAN were found highly expressed in nonclassical monocytes (Wong et al., 2011). In pathological conditions, monocyte functions are finely tuned by the microenvironment. In this regard, hypoxic conditions found in tumors affect gene expression. Transcriptome analysis of hypoxic primary human monocytes revealed modulation of a significant cluster of genes with immunological relevance (Bosco et al., 2006). These included scavenger receptors: CD163, also found highly upregulated in CD16- subsets as well as MARCO , stabilin-1 (STAB1), macrophage scavenger receptor-1 (MSR1) (Mobley et al., 2007). Toll like receptor-7 (TLR7), immunoregulatory, costimulatory, and adhesion molecules: CD32, CD64, CD69, CD89, leukocyte membrane Ag (CMRF-35H), integrin β-5 (ITGB5), chemokines/cytokines receptors (CCL23, CCL15, CCL8, CCR1, CCR2, RDC1, IL-23A, IL-6ST) were also highly expressed under hypoxia (Bosco et al., 2006). Hypoxia also controlled gene expression of chemokine receptors including CXCL1, CXCL8, CCL3, CXCR4 (Murdoch et al., 2004).

Transcriptome studies are unraveling the complexities of the monocyte populations and provide evidence of the specialized function of specific subsets. High expression of IL-8 and adhesion molecules in CD16- subsets seem to support the role as inflammatory, capable to leave the circulation and infiltrate. In addition, high expression of M-CSF in CD16+ support their role in driving differentiation of CD16-, a more immature pool that could replenish macropahges at inflammatory sites. Studies in gene expression profiles in human monocyte subpopulations as part of tumor biology remain scarce and future studies in this area will thereby help to understand their specific roles as well as define future approaches to re-educate monocytes in the tumor microenvironment.

4. Role of monocyte subsets in tumor progression

4.1 Monocyte deactivation

It has been widely accepted that cancer progression is an inherently proinflammatory process that involves the activation of the innate and adaptive immune system. During tumorigenesis, monocytes are destined to give anti-tumor response of the host and act both as cells presenting tumor-associated antigens to tumor-infiltrating lymphocytes and as cytotoxic effector cells (Mytar et al., 2003). However, cancer cells have developed mechanisms that inhibit immune surveillance (Pardoll, 2003), characterized by the impaired ability of monocytes to produce IFN-γ, TNF-α, IL-12, while enhance IL-10 secretion. IL-10 is immunosuppressive, tumor promoting, and inhibits the production of IL-2, IFNγ, IL-12, TNF-α, resulting in a reduced Th1 response (Sica et al., 2006). Different studies have reported increased IL-10 serum levels in patients with melanoma and other solid tumors

(Fortis et al., 1996; Sato et al., 1996). IL-12 plays central role in activating anti-tumor immunity by stimulating the production of IFN-γ and TNF-α necessary for cytotoxic effects. In many cancers, for instance in colorectal cancer reduced production of IL-12 was accompanied by increased production of IL-10 (O'Hara et al., 1998). Deactivation of monocytes can be reversed with Bovis bacillus Calmette-Guerin (BCG), the prototype immunomodulator, which inhibits IL-10 production, thus reversing monocyte deactivation (Baran et al., 2004).

Deactivation of TIM is also mediated by other mechanisms. Hyaluronan (HA), an important tumor microenvironment matrix structure, produced by tumor cells, is now emerging as a key factor in monocyte deactivation and tumor progression (Mytar et al., 2003; Toole, 2004). Ligation of CD44 by HA is a proinflammatory event that regulates monocyte adhesion and cytokine production and was found to stimulate the expression of IRAK (IL-1 receptor-associated kinase)-M. High levels of IRAK-M were reported in patients of chronic myeloid leukemia and metastasis (del Fresno et al., 2005). Co-culture experiments of $CD14^+$ monocytes with a variety of tumor cells show that tumor cells express high level of prostaglandin (PG) that also contributes to the downregulation of TNF-α, IL-12, IRAK-1 interrupting the inflammatory response against cancer progression. These findings strongly suggest that the functional activity of monocytes is adversely modified by the local tumor microenvironment. Notably, the deactivation mechanisms of monocyte in cancer may not just be limited to tumor microenvironment but also players in other inflammatory diseases such as atherosclerosis, arthritis, and obesity.

4.2 Angiogenesis

Once the tumor cells escape recognition and destruction by infiltrating monocyte, these infiltrating cells participate in tumor growth by promoting angiogenesis (Lin et al., 2001), an essential process in the tumor progression and growth. High numbers of human vascular leukocytes found in human ovarian cancer have been suggested to form neovessels in mouse xenotransplantations (Conejo-Garcia et al., 2005). $Gr\text{-}1^+$ monocytes promote angiogenesis via paracrine mechanisms (Yang et al., 2004). Vascular leukocytes, a subset of $CD11C^+$ $MHC\text{-}II^+$ dendritic-cell precursors expressing endothelial vascular markers VE-cadherin, CD34, and CD146 also contribute to tumor angiogenesis (Conejo-Garcia et al., 2005; Yang et al., 2004). Circulating TEM derived from non-classical monocytes contributes to tumor angiogenesis, migrating towards Ang-2, released at high levels by activated endothelial cells and angiogenic vessels at tumor sites (Venneri et al., 2007). Ang-2 also inhibits TNF-α release (Lewis et al., 2007; Murdoch et al., 2007), normally responsible for promoting apoptosis of both tumor and endothelial cells (Petrache et al., 2001). Hence, Ang-2-mediated down-regulation of TNF-α may increase metastasis and angiogenesis contributing to tumor growth. The molecular basis of factors that render proangiogenic activity in TEM are still not well understood. But elimination of TEMs in mouse glioma models was shown to reduce tumor growth and vascularity (De Palma et al., 2005), supporting the role of TEM in tumor blood vessels formation. In human tumor models, $CD14^+$ TIM monocytes can develop endothelial phenotype (Schmeisser et al., 2001) and actively participate in neovascularization during tumor growth (Urbich et al., 2003).

Recent studies indicated that CCL2 synthesized by metastatic tumor cells and by the target-site tissue stroma is critical for the recruitment of CCR2-expressing monocyte subsets. Activation of the CCL2-CCR2 signaling axis promotes extravasation and recruitment of inflammatory monocyte subsets into metastatic tumor sites and helps promote differentiation of these monoyctes into non-proliferating TAMs (Qian et al., 2011). Transcriptome studies in both resident and inflammatory monocytes show higher expression of VegfA, a potent angiogenic factor in inflammatory monocytes $CD14^{+}CD16^{-}$ subsets, recruited in large numbers to metastatic areas (Qian et al., 2011). Future comprehensive trsancriptome analysis in purified monocyte populations under pathophysiological conditions should be helpful to gain a further understanding of the functional roles of different monocyte populations in tumor progression.

5. Regulation of monocyte subsets

5.1 Regulation of survival and cell death of monocytes in tumors

A complex network of survival and apoptotic pathways determines monocyte fate. Several kinases, transcription factors and anti- and pro-apoptotic proteins play key roles in determining monocyte survival and cell death. All circulating monocyte subsets have very short life span of just few days (Fahy et al., 1999; Zeigler et al., 2003). Inflammatory and differentiation stimuli are known to halt apoptosis and inducing prolonged monocyte survival. Among others M-CSF, TNF-α, and IL-1β promote survival by deactivating the apoptotic program lead by caspases (Fahy et al., 1999; Goyal et al., 2002; Kelley et al., 1999). The tumor microenvironment characterized by alterations in cytokine, chemokine, and growth factor expression contributes to mediate prolonged monocyte survival (Zou, 2005). In fact, increase levels of TGF-β, IL-10, and VEGF alter TIM and TEM from anti-tumoral to immunosuppressor and proangiogenic in part by switching their cytokine and growth factors expressions (Whiteside, 2008) (Fig. 1).

Among the signaling molecules involved in activation and survival, the phosphatidylinositol 3-kinase (PI3K)-AKT axis has a central role in regulating a multitude of essential myelogenous events, such as differentiation, phagocytosis, oxidative burst, and TLR-mediated responses (Franke et al., 1997; Parihar et al., 2010). PI3K activation was also shown to direct infiltration (Funamoto et al., 2002; Wang et al., 2002). M-CSF-induced activation of AKT through caspase-9 phosphorylation inhibits apoptosis (Kelley et al., 1999), promoting prolonged survival and sustaining the differentiation program (Gonzalez-Mejia & Doseff, 2009). In addition, PI3K activates protein kinase C (PKC) in monocytes (Herrera-Velit et al., 1997) leading to the induction of the activated mitogen-activated protein kinase (MAPK) pathway (Rao, 2001), including the extracellular signal-regulated kinase (ERK), the c-JNK and p38 which are hubs to multiple networks of survival (Parihar et al., 2010). Pro-inflammatory mediators induce the PI3K/AKT and MAPK/ERK pathways that in turn are responsible in determining the balance of inflammatory versus anti-inflammatory cytokines.

In the hypoxic regions of a tumor, activation of PI3K/AKT leads to HIF (hypoxia inducing factor)-1 activity which in turn regulates tumor growth, angiogenesis, metastasis, and monocytes/macrophages recruitment (Semenza, 2003). While the role of HIF-1 in different monocyte subsets and macrophages is not fully understood, increased HIF-1 expression in TAMs was found to contribute to tumor angiogenesis and invasiveness (Werno et al., 2010).

The transcription factor nuclear factor-κB (NF-κB), plays a critical role in tumor biology (Karin & Greten, 2005). While in other cell types NF-κB has various tumor-promoting functions, in monocytes the activation of NF-κB results in the release of cytokines, such as TNF-α and IL-6 which not only trigger prosurvival signals in tumor cells but also support growth and progression, and importantly sustain a dysregulated immune function (Hagemann et al., 2009; Pikarsky et al., 2004). Activation of NF-κB leads to increase expression of angiogenic factors such as VEGF, CXCL1 and CXCL8 and anti-apoptotic molecules including the inhibitor of apoptotic proteins (IAPs), and bcl-2 (Richmond, 2002). The relevance of the NF-κB signaling pathway is illustrated in a mouse model of colitis associated cancer, where deletion of IKK-β reduced the production of tumor promoting paracrine factors and subsequently decreased carcinoma growth (Greten et al., 2004). In hepatocellular carcinomas the NF-κB activating kinase IKK-β suppresses early chemically-induced liver tumorigenesis by inhibiting hepatocyte death and compensatory proliferation. This anti-tumorigenic activity of hepatocyte IKK-β was suggested to be due to the induction of NF-κB-dependent pro-survival and anti-oxidant genes (He et al., 2010). Deletion of IKK-β in myeloid cells resulted in a significant decrease in tumor size and diminished the expression of proinflammatory cytokines that may serve as tumor growth factors (Yoshimura, 2006).

Caspases, the cysteine proteases central to programmed cell death, including "activators" (caspases-1, 2, 8, 9, and 10) and 'executioners' (caspases-3, 6, and 7) play fundamental roles in myelogenous cells through the activation of the extrinsic and intrinsic apoptotic cascade (Riedl & Shi, 2004). Fas receptor-induced apoptosis has a key role in monocyte biology as both homozygous FasR deficient (*lpr/lpr*) and heterozygous FasR and Fas ligand deficient (*lpr/gld*) mice have increased numbers of inflammatory and resident monocytes resulting in splenomegaly, lymphadenopathy, and accumulation of tissue macrophages (Ashkenazi & Dixit, 1998; Brown et al., 2004). Cytokines, CCL2 and IL-6 abundant in the tumor microenvironment have been shown to inhibit caspase-8 and promote enhanced autophagic activity to protect the monocytes recruited to the tumor and, at the same time, induce their differentiation toward M2-type macrophages (Roca et al., 2009). Futhermore, M-CSF induces caspase-9 inhibition leading to reduce apoptosis (Kelley et al., 1999). Several other inhibitors of the apoptotic pathways including members of the Bcl-2 family have been characterized (Youle & Strasser, 2008) and XIAP also play a crucial role in cell survival and tumor development. XIAP directly inhibits activator caspase-9 and also executioner caspases in cancer cells and increase expression of XIAP has been reported in monocyte differentiation (Sasaki et al., 2000). However, the role of XIAP in different monocyte subsets has not been studied. Our studies identified the small heat shock protein (Hsp27) as a direct inhibitor of caspase-3 in monocytes. Notably a significant increase in Hsp27 expression was found to be required during monocyte-macrophage differentiation (Voss et al., 2007). Hsp27 is highly expressed in several tumors and high levels of Hsp27 in plasma have been associated with risk of lung cancer (Wang et al., 2010). Hsp27 was found to have functions in IL-1-induced cell signaling and pro-inflammatory gene expression suggesting its ability to modulate immunity (Alford et al., 2007). Whether the expression of apoptosis inhibitors such as Hsp27 is altered in TIM and TAMs have yet to be studied. These findings suggest that anti-apoptotic factors in plasma can switch monocyte life span contributing to their accumulation into tumors. It is possible to hypothesize that monocyte re-education programs could target molecular networks involved in shifting survival and cell death programs as well as immunoparalysis in monocytes.

5.2 Epigenetics and microRNAs regulation in monocytes and macrophages during tumor progression

During hematopoiesis gradual changes in gene expression orchestrate lineage-specification. The myelomonocytic lineage originates from a ganulocyte-erythrocyte-megakaryocyte-macrophage colony-forming unit (GEMM-CFU) that promotes formation of the GM-CFU or ganulocyte-macrophage colony-forming unit. GM-CFU under the control of G-MCSF, M-CSF and IL-3 regulate the differentiation of this progenitor to a monocyte precursor (M-CFU) that becomes a promonocyte in the bone marrow. Differentiation of precursor cells is controlled by transcription factors that regulate differentation and survival. A combination of transcription factors including GATA-2, GATA-1, SCL, and members of the homeobox proteins (HOXB) control monocyte survival. Repression of GATA-1, SCL, and c-Myc expression allows monocytic differentiation (Valledor et al., 1998). Earliest stages of myeloid lineage specification involve the activity of Runt-related transcription factor 1 (RUNX1). One of the main targets of RUNX1 is PU.1, a member of the ETS (E-twenty six) family transcription factor (Olson et al., 1995). PU.1 is key in differentiation by controlling the expression of M-CSF and GM-CSF receptors. In addition, PU.1 regulates expression of FCγ receptors involved in phagocytosis. Thus, PU.1 has a critical role in monocytic differentiation by regulating expression of molecules essential for differentiation and function of monocytic lineages. Intermediate stages of differentiation are regulated among others by transcription factor CCAAT enhancer-binding protein (C/EBP) members, c-Myc and HOXB7, the latest induced by GM-CSF (Friedman, 2002; Yeamans et al., 2007). In addition, c-Jun dimmers (AP-1) and STAT members contribute to the induction of monocytic genes (Friedman, 2002). STAT3 is one of the important transcription factors that play an essential role in cell survival, proliferation, and differentiation. Classical monocytes, express high levels of AP-1-axis regulated genes, and it has been suggested that this gene repertoire may be responsible for the plastic behavior of this monocyte subset to recognize self and non-self stimuli (Wong et al., 2011). In non-classical subsets transcription factors controlling apoptosis, differentiation, and proliferation were highly expressed, among them E2F1, ETS1, and FOXO1, well known to regulate proliferation. Intermediate monocyte subsets showed reciprocal increases in transcription factors found in both classical and non-classical subsets (Wong et al., 2011).

Epigenetic changes regulated by histone-modifying enzymes such as histone acetyltransferases (HATs), histone deacetylases (HDAC), and methylases provide additional regulatory mechanisms for monocytic gene expression. Abnormal activity of these enzymes leads to changes in gene expression affecting differentiation and apoptosis and causing neoplasia and other diseases (Haberland et al., 2009). Acetylation of NF-κB induces modifications in a temporal manner leading to recruitment of other co-activator and re-modeling complexes and the induction of inflammatory gene expression (Ito et al., 2000; Lee et al., 2006). In monocytes, histone acetylation of the TNF-α promoter has been shown to be developmentally regulated and is required for TNF-α expression during acute inflammation (Lee et al., 2003). Changes in acetylation of the Decoy Receptor 3 (DcR3) promoter, a member of the TNF receptor superfamily, has been reported in tumors affecting expression of MHC class II (MHC-II)-dependent antigen presentation (Chang et al., 2008). Recent studies found distinct DNA methylation profiles in $CD34^{+}$ hematopoietic progenitor cells and differentiated myeloid cells with pronounced DNA hypomethylation in monocytes (Bocker et al., 2011).

Interestingly, age-related methylation changes in CD34+ cells were found. Older progenitor cells showed a bimodal pattern with hypomethylation of differentiation associated genes and de novo methylation events resembling epigenetic mutations, thus providing an important insight into the methylation dynamics during differentiation and suggest that epigenetic changes contribute to hematopoietic progenitor cell aging (Bocker et al., 2011). Induction of inflammatory genes IL-6, IL-8 and IL-12 were found to depend on HAT/HDAC activity (Lu et al., 2005; Schmeck et al., 2008). Treatment of monocytic leukemia cell lines and patient samples with demethylating and HDAC inhibitors induced reversion to gene profiles found in normal subjects, highlighting the role of chromatin remodeling in monocyte behavior (Serrano et al., 2008). Treatment of macrophages with broad-spectrum HDACs inhibitors showed anti- and pro-inflammatory effects, HDACs suppressed LPS-induced expression of the pro-inflammatory MCP-3, and IL-12 but amplified the expression of the pro-atherogenic factors Cox-2 (Halili et al., 2010). Dietary compounds with HDAC inhibitory activities, including garcinol, curcumin, and anacardic acid, modulate epigenetic status and are being investigated as potential anti-cancer agents (Bolden et al., 2006; Inoue et al., 2004). It will be of interest to evaluate how these therapies influence monocytes epigenomes. Future studies to evaluate the epigenetic dynamics of monocyte subsets will be of great value to further understand their unique functional contributions.

MicroRNAs (miRNAs) are small non-coding RNAs emerging as new post-trancriptional regulators and have been found to contribute in several monocyte functions. The overall relevance of miRNA in hematopoiesis has been discussed in detail elsewhere (Baltimore et al., 2008). Based on the epidemiological studies inflammation contributes to 25% of all cancers by increasing cancer risk and cancer development (Mantovani et al., 2008). Several miRNAs were found to be elevated in inflammation and cancer. In particular, miRNA-155, miRNA-125b, and miRNA-21 have emerged as important miRNAs regulating immune responses. MiRNA-155 is elevated in leukemia and lymphoma and transgenic mice overexpressing miRNA-155 in B cells, develop B-cell leukemia and sustained expression of miRNA-155 in hematopoietic stem cells causes myeloproliferative disorders (O'Connell et al., 2008). MiRNA-155 targets among others suppressors of cytokine signaling (SOCS1) and SH2-domain-containing inositol-5-phosphatase 1 (SHIP-1), both negative regulators of TLR signaling in monocyte/macrophage inflammatory response. Recent studies showed that tumor environment causes a sustained reduction of miRNA-155 in monocytes/macrophages, which in turn activates the C/EBPβ (He et al., 2009). C/EBPβ, a member of C/EBP family of leucine zipper transcription factors, plays pivotal roles in coordinating the expression of a wide variety of genes that control immune responses including COX-2 (Li et al., 2007). C/EBPβ-deficient mice exhibit defects in macrophage activation and differentiation (He et al., 2009). Monocytes exposed to tumor microenvironment showed C/EBPβ expression inversely correlated with miR-155 expression and it was found that miRNA-155 could suppress the C/EBPβ. Furthermore, over-expression of miRNA-155 significantly attenuated the cytokine production in tumor-activated monocytes (He et al., 2009). Expression of miRNA-146 affects downstream TLR signaling molecules such IRAK1 and 2 or TNF receptor-associated factor (TRAF) 6, all involved in the activation of the NF-κB axis (O'Connell et al., 2010). MiRNA-21 and miRNA-125b are also elevated in inflammatory conditions and cancer (Esquela-Kerscher & Slack, 2006).

Recent studies highlighted different miRNAs profile in circulating monocytes when compared with dendritic cells or macrophages (Tserel et al., 2011). However, it is presently unknown whether miRNAs expression is altered in different monocytes subsets in normal conditions or in tumorigenesis.

6. Molecular pathways involved in monocyte fate and re-education programming

Reprogramming implies the conversion of a fully differentiated cell type into another cell type without pluripotent intermediate and generally achieved by overexpressing key transcription-factors (Zhou & Melton, 2008). Recent studies have reported that various cells including fibroblasts can be reprogrammed into blood-cell progenitors (Szabo et al., 2010), neurons (Vierbuchen et al., 2010), and cardiomyocytes (Ieda et al., 2010), demonstrating the ample applicability of this approach for therapeutic uses.

Myelomonocytic cells re-education programs have been described. TAMs have been suggested to be programmed to specific subtypes such as M1 and M2 upon arrival to the tumor microenvironment. It has been shown that administration of GM-CSF in murine breast cancer models induces soluble VEGFR-1 resulting in the suppression of VEGF and angiogenesis (Eubank et al., 2009). Cytokine-dependent reprogramming using IL-12, which impacts innate and adaptive immune systems, has proven the most interesting (Trinchieri, 1995). IL-12 in its soluble or lipid-encapsulated forms injected into tumor-bearing mice resulted in a strong cytotoxic anti-tumor response (Hill et al., 2002), suggesting its capability to restore normal immune functions. Inflammatory monocytes expressing high levels of the chemokine receptor CCR2 but not $CD14^{-}CD16^{+}$ were found in increased numbers in several chronic inflammatory conditions including atherosclerosis and asthma (Parihar et al., 2010). Recent studies showed that administration of lipid nanoparticles containing a CCR2-silencing short interfering RNA in mice, prevents monocyte accumulation at inflammatory sites (Leuschner et al., 2011). Ectopic expression of PU.1 in lymphocytes and neural stem cells induced transdifferentiation to the myeloid lineage with functional chemotactic and immune functions characteristic of monocytes (Forsberg et al., 2010; Laiosa et al., 2006). Transcriptome analysis showed that PU. 1 expression affects chromatin remodeling leading to epigenetic changes that ensure macrophage specification (Ostuni & Natoli, 2011). These monocytes may serve as vehicles to modulate microenvironments with dysregulated immunity such as found in the tumor. Hence, alteration of epigenetic dynamics may also be a potential approach to alter monocyte re-programming. It is recognized that macrophages adapt in response to the microenvironment (referred to other Chapters in this book). Part of this adaptation is based on changes in their transcriptomes (Lawrence & Natoli, 2011). However, the molecular mechanisms determining macrophage genetic adaptations remain mostly unknown. In the case of monocyte subsets similar studies have not yet been conducted. Thus, dissecting the genomic determinants in normal and pathophysiological conditions of functional distinct monocyte subsets and TEMs will provide possibilities to re-educate these cells towards an anti-tumor phenotype, re-establishing apoptotic programs or halting their extravasation activities.

7. Conclusion

Tumor progression is marked by dynamic changes of the tumor microenvironment from early neoplastic events to advanced tumor stages. Recruitment of circulating monocytes to specific tumor sites contributes to progressive modulation of signaling molecules such as chemokines, cytokines, growth factors, and transcription factors. Specific contributions of different monocyte subsets to the tumor associated myelogenous populations of TEM, TIM, and TAMs are starting to emerge. Advances in understanding the molecular networks regulating myelomonocytic cells functions and fate provide opportunities to implement re-education programs to rehabilitate normal anti-tumor monocyte behavior. These strategies should help limiting myelomonocytic cell survival, halting recruitment to tumor sites, and increasing cytotoxic functions providing novel approaches for cancer treatment. Advances in this area will not be limited to tumor biology but will also impact our understanding of other chronic inflammatory diseases.

8. Acknowledgements

Work in Dr. Doseff's lab is supported by grant NIH (RO1-HL075040) and NSF-MCB (0542244). We thank Dr. Oliver Voss for help with some illustrations and Mrs. Malavez for comments. We apologize to those of our colleagues who made important contributions but which were omitted due to space limitations.

9. References

Alford, K. A.; Glennie, S.; Turrell, B. R.; Rawlinson, L.; Saklatvala, J. & Dean, J. L. (2007). Heat shock protein 27 functions in inflammatory gene expression and transforming growth factor-beta-activated kinase-1 (TAK1)-mediated signaling. *J Biol Chem.* 282(9):6232-6241.

Almand, B.; Clark, J. I.; Nikitina, E.; van Beynen, J.; English, N. R.; Knight, S. C.; Carbone, D. P. & Gabrilovich, D. I. (2001). Increased production of immature myeloid cells in cancer patients: a mechanism of immunosuppression in cancer. *J Immunol.* 166(1):678-689.

Ancuta, P.; Liu, K. Y.; Misra, V.; Wacleche, V. S.; Gosselin, A.; Zhou, X. & Gabuzda, D. (2009). Transcriptional profiling reveals developmental relationship and distinct biological functions of CD16+ and CD16- monocyte subsets. *BMC Genomics.* 10(403.

Ashkenazi, A. & Dixit, V. M. (1998). Death receptors: signaling and modulation. *Science.* 281(5381):1305-1308.

Auffray, C.; Sieweke, M. H. & Geissmann, F. (2009). Blood monocytes: development, heterogeneity, and relationship with dendritic cells. *Annu Rev Immunol.* 27(669-692.

Azenshtein, E.; Luboshits, G.; Shina, S.; Neumark, E.; Shahbazian, D.; Weil, M.; Wigler, N.; Keydar, I. & Ben-Baruch, A. (2002). The CC chemokine RANTES in breast carcinoma progression: regulation of expression and potential mechanisms of promalignant activity. *Cancer Res.* 62(4):1093-1102.

Baltimore, D.; Boldin, M. P.; O'Connell, R. M.; Rao, D. S. & Taganov, K. D. (2008). MicroRNAs: new regulators of immune cell development and function. *Nat Immunol.* 9(8):839-845.

Baran, J.; Baj-Krzyworzeka, M.; Weglarczyk, K.; Ruggiero, I. & Zembala, M. (2004). Modulation of monocyte-tumour cell interactions by Mycobacterium vaccae. *Cancer Immunol Immunother.* 53(12):1127-1134.

Bocker, M. T.; Hellwig, I.; Breiling, A.; Eckstein, V.; Ho, A. D. & Lyko, F. (2011). Genome-wide promoter DNA methylation dynamics of human hematopoietic progenitor cells during differentiation and aging. *Blood*. 117(19):e182-189.

Bolden, J. E.; Peart, M. J. & Johnstone, R. W. (2006). Anticancer activities of histone deacetylase inhibitors. *Nat Rev Drug Discov*. 5(9):769-784.

Bosco, M. C.; Puppo, M.; Santangelo, C.; Anfosso, L.; Pfeffer, U.; Fardin, P.; Battaglia, F. & Varesio, L. (2006). Hypoxia modifies the transcriptome of primary human monocytes: modulation of novel immune-related genes and identification of CC-chemokine ligand 20 as a new hypoxia-inducible gene. *J Immunol*. 177(3):1941-1955.

Bronte, V.; Apolloni, E.; Cabrelle, A.; Ronca, R.; Serafini, P.; Zamboni, P.; Restifo, N. P. & Zanovello, P. (2000). Identification of a CD11b(+)/Gr-1(+)/CD31(+) myeloid progenitor capable of activating or suppressing CD8(+) T cells. *Blood*. 96(12):3838-3846.

Brown, N. J.; Hutcheson, J.; Bickel, E.; Scatizzi, J. C.; Albee, L. D.; Haines, G. K., 3rd; Eslick, J.; Bradley, K.; Taricone, E. & Perlman, H. (2004). Fas death receptor signaling represses monocyte numbers and macrophage activation in vivo. *J Immunol*. 173(12):7584-7593.

Chang, Y. C.; Chen, T. C.; Lee, C. T.; Yang, C. Y.; Wang, H. W.; Wang, C. C. & Hsieh, S. L. (2008). Epigenetic control of MHC class II expression in tumor-associated macrophages by decoy receptor 3. *Blood*. 111(10):5054-5063.

Conejo-Garcia, J. R.; Buckanovich, R. J.; Benencia, F.; Courreges, M. C.; Rubin, S. C.; Carroll, R. G. & Coukos, G. (2005). Vascular leukocytes contribute to tumor vascularization. *Blood*. 105(2):679-681.

Cros, J.; Cagnard, N.; Woollard, K.; Patey, N.; Zhang, S. Y.; Senechal, B.; Puel, A.; Biswas, S. K.; Moshous, D.; Picard, C.; Jais, J. P.; D'Cruz, D.; Casanova, J. L.; Trouillet, C. & Geissmann, F. (2010). Human CD14dim monocytes patrol and sense nucleic acids and viruses via TLR7 and TLR8 receptors. *Immunity*. 33(3):375-386.

De Palma, M.; Venneri, M. A.; Galli, R.; Sergi Sergi, L.; Politi, L. S.; Sampaolesi, M. & Naldini, L. (2005). Tie2 identifies a hematopoietic lineage of proangiogenic monocytes required for tumor vessel formation and a mesenchymal population of pericyte progenitors. *Cancer Cell*. 8(3):211-226.

del Fresno, C.; Otero, K.; Gomez-Garcia, L.; Gonzalez-Leon, M. C.; Soler-Ranger, L.; Fuentes-Prior, P.; Escoll, P.; Baos, R.; Caveda, L.; Garcia, F.; Arnalich, F. & Lopez-Collazo, E. (2005). Tumor cells deactivate human monocytes by up-regulating IL-1 receptor associated kinase-M expression via CD44 and TLR4. *J Immunol*. 174(5):3032-3040.

Dineen, S. P.; Lynn, K. D.; Holloway, S. E.; Miller, A. F.; Sullivan, J. P.; Shames, D. S.; Beck, A. W.; Barnett, C. C.; Fleming, J. B. & Brekken, R. A. (2008). Vascular endothelial growth factor receptor 2 mediates macrophage infiltration into orthotopic pancreatic tumors in mice. *Cancer Res*. 68(11):4340-4346.

Esquela-Kerscher, A. & Slack, F. J. (2006). Oncomirs - microRNAs with a role in cancer. *Nat Rev Cancer*. 6(4):259-269.

Eubank, T. D.; Roberts, R. D.; Khan, M.; Curry, J. M.; Nuovo, G. J.; Kuppusamy, P. & Marsh, C. B. (2009). Granulocyte macrophage colony-stimulating factor inhibits breast cancer growth and metastasis by invoking an anti-angiogenic program in tumor-educated macrophages. *Cancer Res*. 69(5):2133-2140.

Fahy, R. J.; Doseff, A. I. & Wewers, M. D. (1999). Spontaneous human monocyte apoptosis utilizes a caspase-3-dependent pathway that is blocked by endotoxin and is independent of caspase-1. *J Immunol*. 163(4):1755-1762.

Forsberg, M.; Carlen, M.; Meletis, K.; Yeung, M. S.; Barnabe-Heider, F.; Persson, M. A.; Aarum, J. & Frisen, J. (2010). Efficient reprogramming of adult neural stem cells to monocytes by ectopic expression of a single gene. *Proc Natl Acad Sci U S A*. 107(33):14657-14661.

Fortis, C.; Foppoli, M.; Gianotti, L.; Galli, L.; Citterio, G.; Consogno, G.; Gentilini, O. & Braga, M. (1996). Increased interleukin-10 serum levels in patients with solid tumours. *Cancer Lett*. 104(1):1-5.

Franke, T. F.; Kaplan, D. R.; Cantley, L. C. & Toker, A. (1997). Direct regulation of the Akt proto-oncogene product by phosphatidylinositol-3,4-bisphosphate. *Science*. 275(5300):665-668.

Friedman, A. D. (2002). Transcriptional regulation of granulocyte and monocyte development. *Oncogene*. 21(21):3377-3390.

Funamoto, S.; Meili, R.; Lee, S.; Parry, L. & Firtel, R. A. (2002). Spatial and temporal regulation of 3-phosphoinositides by PI 3-kinase and PTEN mediates chemotaxis. *Cell*. 109(5):611-623.

Geissmann, F.; Manz, M. G.; Jung, S.; Sieweke, M. H.; Merad, M. & Ley, K. (2010). Development of monocytes, macrophages, and dendritic cells. *Science*. 327(5966):656-661.

Gonzalez-Mejia, M. E. & Doseff, A. I. (2009). Regulation of monocytes and macrophages cell fate. *Front Biosci*. 14(2413-2431.

Goyal, A.; Wang, Y.; Graham, M. M.; Doseff, A. I.; Bhatt, N. Y. & Marsh, C. B. (2002). Monocyte survival factors induce Akt activation and suppress caspase-3. *Am J Respir Cell Mol Biol*. 26(2):224-230.

Greten, F. R.; Eckmann, L.; Greten, T. F.; Park, J. M.; Li, Z. W.; Egan, L. J.; Kagnoff, M. F. & Karin, M. (2004). IKKβ links inflammation and tumorigenesis in a mouse model of colitis-associated cancer. *Cell*. 118(3):285-296.

Gu, L.; Tseng, S. C. & Rollins, B. J. (1999). Monocyte chemoattractant protein-1. *Chem Immunol*. 72(7-29.

Haberland, M.; Montgomery, R. L. & Olson, E. N. (2009). The many roles of histone deacetylases in development and physiology: implications for disease and therapy. *Nat Rev Genet*. 10(1):32-42.

Hagemann, T.; Biswas, S. K.; Lawrence, T.; Sica, A. & Lewis, C. E. (2009). Regulation of macrophage function in tumors: the multifaceted role of NF-κB. *Blood*. 113(14):3139-3146.

Halili, M. A.; Andrews, M. R.; Labzin, L. I.; Schroder, K.; Matthias, G.; Cao, C.; Lovelace, E.; Reid, R. C.; Le, G. T.; Hume, D. A.; Irvine, K. M.; Matthias, P.; Fairlie, D. P. & Sweet, M. J. (2010). Differential effects of selective HDAC inhibitors on macrophage inflammatory responses to the Toll-like receptor 4 agonist LPS. *J Leukoc Biol*. 87(6):1103-1114.

Hanahan, D. & Weinberg, R. A. (2011). Hallmarks of cancer: the next generation. *Cell*. 144(5):646-674.

Hanninen, A.; Jaakkola, I.; Salmi, M.; Simell, O. & Jalkanen, S. (1997). Ly-6C regulates endothelial adhesion and homing of CD8(+) T cells by activating integrin-dependent adhesion pathways. *Proc Natl Acad Sci U S A*. 94(13):6898-6903.

He, G.; Yu, G. Y.; Temkin, V.; Ogata, H.; Kuntzen, C.; Sakurai, T.; Sieghart, W.; Peck-Radosavljevic, M.; Leffert, H. L. & Karin, M. (2010). Hepatocyte IKKβ/NF-κB inhibits tumor promotion and progression by preventing oxidative stress-driven STAT3 activation. *Cancer Cell*. 17(3):286-297.

He, M.; Xu, Z.; Ding, T.; Kuang, D. M. & Zheng, L. (2009). MicroRNA-155 regulates inflammatory cytokine production in tumor-associated macrophages via targeting C/EBPβ. *Cell Mol Immunol*. 6(5):343-352.

Herrera-Velit, P.; Knutson, K. L. & Reiner, N. E. (1997). Phosphatidylinositol 3-kinase-dependent activation of protein kinase C-ζ in bacterial lipopolysaccharide-treated human monocytes. *J Biol Chem*. 272(26):16445-16452.

Hill, H. C.; Conway, T. F., Jr.; Sabel, M. S.; Jong, Y. S.; Mathiowitz, E.; Bankert, R. B. & Egilmez, N. K. (2002). Cancer immunotherapy with interleukin 12 and granulocyte-macrophage colony-stimulating factor-encapsulated microspheres: coinduction of innate and adaptive antitumor immunity and cure of disseminated disease. *Cancer Res*. 62(24):7254-7263.

Ieda, M.; Fu, J. D.; Delgado-Olguin, P.; Vedantham, V.; Hayashi, Y.; Bruneau, B. G. & Srivastava, D. (2010). Direct reprogramming of fibroblasts into functional cardiomyocytes by defined factors. *Cell*. 142(3):375-386.

Inoue, S.; MacFarlane, M.; Harper, N.; Wheat, L. M.; Dyer, M. J. & Cohen, G. M. (2004). Histone deacetylase inhibitors potentiate TNF-related apoptosis-inducing ligand (TRAIL)-induced apoptosis in lymphoid malignancies. *Cell Death Differ*. 11 Suppl 2(S193-206.

Ito, K.; Barnes, P. J. & Adcock, I. M. (2000). Glucocorticoid receptor recruitment of histone deacetylase 2 inhibits interleukin-1beta-induced histone H4 acetylation on lysines 8 and 12. *Mol Cell Biol*. 20(18):6891-6903.

Karin, M. & Greten, F. R. (2005). NF-κB: linking inflammation and immunity to cancer development and progression. *Nat Rev Immunol*. 5(10):749-759.

Kelley, T. W.; Graham, M. M.; Doseff, A. I.; Pomerantz, R. W.; Lau, S. M.; Ostrowski, M. C.; Franke, T. F. & Marsh, C. B. (1999). Macrophage colony-stimulating factor promotes cell survival through Akt/protein kinase B. *J Biol Chem*. 274(37):26393-26398.

Laiosa, C. V.; Stadtfeld, M.; Xie, H.; de Andres-Aguayo, L. & Graf, T. (2006). Reprogramming of committed T cell progenitors to macrophages and dendritic cells by C/EBPα and PU.1 transcription factors. *Immunity*. 25(5):731-744.

Lawrence, T. & Natoli, G. (2011). Transcriptional regulation of macrophage polarization: enabling diversity with identity. *Nat Rev Immunol*. 11(11):750-761.

Lee, J. Y.; Kim, N. A.; Sanford, A. & Sullivan, K. E. (2003). Histone acetylation and chromatin conformation are regulated separately at the TNF-α promoter in monocytes and macrophages. *J Leukoc Biol*. 73(6):862-871.

Lee, K. Y.; Ito, K.; Hayashi, R.; Jazrawi, E. P.; Barnes, P. J. & Adcock, I. M. (2006). NF-κB and activator protein 1 response elements and the role of histone modifications in IL-1β-induced TGF-β1 gene transcription. *J Immunol*. 176(1):603-615.

Leuschner, F.; Dutta, P.; Gorbatov, R.; Novobrantseva, T. I.; Donahoe, J. S.; Courties, G.; Lee, K. M.; Kim, J. I.; Markmann, J. F.; Marinelli, B.; Panizzi, P.; Lee, W. W.; Iwamoto, Y.; Milstein, S.; Epstein-Barash, H.; Cantley, W.; Wong, J.; Cortez-Retamozo, V.; Newton, A.; Love, K.; Libby, P.; Pittet, M. J.; Swirski, F. K.; Koteliansky, V.; Langer, R.; Weissleder, R.; Anderson, D. G. & Nahrendorf, M. (2011). Therapeutic siRNA silencing in inflammatory monocytes in mice. *Nat Biotechnol*. 29(11):1005-1010.

Lewis, C. E.; De Palma, M. & Naldini, L. (2007). Tie2-expressing monocytes and tumor angiogenesis: regulation by hypoxia and angiopoietin-2. *Cancer Res*. 67(18):8429-8432.

Li, H.; Gade, P.; Xiao, W. & Kalvakolanu, D. V. (2007). The interferon signaling network and transcription factor C/EBP-β. *Cell Mol Immunol*. 4(6):407-418.

Lin, E. Y.; Nguyen, A. V.; Russell, R. G. & Pollard, J. W. (2001). Colony-stimulating factor 1 promotes progression of mammary tumors to malignancy. *J Exp Med*. 193(6):727-740.

Lu, J.; Sun, H.; Wang, X.; Liu, C.; Xu, X.; Li, F. & Huang, B. (2005). Interleukin-12 p40 promoter activity is regulated by the reversible acetylation mediated by HDAC1 and p300. *Cytokine*. 31(1):46-51.

Mantovani, A.; Allavena, P.; Sica, A. & Balkwill, F. (2008). Cancer-related inflammation. *Nature*. 454(7203):436-444.

Martinez, F. O. (2009). The transcriptome of human monocyte subsets begins to emerge. *J Biol*. 8(11):99.

Mobley, J. L.; Leininger, M.; Madore, S.; Baginski, T. J. & Renkiewicz, R. (2007). Genetic evidence of a functional monocyte dichotomy. *Inflammation*. 30(6):189-197.

Movahedi, K.; Laoui, D.; Gysemans, C.; Baeten, M.; Stange, G.; Van den Bossche, J.; Mack, M.; Pipeleers, D.; In't Veld, P.; De Baetselier, P. & Van Ginderachter, J. A. (2010). Different tumor microenvironments contain functionally distinct subsets of macrophages derived from Ly6C(high) monocytes. *Cancer Res*. 70(14):5728-5739.

Murdoch, C.; Giannoudis, A. & Lewis, C. E. (2004). Mechanisms regulating the recruitment of macrophages into hypoxic areas of tumors and other ischemic tissues. *Blood*. 104(8):2224-2234.

Murdoch, C.; Tazzyman, S.; Webster, S. & Lewis, C. E. (2007). Expression of Tie-2 by human monocytes and their responses to angiopoietin-2. *J Immunol*. 178(11):7405-7411.

Murdoch, C.; Muthana, M.; Coffelt, S. B. & Lewis, C. E. (2008). The role of myeloid cells in the promotion of tumour angiogenesis. *Nat Rev Cancer*. 8(8):618-631.

Mytar, B.; Woloszyn, M.; Szatanek, R.; Baj-Krzyworzeka, M.; Siedlar, M.; Ruggiero, I.; Wieckiewicz, J. & Zembala, M. (2003). Tumor cell-induced deactivation of human monocytes. *J Leukoc Biol*. 74(6):1094-1101.

Negus, R. P.; Stamp, G. W.; Relf, M. G.; Burke, F.; Malik, S. T.; Bernasconi, S.; Allavena, P.; Sozzani, S.; Mantovani, A. & Balkwill, F. R. (1995). The detection and localization of monocyte chemoattractant protein-1 (MCP-1) in human ovarian cancer. *J Clin Invest*. 95(5):2391-2396.

Negus, R. P.; Stamp, G. W.; Hadley, J. & Balkwill, F. R. (1997). Quantitative assessment of the leukocyte infiltrate in ovarian cancer and its relationship to the expression of C-C chemokines. *Am J Pathol*. 150(5):1723-1734.

Negus, R. P.; Turner, L.; Burke, F. & Balkwill, F. R. (1998). Hypoxia down-regulates MCP-1 expression: implications for macrophage distribution in tumors. *J Leukoc Biol.* 63(6):758-765.

O'Connell, R. M.; Rao, D. S.; Chaudhuri, A. A.; Boldin, M. P.; Taganov, K. D.; Nicoll, J.; Paquette, R. L. & Baltimore, D. (2008). Sustained expression of microRNA-155 in hematopoietic stem cells causes a myeloproliferative disorder. *J Exp Med.* 205(3):585-594.

O'Connell, R. M.; Rao, D. S.; Chaudhuri, A. A. & Baltimore, D. (2010). Physiological and pathological roles for microRNAs in the immune system. *Nat Rev Immunol.* 10(2):111-122.

O'Hara, R. J.; Greenman, J.; MacDonald, A. W.; Gaskell, K. M.; Topping, K. P.; Duthie, G. S.; Kerin, M. J.; Lee, P. W. & Monson, J. R. (1998). Advanced colorectal cancer is associated with impaired interleukin 12 and enhanced interleukin 10 production. *Clin Cancer Res.* 4(8):1943-1948.

Olson, M. C.; Scott, E. W.; Hack, A. A.; Su, G. H.; Tenen, D. G.; Singh, H. & Simon, M. C. (1995). PU. 1 is not essential for early myeloid gene expression but is required for terminal myeloid differentiation. *Immunity.* 3(6):703-714.

Ostuni, R. & Natoli, G. (2011). Transcriptional control of macrophage diversity and specialization. *Eur J Immunol.* 41(9):2486-2490.

Pardoll, D. (2003). Does the immune system see tumors as foreign or self? *Annu Rev Immunol.* 21(807-839.

Parihar, A.; Eubank, T. D. & Doseff, A. I. (2010). Monocytes and macrophages regulate immunity through dynamic networks of survival and cell death. *J Innate Immun.* 2(3):204-215.

Petrache, I.; Verin, A. D.; Crow, M. T.; Birukova, A.; Liu, F. & Garcia, J. G. (2001). Differential effect of MLC kinase in TNF-α-induced endothelial cell apoptosis and barrier dysfunction. *Am J Physiol Lung Cell Mol Physiol.* 280(6):L1168-1178.

Pikarsky, E.; Porat, R. M.; Stein, I.; Abramovitch, R.; Amit, S.; Kasem, S.; Gutkovich-Pyest, E.; Urieli-Shoval, S.; Galun, E. & Ben-Neriah, Y. (2004). NF-κB functions as a tumour promoter in inflammation-associated cancer. *Nature.* 431(7007):461-466.

Pollard, J. W. (2004). Tumour-educated macrophages promote tumour progression and metastasis. *Nat Rev Cancer.* 4(1):71-78.

Qian, B. Z.; Li, J.; Zhang, H.; Kitamura, T.; Zhang, J.; Campion, L. R.; Kaiser, E. A.; Snyder, L. A. & Pollard, J. W. (2011). CCL2 recruits inflammatory monocytes to facilitate breast-tumour metastasis. *Nature.* 475(7355):222-225.

Rao, K. M. (2001). MAP kinase activation in macrophages. *J Leukoc Biol.* 69(1):3-10.

Richmond, A. (2002). Nf-κB, chemokine gene transcription and tumour growth. *Nat Rev Immunol.* 2(9):664-674.

Riedl, S. J. & Shi, Y. (2004). Molecular mechanisms of caspase regulation during apoptosis. *Nat Rev Mol Cell Biol.* 5(11):897-907.

Roca, H.; Varsos, Z. S.; Sud, S.; Craig, M. J.; Ying, C. & Pienta, K. J. (2009). CCL2 and interleukin-6 promote survival of human CD11b+ peripheral blood mononuclear cells and induce M2-type macrophage polarization. *J Biol Chem.* 284(49):34342-34354.

Sasaki, H.; Sheng, Y.; Kotsuji, F. & Tsang, B. K. (2000). Down-regulation of X-linked inhibitor of apoptosis protein induces apoptosis in chemoresistant human ovarian cancer cells. *Cancer Res.* 60(20):5659-5666.

Sato, T.; McCue, P.; Masuoka, K.; Salwen, S.; Lattime, E. C.; Mastrangelo, M. J. & Berd, D. (1996). Interleukin 10 production by human melanoma. *Clin Cancer Res.* 2(8):1383-1390.

Schmeck, B.; Lorenz, J.; N'Guessan P, D.; Opitz, B.; van Laak, V.; Zahlten, J.; Slevogt, H.; Witzenrath, M.; Flieger, A.; Suttorp, N. & Hippenstiel, S. (2008). Histone acetylation and flagellin are essential for Legionella pneumophila-induced cytokine expression. *J Immunol.* 181(2):940-947.

Schmeisser, A.; Garlichs, C. D.; Zhang, H.; Eskafi, S.; Graffy, C.; Ludwig, J.; Strasser, R. H. & Daniel, W. G. (2001). Monocytes coexpress endothelial and macrophagocytic lineage markers and form cord-like structures in Matrigel under angiogenic conditions. *Cardiovasc Res.* 49(3):671-680.

Semenza, G. L. (2003). Targeting HIF-1 for cancer therapy. *Nat Rev Cancer.* 3(10):721-732.

Serrano, E.; Carnicer, M. J.; Lasa, A.; Orantes, V.; Pena, J.; Brunet, S.; Aventin, A.; Sierra, J. & Nomdedeu, J. F. (2008). Epigenetic-based treatments emphasize the biologic differences of core-binding factor acute myeloid leukemias. *Leuk Res.* 32(6):944-953.

Sica, A.; Schioppa, T.; Mantovani, A. & Allavena, P. (2006). Tumour-associated macrophages are a distinct M2 polarised population promoting tumour progression: potential targets of anti-cancer therapy. *Eur J Cancer.* 42(6):717-727.

Szabo, E.; Rampalli, S.; Risueno, R. M.; Schnerch, A.; Mitchell, R.; Fiebig-Comyn, A.; Levadoux-Martin, M. & Bhatia, M. (2010). Direct conversion of human fibroblasts to multilineage blood progenitors. *Nature.* 468(7323):521-526.

Tang, R.; Beuvon, F.; Ojeda, M.; Mosseri, V.; Pouillart, P. & Scholl, S. (1992). M-CSF (monocyte colony stimulating factor) and M-CSF receptor expression by breast tumour cells: M-CSF mediated recruitment of tumour infiltrating monocytes? *J Cell Biochem.* 50(4):350-356.

Toole, B. P. (2004). Hyaluronan: from extracellular glue to pericellular cue. *Nat Rev Cancer.* 4(7):528-539.

Trinchieri, G. (1995). Interleukin-12: a proinflammatory cytokine with immunoregulatory functions that bridge innate resistance and antigen-specific adaptive immunity. *Annu Rev Immunol.* 13(251-276.

Tserel, L.; Runnel, T.; Kisand, K.; Pihlap, M.; Bakhoff, L.; Kolde, R.; Peterson, H.; Vilo, J.; Peterson, P. & Rebane, A. (2011). MicroRNA expression profiles of human blood monocyte-derived dendritic cells and macrophages reveal miR-511 as putative positive regulator of Toll-like receptor 4. *J Biol Chem.* 286(30):26487-26495.

Urbich, C.; Heeschen, C.; Aicher, A.; Dernbach, E.; Zeiher, A. M. & Dimmeler, S. (2003). Relevance of monocytic features for neovascularization capacity of circulating endothelial progenitor cells. *Circulation.* 108(20):2511-2516.

Valledor, A. F.; Borras, F. E.; Cullell-Young, M. & Celada, A. (1998). Transcription factors that regulate monocyte/macrophage differentiation. *J Leukoc Biol.* 63(4):405-417.

Venneri, M. A.; De Palma, M.; Ponzoni, M.; Pucci, F.; Scielzo, C.; Zonari, E.; Mazzieri, R.; Doglioni, C. & Naldini, L. (2007). Identification of proangiogenic TIE2-expressing monocytes (TEMs) in human peripheral blood and cancer. *Blood.* 109(12):5276-5285.

Vierbuchen, T.; Ostermeier, A.; Pang, Z. P.; Kokubu, Y.; Sudhof, T. C. & Wernig, M. (2010). Direct conversion of fibroblasts to functional neurons by defined factors. *Nature.* 463(7284):1035-1041.

Voss, O. H.; Batra, S.; Kolattukudy, S. J.; Gonzalez-Mejia, M. E.; Smith, J. B. & Doseff, A. I. (2007). Binding of caspase-3 prodomain to heat shock protein 27 regulates monocyte apoptosis by inhibiting caspase-3 proteolytic activation. *J Biol Chem.* 282(34):25088-25099.

Wang, F.; Herzmark, P.; Weiner, O. D.; Srinivasan, S.; Servant, G. & Bourne, H. R. (2002). Lipid products of PI(3)Ks maintain persistent cell polarity and directed motility in neutrophils. *Nat Cell Biol.* 4(7):513-518.

Wang, H.; Xing, J.; Wang, F.; Han, W.; Ren, H.; Wu, T. & Chen, W. (2010). Expression of Hsp27 and Hsp70 in lymphocytes and plasma in healthy workers and coal miners with lung cancer. *J Huazhong Univ Sci Technolog [Med Sci].* 30(4):415-420.

Werno, C.; Menrad, H.; Weigert, A.; Dehne, N.; Goerdt, S.; Schledzewski, K.; Kzhyshkowska, J. & Brune, B. (2010). Knockout of HIF-1alpha in tumor-associated macrophages enhances M2 polarization and attenuates their pro-angiogenic responses. *Carcinogenesis.* 31(10):1863-1872.

Whiteside, T. L. (2008). The tumor microenvironment and its role in promoting tumor growth. *Oncogene.* 27(45):5904-5912.

Wong, K. L.; Tai, J. J.; Wong, W. C.; Han, H.; Sem, X.; Yeap, W. H.; Kourilsky, P. & Wong, S. C. (2011). Gene expression profiling reveals the defining features of the classical, intermediate, and nonclassical human monocyte subsets. *Blood.* 118(5):e16-31.

Yang, L.; DeBusk, L. M.; Fukuda, K.; Fingleton, B.; Green-Jarvis, B.; Shyr, Y.; Matrisian, L. M.; Carbone, D. P. & Lin, P. C. (2004). Expansion of myeloid immune suppressor Gr+CD11b+ cells in tumor-bearing host directly promotes tumor angiogenesis. *Cancer Cell.* 6(4):409-421.

Yeamans, C.; Wang, D.; Paz-Priel, I.; Torbett, B. E.; Tenen, D. G. & Friedman, A. D. (2007). C/EBPα binds and activates the PU.1 distal enhancer to induce monocyte lineage commitment. *Blood.* 110(9):3136-3142.

Yoshimura, A. (2006). Signal transduction of inflammatory cytokines and tumor development. *Cancer Sci.* 97(6):439-447.

Youle, R. J. & Strasser, A. (2008). The BCL-2 protein family: opposing activities that mediate cell death. *Nat Rev Mol Cell Biol.* 9(1):47-59.

Zeigler, M. M.; Doseff, A. I.; Galloway, M. F.; Opalek, J. M.; Nowicki, P. T.; Zweier, J. L.; Sen, C. K. & Marsh, C. B. (2003). Presentation of nitric oxide regulates monocyte survival through effects on caspase-9 and caspase-3 activation. *J Biol Chem.* 278(15):12894-12902.

Zhao, C.; Zhang, H.; Wong, W. C.; Sem, X.; Han, H.; Ong, S. M.; Tan, Y. C.; Yeap, W. H.; Gan, C. S.; Ng, K. Q.; Koh, M. B.; Kourilsky, P.; Sze, S. K. & Wong, S. C. (2009). Identification of novel functional differences in monocyte subsets using proteomic and transcriptomic methods. *J Proteome Res.* 8(8):4028-4038.

Zhou, Q. & Melton, D. A. (2008). Extreme makeover: converting one cell into another. *Cell Stem Cell.* 3(4):382-388.

Ziegler-Heitbrock, L.; Ancuta, P.; Crowe, S.; Dalod, M.; Grau, V.; Hart, D. N.; Leenen, P. J.; Liu, Y. J.; MacPherson, G.; Randolph, G. J.; Scherberich, J.; Schmitz, J.; Shortman, K.; Sozzani, S.; Strobl, H.; Zembala, M.; Austyn, J. M. & Lutz, M. B. (2010). Nomenclature of monocytes and dendritic cells in blood. *Blood*. 116(16):e74-80.

Zou, W. (2005). Immunosuppressive networks in the tumour environment and their therapeutic relevance. *Nat Rev Cancer*. 5(4):263-274.

4

Myeloid Derived Suppressor Cells: Subsets, Expansion, and Role in Cancer Progression

Liang Zhi, Benjamin Toh and Jean-Pierre Abastado
Singapore Immunology Network, BMSI, A-STAR
Singapore

1. Introduction

Cancer immunotherapies have shown considerable promise in pre-clinical studies, but the potency of these interventions has often proved disappointing *in vivo*. This is in part due to tumor infiltration by myeloid cells, which are usually associated with less favorable clinical outcomes. In the past decade, several distinct subsets of tumor-infiltrating myeloid cells have been described (Movahedi et al., 2010), among which myeloid-derived suppressor cells (MDSC) have been subject to particular scrutiny for exerting a critical role in cancer progression (Bronte, 2009; Gabrilovich and Nagaraj, 2009; Ostrand-Rosenberg and Sinha, 2009; Ribechini et al., 2010). MDSC have been studied intensively in the context of cancer, and the weight of evidence indicates that these cells accumulate in most human cancers and also in experimental animal models with transplanted or spontaneous tumors (Eruslanov et al., 2011; Gabitass et al., 2011; Movahedi et al., 2008; Peranzoni et al., 2010; Raychaudhuri et al., 2011; Youn et al., 2008). MDSC also have significant roles to play in numerous other pathologies, including bacterial infections (Delano et al., 2007), parasitic infections (Brys et al., 2005; Goni et al., 2002), chemotherapy outcomes (Angulo et al., 2000), experimental autoimmunity (Arora et al., 2011; Kerr et al., 2008; Moline-Velazquez et al., 2011; Zhu et al., 2007), inflammatory bowel diseases (Haile et al., 2008), obesity (Xia et al., 2011), transplant rejection (Hock et al., 2011), and stress responses (Makarenkova et al., 2006).

MDSC are a heterogeneous population of myeloid lineage cells that comprises progenitor cells, immature macrophages, immature granulocytes and immature dendritic cells (Gabrilovich and Nagaraj, 2009). MDSC lack specific phenotypic markers of macrophages, dendritic cells and monocytes, but instead exist as two morphologically distinct subsets: monocytic (MO)-MDSC and granulocytic/polymorphonuclear (PMN)-MDSC (Movahedi et al., 2008; Youn et al., 2008). MDSC populations accumulate and become activated in response to various factors released by tumor cells and/or by host cells in the tumor microenvironment, where they suppress both innate and adaptive anti-tumor immunity through a variety of different mechanisms. MDSC are therefore considered to be a major contributor to tumor immune evasion. However, the pro-tumor action of MDSC is not limited to their direct immunosuppressive properties - these cells have also been shown to favor cancer progression by promoting angiogenesis, cancer cell proliferation, invasion, and metastasis. The induction of MDSC by pro-inflammatory mediators and by tumor-derived soluble factors highlights key contributions from chronic inflammation and from the tumor microenvironment to the onset and progression of cancer.

In this chapter, we will review the recent literature on MDSC expansion, their role in cancer progression, their proposed mechanisms of action, and the therapeutic challenges of targeting MDSC. We will focus more specifically on mouse MDSC and their role in melanoma.

2. Origin, distribution and expansion of MDSC

Hematopoietic stem cells give rise to myeloid progenitor and precursor cells in bone marrow. Then these immature myeloid cells (IMC) migrate into peripheral lymphoid organs and differentiate into mature granulocytes, macrophages, or dendritic cells. Various sources of immunological stress, including cancer, inflammation, trauma, and autoimmune disorder, can inhibit the differentiation of IMC and thus promote the expansion of this population. IMC can subsequently become activated by tumor-derived factors and host cytokines which results in the generation of MDSC with potent immunosuppressive potential (Ribechini et al., 2010). In the steady state, IMC primarily reside in the bone marrow, but in pathological settings (cancer being the most well studied), MDSC can be detected in the bone marrow, spleen, blood, tumor, and also in lymph nodes (Haile et al., 2008; Kusmartsev et al., 2005; Serafini et al., 2004; Sinha et al., 2008).

The expansion, activation and accumulation of MDSC in peripheral tissues can be driven by multiple factors produced by tumor cells, tumor stromal cells, or by activated T cells. These mediators include prostaglandins; matrix metalloproteinases (MMPs); growth factors such as granulocyte-macrophage colony-stimulating factor (GM-CSF), granulocyte colony-stimulating factor (G-CSF), macrophage colony-stimulating factor (M-CSF), vascular endothelial growth factor (VEGF), stem-cell factor (SCF); cytokines such as transforming growth factor (TGF)-β, tumor necrosis factor (TNF)-α, interferon γ (IFN-γ), IL-1β, IL-4, IL-6, IL-10, IL-12, IL-13; chemokines CCL2, CXCL5, CXCL12; and various other pro-inflammatory molecules including S100A8/9 proteins, toll-like receptor agonists, tumor-derived exosome-associated Hsp72, inflammasome component NLRP3, and complement component C5a (Chalmin et al., 2010; Gabrilovich and Nagaraj, 2009; Ostrand-Rosenberg and Sinha, 2009; Ribechini et al., 2010; van Deventer et al., 2010). These agents either promote MDSC expansion through the JAK2/STAT3 signaling pathway or induce the activation of MDSC via STAT1, STAT6, or through NF-κB-dependent mechanisms (Gabrilovich and Nagaraj, 2009; Kusmartsev and Gabrilovich, 2006).

3. Subsets of murine MDSC

MDSC comprise numerous different types of myeloid precursor cells. In mice, MDSC are characterized by the co-expression of surface markers Gr-1 and CD11b. In healthy mice, cells with this phenotype constitute around 20-30% of cells in bone marrow, approximately 2-4% of cells in the spleen, and fewer still in the lymph nodes (Kusmartsev and Gabrilovich, 2006), although the frequency of these cells can increase dramatically in tumor-bearing mice (Movahedi et al., 2008). Since Gr-1 antibodies can bind to two separate epitopes, Ly6G and Ly6C, it has recently become possible to further delineate MDSC subsets using antibodies that specifically target these distinct antigens. The Ly6G molecule is expressed primarily by granulocytes, whereas Ly6C is highly expressed by monocytes (Fleming et al., 1993; Sunderkotter et al., 2004). Among murine MDSC, the $CD11b^{+}Ly6G^{+}Ly6C^{low}$ subset (PMN-MDSC), exhibits a polymorphonulear phenotype, while the $CD11b^{+}Ly6G^{-}Ly6C^{high}$ subset (MO-MDSC), displays a monocytic phenotype. More recently, some new features of MDSC have emerged that provide further insights into the diversity of these cells. Using a simple staining strategy, Greifenberg and colleagues were able to divide mouse splenocytes into six distinct sub-populations with regard to their size, granularity, morphology, and relative expression of CD11b and Gr-1 (Greifenberg et al., 2009). Among these various populations, Gr-1^{low}CD11b^{high}Ly6C^{high}SSC^{low} and Gr-1^{high}CD11b^{low} (with ring-shaped nuclei) MDSC possessed suppressive potential. Additionally, Elkabets *et al.* identified a novel sub-population of murine MDSC that lacks Ly6C expression and predominates during IL-1β-induced inflammatory responses. Ly6C^{neg} MDSC and Ly6C^{low} MDSC may constitute separate lineages of MDSC, or could perhaps represent distinct states of differentiation within a single MDSC lineage (Elkabets et al., 2010). In addition to Gr-1 and CD11b, several other surface molecules have been reported to discriminate between sub-populations of MDSC, including the co-stimulatory molecule CD80 (B7.1) (Yang et al., 2006), macrophage marker F4/80 (Huang et al., 2006), the M-CSF receptor (CSF1R/CD115) (Huang et al., 2006), and the α-chain of the receptor for IL-4 and IL-13 (IL-4Rα/CD124) (Gallina et al., 2006). MO-MDSC express higher levels of F4/80, CD115, 7/4, and CCR2 when compared with PMN-MDSC, which suggests a monocytic origin for these cells. However, further studies have demonstrated that, although these additional markers are undoubtedly expressed by MDSC, they do not specifically define a population of immunosuppressive cells (Youn et al., 2008). Indeed, while useful for analytical purposes, the Ly6G and Ly6C antibodies are not essential for identifying MDSC populations by flow-cytometry: differential expression of Gr-1 and F4/80 alone can suffice to distinguish PMN-MDSC (CD11b^+Gr-1^{high}F4/80^-) from MO-MDSC (CD11b^+Gr-1^{int}F4/80^{int}). The use of Ly6G-specific antibodies is therefore only required when attempting to isolate a pure PMN-MDSC subset from a mixed cell population that also includes MO-MDSC (Toh et al., 2011). A summary of MDSC subsets can be found in Table 1.

PMN-MDSC	MO-MDSC
CD11b^+Ly6G^+Ly6C^{low}	CD11b^+Ly6G^-Ly6C^{high} Higher expression of F4/80, CCR2 and CD115
Cell contact-dependent Antigen-specific immunosuppression	Cell contact-independent Antigen-specific and antigen-independent immunosuppression
Immune suppression via ROS-mediated mechanisms	Immune suppression via arginase and NOS-mediated mechanisms
Terminally differentiated	Capable in differentiating into macrophages

Table 1. Main characteristics of two well-accepted MDSC subsets (Movahedi et al., 2008; Youn et al., 2008). It should be noted that some novel sub-populations of MDSC have recently been identified.

4. MDSC in cancer progression

There is ample evidence from the literature that MDSC are associated with tumor progression. Adoptive transfer of MDSC in murine tumor models has been found to significantly promote tumor growth (Balwit et al., 2011; Yang et al., 2004), and administration of MDSC after 5-Fluorouracil (5FU) injection blunted the anti-tumor effect of 5FU in tumor-bearing mice (Vincent et al., 2010). Depletion of Gr-1$^+$ cells in tumor-bearing mice by injection of anti-Gr-1 antibody strikingly inhibited tumor growth, reduced cancer cell dissemination and metastasis, and prolonged survival (Li et al., 2009; Pekarek et al., 1995; Zhang et al., 2009). Treatment of tumor-bearing mice with drugs that target MDSC, such as gemcitabine chemotherapeutic agent, all-trans-retinoic acid, and phosphodiesterase-5 inhibitors led to delayed tumor progression, improved survival, and enhanced efficacy of cancer vaccines and immunotherapies (Kusmartsev et al., 2003; Serafini et al., 2006; Suzuki et al., 2005). Reduction of murine MDSC numbers has also been shown to facilitate the rejection of established metastatic disease after the removal of primary tumors (Sinha et al., 2005).

5. MDSC use multiple mechanisms to suppress T-cell function

MDSC use a variety of different mechanisms to suppress anti-tumor immunity. Multiple lines of evidence indicate that MDSC are potent inhibitors of both antigen-specific and non-specific T-cell activation.

5.1 Arginase

L-arginine is a conditionally essential amino acid and is primarily metabolized by arginases (ARGs) and nitric oxide synthases (NOSs) to produce either L-ornithine and urea, or to provide L-citrulline and nitric oxide (NO) (Bogdan, 2001; Morris, 2002; Wu and Morris, 1998). The suppressive activity of MDSC was initially thought to be associated with the metabolism of L-arginine since depletion of this amino acid is accompanied by marked suppression of T-cell function and proliferation (Bronte et al., 2003; Bronte and Zanovello, 2005; Rodriguez et al., 2005; Rodriguez and Ochoa, 2008). L-arginine deprivation has been reported to induce T-cell dysfunction via two distinct pathways, the first being loss of CD3ζ chain expression by these cells (Ezernitchi et al., 2006; Rodriguez et al., 2004; Rodriguez et al., 2002; Rodriguez et al., 2003a). CD3ζ is a key component of the T-cell receptor (TCR) and contains three immunoreceptor tyrosine-based activation motifs (ITAM) that generate an activation signal in T cells upon antigen recognition (Pitcher and van Oers, 2003). Lack of L-arginine may therefore decrease the propensity for T cells to become activated by down-regulating the CD3ζ signal transduction machinery. Alternatively, shortage of L-arginine may prevent the up-regulation of cell cycle regulators cyclin D3 and cyclin-dependent kinase 4 (CDK4) to arrest T cells in the G_0-G_1 phase of the cell cycle (Rodriguez et al., 2007). MDSC produce high levels of arginase, which depletes L-arginine in the local microenvironment, and can also uptake excess arginine through the CAT-2B transporter (Rodriguez et al., 2004; Rodriguez et al., 2003b). MDSC may therefore deprive T cells of L-arginine to limit their proliferative potential, as well as decreasing TCR signaling, to induce broad suppression of T-cell function. These mechanisms seem to contribute to the pro-tumor function of MDSC, since injection of the arginase I inhibitor *N*-hydroxy-nor-l-arginine (Nor-NOHA) in tandem with tumor implantation has been shown to significantly slow the growth of lung carcinoma in a dose-dependent manner. However, inhibition of tumor growth upon Nor-NOHA treatment was not observed in tumor-laden SCID mice (severe combined immunodeficient animals), suggesting that the anti-tumor effect of arginase inhibition was dependent on lymphocyte function (Rodriguez et al., 2004).

5.2 Nitric oxide

L-arginine is a substrate for inducible nitric oxide synthase (iNOS) which is highly expressed in MDSC. Nitric oxide (NO) production via this pathway is a powerful modulator of inflammation and has been reported to preferentially inhibit Th1-mediated immune responses (Bauer et al., 1997; Sosroseno et al., 2009). NO potently suppresses T-cell activation, proliferation, adhesion, and migration (Bingisser et al., 1998; Bobe et al., 1999; Lejeune et al., 1994; Mazzoni et al., 2002; Medot-Pirenne et al., 1999; Sato et al., 2007). It suppresses T-cell function through blocking the activation of several important signaling molecules in T cells, including Janus-activated kinase 1 (JAK1), JAK3, signal transducer and activator of transcription 5 (STAT5), extracellular signal-regulated kinase (ERK), and AKT (Bingisser et al., 1998; Mazzoni et al., 2002). NO has also been shown to inhibit MHC class II expression and promote T-cell apoptosis (Harari and Liao, 2004; Rivoltini et al., 2002).

5.3 Reactive oxygen species

Reactive oxygen species (ROS) have emerged as a potential key mechanism of MDSC-induced immunosuppression in tumor-bearing hosts. Hyper-production of ROS is an archetypal feature of MDSC in both mouse tumor models and in human cancer patients (Greten et al., 2011; Kusmartsev et al., 2004; Youn et al., 2008). Elevated ROS production by MDSC is mediated primarily by increased NADPH oxidase NOX2 activity (Corzo et al., 2009). In a previous report, lack of NOX2 activity abrogated the ability of MDSC to suppress T-cell responses (Corzo et al., 2009). Arginases and NOS can also contribute to the generation of ROS in MDSC: arginase depletion of L-arginine in the local environment triggers superoxide (O_2^-) generation from iNOS (Bronte et al., 2003; Xia et al., 1998). The unstable O_2^- anion can then react with protons in water to generate hydrogen peroxide. ROS appear then to exert a major role in MDSC-mediated T-cell suppression (Kusmartsev et al., 2008; Markiewski et al., 2008; Nagaraj et al., 2007) and have been implicated in the inhibition of antigen-specific $CD8^+$ T-cell responses in tumor-bearing mice (Kusmartsev et al., 2004). ROS are also thought to play a direct role in inducing apoptosis of activated T cells by decreasing Bcl-2 expression (Hildeman et al., 2003). Accordingly, inhibition of ROS production in MDSC by the addition of ROS scavengers can reverse MDSC-mediated immune suppression and rescues IFN-γ production (Kusmartsev et al., 2004; Kusmartsev et al., 2008).

5.4 Peroxynitrite

Peroxynitrite ($ONOO^-$) is a reactive nitrogen-oxide species (RNOS) formed from the reaction between NO and O_2^- (Squadrito and Pryor, 1995). A major action of peroxynitrite is the modification of proteins by oxidation or nitration of the amino acids tyrosine, cystine, methionine, and tryptophan (Gabrilovich and Nagaraj, 2009). MDSC are copious producers of peroxynitrite, and increased levels of this species are associated with tumor progression (Cobbs et al., 2003; Ekmekcioglu et al., 2000; Nakamura et al., 2006). Hyper-production of peroxynitrite during direct contact with T cells allows MDSC to induce nitration of tyrosine residues in the TCR and CD8 co-receptor, leading to decreased conformational flexibility of the TCR chains and impaired interactions with MHC, thus inhibiting antigen-specific, cytotoxic T-cell responses (Nagaraj et al., 2007). Peroxynitrite-driven nitration of tyrosine residues in human lymphocytes is also able to promote apoptotic cell death by inhibiting activation-induced tyrosine phosphorylation in these cells (Brito et al., 1999).

5.5 Cysteine

Recent work has demonstrated that murine MDSC block T-cell activation by depleting cysteine from the local microenvironment (Srivastava et al., 2010). Cysteine is an essential amino acid required for T-cell activation, differentiation and proliferation. Cells generate cysteine through two distinct pathways: the cystathionase enzyme can convert intracellular methionine into cysteine (Gout et al., 2001; Ishii et al., 2004), or alternatively, the plasma membrane cystine transporter x_c^- can import the oxidized form of the acid (cystine) from the extracellular environment. Imported cystine can then be reduced to form cysteine (Arner and Holmgren, 2000; Mansoor et al., 1992). Since T cells lack both cystathionase and an intact x_c^- transporter, they are unable to generate cysteine independently. Under homeostatic conditions, antigen-presenting cells (APC) provide cysteine to T cells by importing cystine, converting it to cysteine, and then exporting the cysteine through their plasma membrane ASC transporters (Sato et al., 1987; Angelini et al., 2002). Like T cells, MDSC lack cystathionase and depend on extracellular cystine for the synthesis of cysteine, but they lack the APC-expressed ASC transporter required to export cysteine. This results in MDSC readily importing cystine at a rate similar to that of macrophages and DC, but they do not export cysteine. This action depletes the environment of cysteine and results in the inhibition of T-cell activation and function (Srivastava et al., 2010).

5.6 Alternative immunosuppressive mechanisms

Alternative pathways have been identified through which MDSC might exert their suppressive functions. The immunoregulatory cytokine TGF-β has been implicated in MDSC function. It is regulated in MDSC by IL-13 and $CD4^+$ CD1d-restricted T cells. Blocking IL-13 or TGF-β limited tumor incidence in murine transplanted tumor models (Fichtner-Feigl et al., 2008; Terabe et al., 2003). MDSC also have the ability to systemically down-regulate CD62L (L-selectin) on T cells in tumor-bearing mice. This action impairs naïve $CD4^+$ and $CD8^+$ T-cell homing to lymph nodes. Therefore, these T cells are not able to be activated by tumor antigens (Hanson et al., 2009). Down-regulation of CD62L was not due to general T-cell activation and could even be observed in tumor-free mice that exhibited high numbers of MDSC, (a common profile in aged animals). MDSC also constitutively express a disintegrin and metalloproteinase domain 17 (ADAM17, also known as TACE/TNFα-converting enzyme) on their cell surface, thus allowing the proteolytic cleavage and shedding of the ectodomain of CD62L (Hanson et al., 2009).

Various reports have demonstrated that MDSC can induce the differentiation of regulatory T cells (Treg) in tumor-bearing hosts and indirectly promote immune suppression (Gabrilovich and Nagaraj, 2009). Treg induction can occur through diverse pathways that depend on the tumor model in use (Bianchi et al., 2011). In a mouse lymphoma model, induction of Treg is dependent on arginase and is independent of TGF-β (Serafini et al., 2008), but in murine ovarian cancer, cytotoxic T lymphocyte-associated antigen 4 (CTLA-4) expression on MDSC can mediate Treg induction (Yang et al., 2006). Another study by Huang *et al.* using several murine transplanted tumor models showed that IL-10 and IFN-γ, but not NO, were important factors in MDSC-mediated Treg development (Huang et al., 2006). A more recent study has also reported that the immune stimulatory receptor CD40 on MDSC is required to induce tumor-specific Treg expansion in a mouse colon cancer model (Pan et al., 2010).

5.7 Suppressive mechanisms differ between MDSC subsets

In addition to morphological and phenotypic distinctions, PMN-MDSC and MO-MDSC also exert their suppressive activity by different mechanisms. MO-MDSC express high levels of NO and low levels of ROS, and they effectively suppress T-cell function in both antigen-dependent and independent manners without requiring cell-cell contact. Primarily, MO-MDSC inhibit T-cell function through NOS-mediated mechanisms since NOS inhibitors are able to block this suppressive effect. This pathway is IFN-γ/STAT1-dependent (Movahedi et al., 2008; Youn et al., 2008). In contrast, PMN-MDSC produce high levels of ROS but only nominal amounts of NO, indicating that ROS are the primary mediators of their suppressive functions (Movahedi et al., 2008; Youn et al., 2008). PMN-MDSC generally require antigen-specific interactions with T cells to mediate suppression (Nagaraj et al., 2007), although it has also been reported that PMN-MDSC do not require direct MHC I presentation to exert inhibitory effects (Movahedi et al., 2008). In most tumor models, PMN-MDSC are the main MDSC subset to be expanded in the peripheral lymphoid organs (Youn et al., 2008), while the MO-MDSC population possesses more potent inhibitory activity (Dolcetti et al., 2010; Movahedi et al., 2008; Nausch et al., 2008; Priceman et al., 2010).

Murine splenic MDSC have also been shown to differ from their tumor-derived counterparts with regards to T-cell suppression. Tumor MDSC can potently suppress T-cell proliferation in both antigen-specific and non-specific manner, whereas splenic MDSC are comparatively weak suppressor cells and exert only antigen-specific T-cell inhibition. This functional difference is suggested to be due to the different suppressive mechanisms used by splenic and tumor MDSC. Splenic MDSC suppress T cells through ROS production. In contrast, at the tumor site, MDSC, as a result of the effect of hypoxia via HIF-1α, dramatically up-regulate *inos* and *argI* expression and therefore acquire the ability to inhibit antigen-nonspecific T-cell functions (Corzo et al., 2010).

6. Mechanisms by which MDSC disrupt innate immunity

In addition to T-cell suppression, MDSC restrict innate responses via their interactions with macrophages, NK cells, and NKT cells to further impair anti-tumor immunity. Cross-talk between MDSC and macrophages results in increased MDSC production of the type 2 cytokine IL-10, and decreased macrophage production of type 1 cytokine IL-12, which skews tumor immunity towards a tumor-promoting type 2 response (Sinha et al., 2007).

The role of MDSC in regulating NK-cell function remains controversial. Some studies have shown that MDSC impair NK-cell development, IFN-γ production and cytotoxicity against tumor cells. This suppression is mediated by membrane-bound TGF-β1 and through down-modulation of NKG2D (the primary activating receptor for NK cells) (Elkabets et al., 2010; Li et al., 2009; Liu et al., 2007; Suzuki et al., 2005). However, in a separate mouse study, MO-MDSC isolated from RMA-S tumor-bearing mice failed to suppress NK-cell function, and instead elicited high production of IFN-γ by these cells. These effects partially depended on the interaction of NKG2D on NK cells with ligand RAE-1 on MDSC. Following activation, the NK cells eliminated the MDSC (Nausch et al., 2008).

7. Non-immunosuppressive pro-tumor functions

MDSC support for tumor growth does not depend solely on immunosuppression - these cells also promote tumor progression by augmenting blood vessel development and enhancing tumor-cell invasion and metastasis. In a murine colorectal cancer model (MC26), tumors co-injected with MDSC from mice bearing large tumors exhibited increased vascular density and maturation, as well as decreased necrosis (Yang et al., 2004). Tumor growth was markedly facilitated when co-injected with tumor-derived MDSC, but not when co-injected with MDSC from normal mice. This increased vasculature was attributed to the production of MMP9, a critical mediator of tumor angiogenesis, vasculogenesis, and metastasis. MDSC-derived MMP9 was shown to increase the bioavailability of VEGF in tumors and promote tumor angiogenesis and vascular stability. Accordingly, selective deletion of MMP9 in MDSC completely abolished their tumor-promoting activity (Yang et al., 2004). In a separate study using the mouse MT1A2 mammary cancer model, it was demonstrated that bone marrow-derived $CD11b^+$ myelomonocytic cells significantly contributed to tumor vasculogenesis by producing MMP9 (Ahn and Brown, 2008). Various other MMPs, including MMP14, MMP13, and MMP2, were also found to be highly expressed in tumor-resident MDSC (Yang et al., 2008). These MDSC were recruited to the invasive front of mammary carcinomas with conditional deletion of the type II TGF-β receptor gene. The MDSC infiltrate directly facilitated tumor invasion and metastasis through enhanced MMP and TGF-β production (Yang et al., 2008). Furthermore, Bv8 protein (also known as prokineticin 2, or Prok2) has also been reported to contribute to MDSC-dependent tumor angiogenesis. Transplantation of tumor cells in mice resulted in significant up-regulation of Bv8 in MDSC, while treatment with neutralizing anti-Bv8 antibodies suppressed tumor angiogenesis and inhibited tumor growth (Shojaei et al., 2007). In addition, murine tumor-associated MDSC were shown to confer tumor resistance to anti-angiogenic therapy (anti-VEGF antibody) that was mediated by G-CSF and depended on Bv8 expression. Combining anti-VEGF treatment with anti-Gr-1, anti-G-CSF, or anti-Bv8 antibody inhibited growth of refractory tumors more effectively that anti-VEGF therapy alone. Anti-G-CSF treatment robustly reduced MDSC frequency in refractory tumors, decreased Bv8 levels, and inhibited tumor angiogenesis (Shojaei et al., 2009). The tumor microenvironment has also been proposed to support MDSC shape change and expression of endothelial markers such as VEGFR2 and VE-Cadherin (Yang et al., 2004), which may allow MDSC to differentiate locally and directly incorporate into the tumor endothelium to contribute to vascular development.

Although MDSC up-regulation of proteases seems to be the primary route by which these cells promote tumor metastasis, a recent study by Boutte and colleagues also highlighted the importance of down-regulating protease inhibitors in tumor dissemination (Boutte et al., 2011). In this study of transplanted tumors, neutrophilic granule protein (NGP: a cathepsin B inhibitor), was down-regulated in MDSC from metastatic tumor-bearing mice compared with non-metastatic controls. Up-regulation of NGP in tumors delayed primary tumor growth and greatly reduced tumor vasculature, invasiveness, and metastasis.

MDSC have been further implicated in pre-metastatic niche formation in the lungs of tumor-bearing mice. The concept of the pre-metastatic niche arises from the observation that many tumors have a pre-disposition to metastasize certain organs. Various leukocyte populations and secreted inflammatory factors have been shown to "prepare" distal organs for metastatic cells (Hiratsuka et al., 2006; Kaplan et al., 2006; Kaplan et al., 2005), and MDSC can infiltrate the lungs of tumor-bearing mice before the arrival of tumor cells. These MDSC create a proliferative and immunosuppressive lung environment that is permissive for the growth of metastatic tumor cells. Pre-metastatic lungs with elevated MDSC have increased levels of basic fibroblast growth factor (bFGF), insulin growth factor 1 (IGF1), IL-4, IL-5, IL-9, IL-10, and MMP9, whereas IFN-γ is down-regulated in these lungs. Up-regulation of MMP9 in pulmonary MDSC drives abnormal vasculature development in the pre-metastatic lung (Yan et al., 2010), while myeloid cell-derived S100A8 and S100A9 pre-dispose the lung microenvironment towards eventual tumor metastasis (Hiratsuka et al., 2006).

Finally, our own data reveal that PMN-MDSC promote melanoma cell proliferation by secreting soluble factors while also supporting cancer cell dissemination and metastasis by inducing epithelial-mesenchymal transition (Toh et al., 2011). These novel MDSC functions are discussed in more detail in the subsequent sections.

8. Melanoma and the immune system

Malignant melanoma is one of the most immunogenic forms of cancer and hundreds of immunotherapeutic trials have been conducted in melanoma patients to date. Substantial knowledge has been accumulated on the immunosuppressive pathways at work in melanoma and the role played by MDSC in disease progression. Tumor infiltrating lymphocytes (TIL) have been correlated with better prognoses and improved five-year survival rates (Day et al., 1981), and TIL isolated from melanoma patients are able to lyse MHC-matched allogeneic tumors (Degiovanni et al., 1988; Oble et al., 2009). However, the prognostic value of TIL is only valid in the early stages of melanoma, since TIL numbers in thick lesions do not predict clinical outcomes. Many melanoma-associated antigens are non-mutated proteins that contribute to melanin synthesis, such as MelanA/MART-1, tyrosinase related protein (TRP)-1, TRP-2, gp100 and tyrosinase (Kawakami, 2000). Unfortunately, there has been only limited success in vaccinating patients with these antigens (Linette et al., 2005). Large numbers of MelanA/MART-1 specific T cells have been found in the blood and tumors of melanoma patients (Salcedo et al., 2006), but only the circulating T cells were able to produce IFN-γ and granzyme B upon antigen stimulation (Zippelius et al., 2004). These data indicate potent local immunosuppression at the tumor site which is most likely driven by immune cells recruited into the tumor itself. Accordingly, lymphocyte depletion has been shown to be effective method of enhancing adoptive T-cell transfer therapy in melanoma patients (Hershkovitz et al., 2010). In a clinical trial to test the efficacy of adoptive T-cell transfer in combination with lympho-depletion (non-myeloablative chemotherapy; NMC), better objective responses and complete remission could be achieved when NMC was combined with total body irradiation or high dose irradiation alone (Dudley et al., 2008). These findings suggest that tumor-induced immunosuppression does not arise from lymphocytes alone but also from myeloid cells.

To study the complex interactions between tumors and the immune system, investigators are progressively turning to transgenic mice that develop spontaneous tumors and replicate human cancers more closely than transplanted tumor models. RETAAD mice are transgenic for the activated *RET* oncogene which is specifically expressed in melanocytes of the skin and eyes, leading to spontaneous skin tumors and primary uveal melanomas that are clinically detectable by four to eight weeks of age. While exophthalmos eventually presents in adult RETAAD mice, microscopic eye tumors can be detected as early as ten days after birth, and cancer cells disseminate from the primary eye tumor throughout the body within three weeks (Eyles et al., 2010; Kato et al., 1998). Disseminated RETAAD cancer cells remain dormant for months before developing into cutaneous and visceral metastases, and the stepwise evolution of melanoma in these mice closely mimics the histopathology and natural history of human cancers (Eskelin et al., 2000; Kato et al., 1998; Kato et al., 2004). The RETAAD melanoma model is therefore particularly suitable for dissecting the role of host immune cells in metastatic processes.

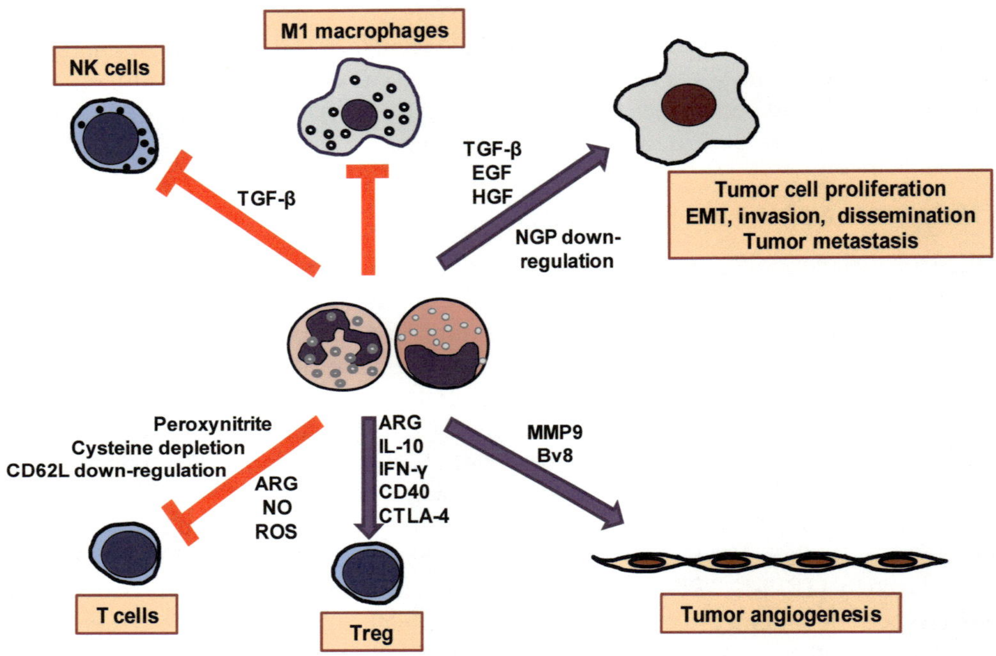

Fig. 1. Immunosuppressive and non-immunosuppressive tumor-promoting functions of MDSC. —┤: Inhibition. ➡: Induction or promotion.

Similar to human melanoma patients, tumors in RETAAD mice grow despite the induction of a broad melanoma-specific CD8+ T-cell response (Lengagne et al., 2008). It is surprising then that cutaneous tumor cell lines derived from RETAAD mice are still recognized by tumor-specific T cells, indicating that they are indeed antigenic (Lengagne et al., 2008). Functionally active, melanoma-specific, memory T lymphocytes can be detected at the early stages of melanoma progression, in the absence of clinically visible cutaneous tumors (Lengagne et al., 2008; Umansky et al., 2008). However, tumor progression continues despite the presence of these antigen-specific CD8+ T cells, suggesting that potent suppressive mechanisms shield the developing tumor from immune destruction.

Even though a pathological role for Treg cells has been implicated in several tumor models, depletion of Treg in RET transgenic melanoma mice neither delayed nor inhibited tumor development (Kimpfler et al., 2009). In RET mice, intra-tumoral dendritic cell (DC) numbers correlated with tumor size, and DC from mice with macroscopic tumors secreted significantly less IL-12p70, increased quantities of IL-10, and were impaired in their ability to activate T cells. The tolerogenic properties of these DC were mediated by IL-6, VEGF, and TGF-β_1 secreted in the tumor microenvironment (Zhao et al., 2009). Interestingly, in a separate study, IL-6 ablation in RET mice also reduced the incidence and size of tumors (von Felbert et al., 2005). Relative aggression of cutaneous tumors in RET mice correlated with numbers of tumor-infiltrating CD11b$^+$Gr1^{low} macrophages that displayed an M2-like, pro-tumor phenotype, characterized by high transcript levels of *il10, arginase I, mgl1, fizz1,* and *ccl2.* Tumor- and spleen-derived macrophages in these mice were able to potently inhibit T-cell function. Surprisingly, depletion of T cells from RET mice resulted in the switching of these macrophages towards a M1, anti-tumor phenotype, characterized by secretion of IL-12. In the absence of T cells, macrophages in RET mice also displayed reduced ability to support tumor growth (Lengagne et al., 2011). In our own laboratory, we have further observed that the microenvironment of RETAAD cutaneous tumors supports only limited infiltration of CD4$^+$ and CD8$^+$ T cells compared with transplanted B16 tumors (Hong et al., 2011).

9. MDSC in melanoma

We have observed that CD11b$^+$Gr1^{high} PMN-MDSC are increased in the spleen and blood of RETAAD mice during tumor progression. PMN-MDSC, but not MO-MDSC, preferentially accumulate in the primary tumor compared with metastases, which is due to the expression of CXCL1, CXCL2 and CXCL5 (chemotactic mediators specific for PMN-MDSC) in the primary tumor, but not in metastases. PMN-MDSC notably affect two primary aspects of tumor progression - tumor growth and metastasis. In RETAAD mice, depletion of PMN-MDSC by treatment with anti-Ly6G antibody resulted in a decrease in primary tumor size, but failed to diminish cutaneous tumors (which have low infiltrates of PMN-MDSC). Furthermore, early depletion of PMN-MDSC (before primary tumor development) resulted in decreased proliferation of primary tumors, while *in vitro* assays demonstrated that the ability to induce cancer cell proliferation is specific to PMN-MDSC but not macrophages. These data also indicate that PMN-MDSC are able to directly induce tumor cell proliferation by secreting a soluble factor (Toh et al., 2011).

PMN-MDSC also induce epithelial-mesenchymal transition (EMT) which is the first step towards metastasis in early stage cancers (Toh et al., 2011). Depletion of PMN-MDSC reduced dissemination of tumor cells to distant metastatic sites such as the lungs and the tumor-draining lymph nodes. Primary tumor cells in control mice exhibited higher expression of mesenchymal markers S100A4 and vimentin compared with mice depleted of PMN-MDSC. *In vitro,* PMN-MDSC were also able to down-modulate E-Cadherin, a classical epithelial marker, in both mouse and human melanoma cells. Induction of EMT was dependent on TGF-β, epidermal growth factor and hepatocyte growth factor, since blockade of these molecules either individually or in combination resulted in partial or complete inhibition of EMT (Toh et al., 2011).

The ability of melanomas to evade immune destruction depends on components of the host immune system. While extensive research has already been conducted on immunotherapy strategies that enhance T-cell responses against tumors, improving the efficacy of these interventions will require a better understanding of the interactions between melanoma cells and the immune system, with a particular focus on immunosuppressive MDSC populations.

Additional research will also be required to determine whether MDSC are capable of inducing cancer cell proliferation and epithelial-mesenchymal transition in other types of cancers besides melanoma.

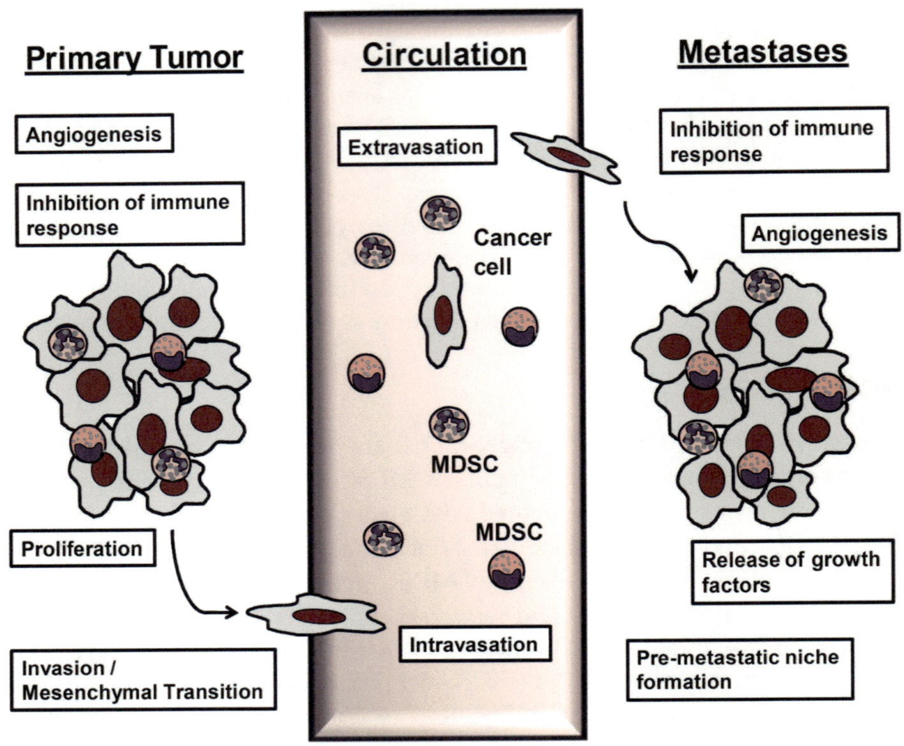

Fig. 2. Roles of MDSC in the growth, invasion, and metastasis of melanoma.

10. Therapeutic strategies targeting MDSC

Recognition that MDSC-mediated immune suppression plays a pivotal role in tumor progression highlights these cells as an appealing target for novel cancer treatments. Agents that modulate MDSC development, differentiation and recruitment, or block the suppressive functions of these cells could represent potent new methods of limiting tumor progression, or could perhaps enhance the efficacy of existing therapies. Limiting the infiltration and activation of MDSC during chronic inflammation may even reduce the risk of *de novo* tumor development.

10.1 Promoting MDSC differentiation

Given the fact that MDSC are immature myeloid cells, a promising approach in cancer immunotherapy would be to drive MDSC differentiation into mature populations that no longer have suppressive activity. Vitamin A has been identified as a candidate agent that possesses this ability, since vitamin A deficiency causes systemic expansion of MDSC in mice (Kuwata et al., 2000). Vitamin A metabolites such as retinoic acid have been found to favor MDSC differentiation into mature DC, macrophages, and granulocytes. Treatment of mouse or human MDSC with all-*trans*-retinoic acid (ATRA) *in vitro* resulted in induction of myeloid cell differentiation (Almand et al., 2001; Gabrilovich et al., 2001; Hengesbach and Hoag, 2004; Kusmartsev et al., 2008). Using adoptive transfer of MDSC into congenic mice, Kusmartsev *et al.* were able to demonstrate that ATRA also induced rapid differentiation of MDSC into mature myeloid cells *in vivo* (Kusmartsev et al., 2003). In tumor-bearing mice, ATRA administration substantially reduced the presence of MDSC and noticeably improved $CD4^+$ and $CD8^+$ T-cell-mediated anti-tumor immune responses. Combination of ATRA with two different types of cancer vaccines significantly prolonged the anti-tumor effect of the vaccination in two different mouse tumor models (Kusmartsev et al., 2003). Moreover, in human patients with metastatic renal cell carcinoma, effective concentrations of ATRA were shown to eliminate MDSC and improve antigen-specific T-cell responses (Kusmartsev et al., 2008; Mirza et al., 2006). Vitamin D derivatives have also been reported to drive myeloid progenitor cell differentiation both *in vitro* and *in vivo* (Duits et al., 1992; Testa et al., 1993). 25-hydroxyvitamin D_3 treatment in patients with head and neck squamous cell carcinoma diminished the number of immuno-suppressive $CD34^+$ progenitor cells and improved numerous parameters of immune responsiveness (Lathers et al., 2004).

10.2 Inhibiting MDSC expansion

As described above, many tumor-derived factors can induce the development and expansion of MDSC from hematopoietic precursors (see also section 2). Neutralization of these mediators is therefore another attractive strategy for novel cancer therapies. For example, stem-cell factor (SCF) has been identified as a vital mediator of MDSC expansion and accumulation, since SCF knockdown using silencing RNA decreased MDSC frequency and reversed tumor-specific T-cell tolerance in the mouse MCA26 colon cancer model. Blocking SCF interactions with its receptor, c-kit, by the use of specific antibodies dramatically reduced the MDSC population and prevented tumor-specific T-cell anergy, Treg development, and tumor angiogenesis, resulting in tumor regression and enhanced efficacy of immune-activating cancer therapy (Pan et al., 2008). Another study also reported that melanoma development is restrained in RET-transgenic mice with impaired c-kit function, or when RET mice are treated with anti-c-kit antibody. Although the authors attributed this phenomenon to the direct function of c-kit in tumor cells, we cannot exclude the possibility that the suppression of tumor development was due to attenuated MDSC expansion caused by c-kit impairment (Kato et al., 2004).

MMP9 inhibition is another logical therapeutic approach in cancer therapy due to the MDSC requirement for MMP9 in supporting their expansion and function. In a spontaneous mouse mammary tumor model, treatment with a MMP9 inhibitor (amino-biphosphonate) was shown to significantly reduce MDSC expansion and impair tumor growth, while simultaneously enhancing tumor necrosis and improving the anti-tumor responses induced by immunotherapy (Melani et al., 2007). Finally, targeting the intracellular signaling pathways that are involved in MDSC expansion is also a promising strategy. Using selective STAT3 inhibitors, such as JSI-124 (cucurbitacin I), or tyrosine kinase inhibitors, such as sunitinib, can augment anti-tumor immune responses by reducing the presence of MDSC. Sunitinib combination therapy with IL-12 and 4-1BB activation significantly improved the long-term survival rate of mice bearing MCA26 colon tumors (Ko et al., 2009; Nefedova et al., 2005; Ozao-Choy et al., 2009). In a more recent study, treating mice with docetaxel antimitotic, chemotherapeutic reagent was found to polarize MDSC towards a M1-like phenotype by inhibiting STAT3 activation, and consequently restored $CD4^+$ and $CD8^+$ T-cell function to reduce 4T1-Neu tumor burden (Kodumudi et al., 2010).

10.3 Eliminating MDSC

Direct elimination of MDSC can be achieved with chemotherapeutic drugs such as gemcitabine, which dramatically and specifically reduces MDSC numbers in tumor-bearing mice, but spares $CD4^+$ T cells, $CD8^+$ T cells, NK cells, macrophages, and B cells. This beneficial loss of MDSC is also accompanied by an increase in the anti-tumor activity of the preserved $CD8^+$ T-cell and NK-cell pool (Suzuki et al., 2005). Treatment with 5-fluorouracil (5FU) has also been shown to induce selective apoptosis of MDSC, thereby decreasing the burden of these cells in murine spleen and tumor beds, but without depleting host T cells, NK cells, dendritic cells, or B cells. The elimination of MDSC by 5FU treatment also increased IFN-γ production by tumor-specific $CD8^+$ T cells and promoted T-cell–dependent anti-tumor responses (Apetoh et al., 2011; Vincent et al., 2010).

10.4 Blocking MDSC suppressive function

Another approach to restricting MDSC support for tumor progression is to block the immunosuppressive function of these cells. Since ARG1 and NOS2 are the primary mediators of MDSC immunosuppression, these enzymes are the most likely targets for novel therapeutic interventions. Various different drugs including nitro-aspirin, COX-2 inhibitors, and phosphodiesterase-5 (PDE5) inhibitors have been shown to profoundly inhibit both ARG1 and NOS2 activity in MDSC. By removing MDSC suppressive mediators, these drugs exhibited a potent ability to restore anti-tumor immune responses and delayed tumor progression in several mouse models (De Santo et al., 2005; Serafini et al., 2006; Talmadge et al., 2007; Zea et al., 2005). Interestingly, in addition to inhibiting MDSC function, COX2 inhibitors also blocked the systemic development of MDSC as well as CCL2-mediated accumulation of these cells in the tumor microenvironment in a mouse model of glioma (Fujita et al., 2011).

11. Conclusion

In recent years, it is becoming increasingly apparent that the immuno-suppressive mechanisms operating in cancer patients significantly contribute to tumor progression and attenuate the efficacy of immunotherapies. The tumor microenvironment incorporates several distinct immunosuppressive cell populations that play dominant roles in this process. MDSC are a heterogeneous population of immature myeloid cells that possess potent ability to inhibit immune responses. These MDSC also have the capacity to promote angiogenesis, cancer cell proliferation, and epithelial-mesenchymal transition, and thus enhance cancer growth, invasion, and metastasis. Controlling the expansion and accumulation of MDSC or blocking their suppressive functions represents promising novel approaches in cancer therapy. However, vital questions remain to be answered if this potential is to be fully realized. What is the predominant mechanism driving the differentiation and activation of MDSC? Which mechanisms primarily contribute to the suppressive activities of MDSC? What are the dynamics of MDSC migration into tumor tissues and peripheral lymphatic organs, and which factors affect their trafficking? Do different subsets of MDSC differ in their function, and does this difference depend on the cancer sub-type? Are there better specific markers that would allow investigators to identify functional MDSC and distinguish various subpopulations of MDSC (particularly in humans)? Solving these questions will advance our understanding of the critical role of MDSC in cancer and could aid the development of novel interventions for cancer treatment.

12. Acknowledgment

We thank Neil McCarthy for editing and proofreading the manuscript and Michelle Hong for providing her unpublished results.

13. References

Ahn, G. O., and Brown, J. M. (2008). Matrix metalloproteinase-9 is required for tumor vasculogenesis but not for angiogenesis: role of bone marrow-derived myelomonocytic cells. Cancer Cell *13*, 193-205.

Almand, B., Clark, J. I., Nikitina, E., van Beynen, J., English, N. R., Knight, S. C., Carbone, D. P., and Gabrilovich, D. I. (2001). Increased production of immature myeloid cells in cancer patients: a mechanism of immunosuppression in cancer. J Immunol *166*, 678-689.

Angelini, G., Gardella, S., Ardy, M., Ciriolo, M. R., Filomeni, G., Di Trapani, G., Clarke, F., Sitia, R., and Rubartelli, A. (2002). Antigen-presenting dendritic cells provide the reducing extracellular microenvironment required for T lymphocyte activation. Proc Natl Acad Sci U S A *99*, 1491-1496.

Angulo, I., de las Heras, F. G., Garcia-Bustos, J. F., Gargallo, D., Munoz-Fernandez, M. A., and Fresno, M. (2000). Nitric oxide-producing CD11b(+)Ly-6G(Gr-1)(+)CD31(ER-MP12)(+) cells in the spleen of cyclophosphamide-treated mice: implications for T-cell responses in immunosuppressed mice. Blood *95*, 212-220.

Apetoh, L., Vegran, F., Ladoire, S., and Ghiringhelli, F. (2011). Restoration of antitumor immunity through selective inhibition of myeloid derived suppressor cells by anticancer therapies. Curr Mol Med *11*, 365-372.

Arner, E. S., and Holmgren, A. (2000). Physiological functions of thioredoxin and thioredoxin reductase. Eur J Biochem *267*, 6102-6109.

Arora, M., Poe, S. L., Ray, A., and Ray, P. (2011). LPS-induced CD11b(+)Gr1(int)F4/80(+) regulatory myeloid cells suppress allergen-induced airway inflammation. Int Immunopharmacol *11*, 825-830.

Balwit, J. M., Hwu, P., Urba, W. J., and Marincola, F. M. (2011). The iSBTc/SITC primer on tumor immunology and biological therapy of cancer: a summary of the 2010 program. J Transl Med *9*, 18.

Bauer, H., Jung, T., Tsikas, D., Stichtenoth, D. O., Frolich, J. C., and Neumann, C. (1997). Nitric oxide inhibits the secretion of T-helper 1- and T-helper 2-associated cytokines in activated human T cells. Immunology *90*, 205-211.

Bianchi, G., Borgonovo, G., Pistoia, V., and Raffaghello, L. (2011). Immunosuppressive cells and tumour microenvironment: Focus on mesenchymal stem cells and myeloid derived suppressor cells. Histol Histopathol *26*, 941-951.

Bingisser, R. M., Tilbrook, P. A., Holt, P. G., and Kees, U. R. (1998). Macrophage-derived nitric oxide regulates T cell activation via reversible disruption of the Jak3/STAT5 signaling pathway. J Immunol *160*, 5729-5734.

Bobe, P., Benihoud, K., Grandjon, D., Opolon, P., Pritchard, L. L., and Huchet, R. (1999). Nitric oxide mediation of active immunosuppression associated with graft-versus-host reaction. Blood *94*, 1028-1037.

Bogdan, C. (2001). Nitric oxide and the immune response. Nat Immunol *2*, 907-916.

Boutte, A. M., Friedman, D. B., Bogyo, M., Min, Y., Yang, L., and Lin, P. C. (2011). Identification of a myeloid-derived suppressor cell cystatin-like protein that inhibits metastasis. FASEB J *25*, 2626-2637.

Brito, C., Naviliat, M., Tiscornia, A. C., Vuillier, F., Gualco, G., Dighiero, G., Radi, R., and Cayota, A. M. (1999). Peroxynitrite inhibits T lymphocyte activation and proliferation by promoting impairment of tyrosine phosphorylation and peroxynitrite-driven apoptotic death. J Immunol *162*, 3356-3366.

Bronte, V. (2009). Myeloid-derived suppressor cells in inflammation: uncovering cell subsets with enhanced immunosuppressive functions. Eur J Immunol *39*, 2670-2672.

Bronte, V., Serafini, P., De Santo, C., Marigo, I., Tosello, V., Mazzoni, A., Segal, D. M., Staib, C., Lowel, M., Sutter, G., *et al.* (2003). IL-4-induced arginase 1 suppresses alloreactive T cells in tumor-bearing mice. J Immunol *170*, 270-278.

Bronte, V., and Zanovello, P. (2005). Regulation of immune responses by L-arginine metabolism. Nat Rev Immunol *5*, 641-654.

Brys, L., Beschin, A., Raes, G., Ghassabeh, G. H., Noel, W., Brandt, J., Brombacher, F., and De Baetselier, P. (2005). Reactive oxygen species and 12/15-lipoxygenase contribute to the antiproliferative capacity of alternatively activated myeloid cells elicited during helminth infection. J Immunol *174*, 6095-6104.

Chalmin, F., Ladoire, S., Mignot, G., Vincent, J., Bruchard, M., Remy-Martin, J. P., Boireau, W., Rouleau, A., Simon, B., Lanneau, D., *et al.* (2010). Membrane-associated Hsp72 from tumor-derived exosomes mediates STAT3-dependent immunosuppressive function of mouse and human myeloid-derived suppressor cells. J Clin Invest *120*, 457-471.

Cobbs, C. S., Whisenhunt, T. R., Wesemann, D. R., Harkins, L. E., Van Meir, E. G., and Samanta, M. (2003). Inactivation of wild-type p53 protein function by reactive oxygen and nitrogen species in malignant glioma cells. Cancer Res *63*, 8670-8673.

Corzo, C. A., Condamine, T., Lu, L., Cotter, M. J., Youn, J. I., Cheng, P., Cho, H. I., Celis, E., Quiceno, D. G., Padhya, T., *et al.* (2010). HIF-1alpha regulates function and differentiation of myeloid-derived suppressor cells in the tumor microenvironment. J Exp Med *207*, 2439-2453.

Corzo, C. A., Cotter, M. J., Cheng, P., Cheng, F., Kusmartsev, S., Sotomayor, E., Padhya, T., McCaffrey, T. V., McCaffrey, J. C., and Gabrilovich, D. I. (2009). Mechanism regulating reactive oxygen species in tumor-induced myeloid-derived suppressor cells. J Immunol *182*, 5693-5701.

Day, C. L., Jr., Sober, A. J., Kopf, A. W., Lew, R. A., Mihm, M. C., Jr., Hennessey, P., Golomb, F. M., Harris, M. N., Gumport, S. L., Raker, J. W., *et al.* (1981). A prognostic model for clinical stage I melanoma of the upper extremity. The importance of anatomic subsites in predicting recurrent disease. Ann Surg *193*, 436-440.

De Santo, C., Salio, M., Masri, S. H., Lee, L. Y., Dong, T., Speak, A. O., Porubsky, S., Booth, S., Veerapen, N., Besra, G. S., *et al.* (2008). Invariant NKT cells reduce the immunosuppressive activity of influenza A virus-induced myeloid-derived suppressor cells in mice and humans. J Clin Invest *118*, 4036-4048.

De Santo, C., Serafini, P., Marigo, I., Dolcetti, L., Bolla, M., Del Soldato, P., Melani, C., Guiducci, C., Colombo, M. P., Iezzi, M., *et al.* (2005). Nitroaspirin corrects immune dysfunction in tumor-bearing hosts and promotes tumor eradication by cancer vaccination. Proc Natl Acad Sci U S A *102*, 4185-4190.

Degiovanni, G., Lahaye, T., Herin, M., Hainaut, P., and Boon, T. (1988). Antigenic heterogeneity of a human melanoma tumor detected by autologous CTL clones. Eur J Immunol *18*, 671-676.

Delano, M. J., Scumpia, P. O., Weinstein, J. S., Coco, D., Nagaraj, S., Kelly-Scumpia, K. M., O'Malley, K. A., Wynn, J. L., Antonenko, S., Al-Quran, S. Z., *et al.* (2007). MyD88-dependent expansion of an immature GR-1(+)CD11b(+) population induces T cell suppression and Th2 polarization in sepsis. J Exp Med *204*, 1463-1474.

Dolcetti, L., Peranzoni, E., Ugel, S., Marigo, I., Fernandez Gomez, A., Mesa, C., Geilich, M., Winkels, G., Traggiai, E., Casati, A., *et al.* (2010). Hierarchy of immunosuppressive strength among myeloid-derived suppressor cell subsets is determined by GM-CSF. Eur J Immunol *40*, 22-35.

Dudley, M. E., Yang, J. C., Sherry, R., Hughes, M. S., Royal, R., Kammula, U., Robbins, P. F., Huang, J., Citrin, D. E., Leitman, S. F., *et al.* (2008). Adoptive cell therapy for patients with metastatic melanoma: evaluation of intensive myeloablative chemoradiation preparative regimens. J Clin Oncol *26*, 5233-5239.

Duits, A. J., Dimjati, W., van de Winkel, J. G., and Capel, P. J. (1992). Synergism of interleukin 6 and 1 alpha,25-dihydroxyvitamin D3 in induction of myeloid differentiation of human leukemic cell lines. J Leukoc Biol *51*, 237-243.

Ekmekcioglu, S., Ellerhorst, J., Smid, C. M., Prieto, V. G., Munsell, M., Buzaid, A. C., and Grimm, E. A. (2000). Inducible nitric oxide synthase and nitrotyrosine in human metastatic melanoma tumors correlate with poor survival. Clin Cancer Res *6*, 4768-4775.

Elkabets, M., Ribeiro, V. S., Dinarello, C. A., Ostrand-Rosenberg, S., Di Santo, J. P., Apte, R. N., and Vosshenrich, C. A. (2010). IL-1beta regulates a novel myeloid-derived suppressor cell subset that impairs NK cell development and function. Eur J Immunol *40*, 3347-3357.

Eruslanov, E., Neuberger, M., Daurkin, I., Perrin, G. Q., Algood, C., Dahm, P., Rosser, C., Vieweg, J., Gilbert, S. M., and Kusmartsev, S. (2011). Circulating and tumor-infiltrating myeloid cell subsets in patients with bladder cancer. Int J Cancer.

Eskelin, S., Pyrhonen, S., Summanen, P., Hahka-Kemppinen, M., and Kivela, T. (2000). Tumor doubling times in metastatic malignant melanoma of the uvea: tumor progression before and after treatment. Ophthalmology *107*, 1443-1449.

Eyles, J., Puaux, A. L., Wang, X., Toh, B., Prakash, C., Hong, M., Tan, T. G., Zheng, L., Ong, L. C., Jin, Y., *et al.* (2010). Tumor cells disseminate early, but immunosurveillance limits metastatic outgrowth, in a mouse model of melanoma. J Clin Invest *120*, 2030-2039.

Ezernitchi, A. V., Vaknin, I., Cohen-Daniel, L., Levy, O., Manaster, E., Halabi, A., Pikarsky, E., Shapira, L., and Baniyash, M. (2006). TCR zeta down-regulation under chronic inflammation is mediated by myeloid suppressor cells differentially distributed between various lymphatic organs. J Immunol *177*, 4763-4772.

Fichtner-Feigl, S., Terabe, M., Kitani, A., Young, C. A., Fuss, I., Geissler, E. K., Schlitt, H. J., Berzofsky, J. A., and Strober, W. (2008). Restoration of tumor immunosurveillance via targeting of interleukin-13 receptor-alpha 2. Cancer Res *68*, 3467-3475.

Fleming, T. J., Fleming, M. L., and Malek, T. R. (1993). Selective expression of Ly-6G on myeloid lineage cells in mouse bone marrow. RB6-8C5 mAb to granulocyte-differentiation antigen (Gr-1) detects members of the Ly-6 family. J Immunol *151*, 2399-2408.

Forman, H. J., and Torres, M. (2001). Redox signaling in macrophages. Mol Aspects Med *22*, 189-216.

Fujita, M., Kohanbash, G., Fellows-Mayle, W., Hamilton, R. L., Komohara, Y., Decker, S. A., Ohlfest, J. R., and Okada, H. (2011). COX-2 blockade suppresses gliomagenesis by inhibiting myeloid-derived suppressor cells. Cancer Res *71*, 2664-2674.

Gabitass, R. F., Annels, N. E., Stocken, D. D., Pandha, H. A., and Middleton, G. W. (2011). Elevated myeloid-derived suppressor cells in pancreatic, esophageal and gastric cancer are an independent prognostic factor and are associated with significant elevation of the Th2 cytokine interleukin-13. Cancer Immunol Immunother.

Gabrilovich, D. I., and Nagaraj, S. (2009). Myeloid-derived suppressor cells as regulators of the immune system. Nat Rev Immunol *9*, 162-174.

Gabrilovich, D. I., Velders, M. P., Sotomayor, E. M., and Kast, W. M. (2001). Mechanism of immune dysfunction in cancer mediated by immature Gr-1+ myeloid cells. J Immunol *166*, 5398-5406.

Gallina, G., Dolcetti, L., Serafini, P., De Santo, C., Marigo, I., Colombo, M. P., Basso, G., Brombacher, F., Borrello, I., Zanovello, P., *et al.* (2006). Tumors induce a subset of inflammatory monocytes with immunosuppressive activity on CD8+ T cells. J Clin Invest *116*, 2777-2790.

Goni, O., Alcaide, P., and Fresno, M. (2002). Immunosuppression during acute Trypanosoma cruzi infection: involvement of Ly6G (Gr1(+))CD11b(+)immature myeloid suppressor cells. Int Immunol *14*, 1125-1134.

Gout, P. W., Buckley, A. R., Simms, C. R., and Bruchovsky, N. (2001). Sulfasalazine, a potent suppressor of lymphoma growth by inhibition of the x(c)- cystine transporter: a new action for an old drug. Leukemia *15*, 1633-1640.

Greifenberg, V., Ribechini, E., Rossner, S., and Lutz, M. B. (2009). Myeloid-derived suppressor cell activation by combined LPS and IFN-gamma treatment impairs DC development. Eur J Immunol *39*, 2865-2876.

Greten, T. F., Manns, M. P., and Korangy, F. (2011). Myeloid derived suppressor cells in human diseases. Int Immunopharmacol *11*, 802-806.

Haile, L. A., von Wasielewski, R., Gamrekelashvili, J., Kruger, C., Bachmann, O., Westendorf, A. M., Buer, J., Liblau, R., Manns, M. P., Korangy, F., and Greten, T. F. (2008). Myeloid-derived suppressor cells in inflammatory bowel disease: a new immunoregulatory pathway. Gastroenterology *135*, 871-881, 881 e871-875.

Hanson, E. M., Clements, V. K., Sinha, P., Ilkovitch, D., and Ostrand-Rosenberg, S. (2009). Myeloid-derived suppressor cells down-regulate L-selectin expression on CD4+ and CD8+ T cells. J Immunol *183*, 937-944.

Harari, O., and Liao, J. K. (2004). Inhibition of MHC II gene transcription by nitric oxide and antioxidants. Curr Pharm Des *10*, 893-898.

Hengesbach, L. M., and Hoag, K. A. (2004). Physiological concentrations of retinoic acid favor myeloid dendritic cell development over granulocyte development in cultures of bone marrow cells from mice. J Nutr *134*, 2653-2659.

Hershkovitz, L., Schachter, J., Treves, A. J., and Besser, M. J. (2010). Focus on adoptive T cell transfer trials in melanoma. Clin Dev Immunol *2010*, 260267.

Hildeman, D. A., Mitchell, T., Aronow, B., Wojciechowski, S., Kappler, J., and Marrack, P. (2003). Control of Bcl-2 expression by reactive oxygen species. Proc Natl Acad Sci U S A *100*, 15035-15040.

Hiratsuka, S., Watanabe, A., Aburatani, H., and Maru, Y. (2006). Tumour-mediated upregulation of chemoattractants and recruitment of myeloid cells predetermines lung metastasis. Nat Cell Biol *8*, 1369-1375.

Hock, B. D., Mackenzie, K. A., Cross, N. B., Taylor, K. G., Currie, M. J., Robinson, B. A., Simcock, J. W., and McKenzie, J. L. (2011). Renal transplant recipients have elevated frequencies of circulating myeloid-derived suppressor cells. Nephrol Dial Transplant.

Hong, M., Puaux, A. L., Huang, C., Loumagne, L., Tow, C., Mackay, C., Kato, M., Prévost-Blondel, A., Avril, M. F., Nardin, A., and Abastado, J. P. (2011). Chemotherapy induces intratumoral expression of chemokines in cutaneous melanoma, favoring T-cell infiltration and tumor control. Cancer Res *71*, 6997-7009.

Huang, B., Pan, P. Y., Li, Q., Sato, A. I., Levy, D. E., Bromberg, J., Divino, C. M., and Chen, S. H. (2006). Gr-1+CD115+ immature myeloid suppressor cells mediate the development of tumor-induced T regulatory cells and T-cell anergy in tumor-bearing host. Cancer Res *66*, 1123-1131.

Ishii, I., Akahoshi, N., Yu, X. N., Kobayashi, Y., Namekata, K., Komaki, G., and Kimura, H. (2004). Murine cystathionine gamma-lyase: complete cDNA and genomic sequences, promoter activity, tissue distribution and developmental expression. Biochem J *381*, 113-123.

Kaplan, R. N., Rafii, S., and Lyden, D. (2006). Preparing the "soil": the premetastatic niche. Cancer Res *66*, 11089-11093.

Kaplan, R. N., Riba, R. D., Zacharoulis, S., Bramley, A. H., Vincent, L., Costa, C., MacDonald, D. D., Jin, D. K., Shido, K., Kerns, S. A., *et al.* (2005). VEGFR1-positive haematopoietic bone marrow progenitors initiate the pre-metastatic niche. Nature *438*, 820-827.

Kato, M., Takahashi, M., Akhand, A. A., Liu, W., Dai, Y., Shimizu, S., Iwamoto, T., Suzuki, H., and Nakashima, I. (1998). Transgenic mouse model for skin malignant melanoma. Oncogene *17*, 1885-1888.

Kato, M., Takeda, K., Kawamoto, Y., Tsuzuki, T., Hossain, K., Tamakoshi, A., Kunisada, T., Kambayashi, Y., Ogino, K., Suzuki, H., *et al.* (2004). c-Kit-targeting immunotherapy for hereditary melanoma in a mouse model. Cancer Res *64*, 801-806.

Kawakami, Y. (2000). New cancer therapy by immunomanipulation: development of immunotherapy for human melanoma as a model system. Cornea *19*, S2-6.

Kerr, E. C., Raveney, B. J., Copland, D. A., Dick, A. D., and Nicholson, L. B. (2008). Analysis of retinal cellular infiltrate in experimental autoimmune uveoretinitis reveals multiple regulatory cell populations. J Autoimmun *31*, 354-361.

Kimpfler, S., Sevko, A., Ring, S., Falk, C., Osen, W., Frank, K., Kato, M., Mahnke, K., Schadendorf, D., and Umansky, V. (2009). Skin melanoma development in ret transgenic mice despite the depletion of CD25+Foxp3+ regulatory T cells in lymphoid organs. J Immunol *183*, 6330-6337.

Ko, J. S., Zea, A. H., Rini, B. I., Ireland, J. L., Elson, P., Cohen, P., Golshayan, A., Rayman, P. A., Wood, L., Garcia, J., *et al.* (2009). Sunitinib mediates reversal of myeloid-derived suppressor cell accumulation in renal cell carcinoma patients. Clin Cancer Res *15*, 2148-2157.

Kodumudi, K. N., Woan, K., Gilvary, D. L., Sahakian, E., Wei, S., and Djeu, J. Y. (2010). A novel chemoimmunomodulating property of docetaxel: suppression of myeloid-derived suppressor cells in tumor bearers. Clin Cancer Res *16*, 4583-4594.

Kusmartsev, S., Cheng, F., Yu, B., Nefedova, Y., Sotomayor, E., Lush, R., and Gabrilovich, D. (2003). All-trans-retinoic acid eliminates immature myeloid cells from tumor-bearing mice and improves the effect of vaccination. Cancer Res *63*, 4441-4449.

Kusmartsev, S., and Gabrilovich, D. I. (2006). Role of immature myeloid cells in mechanisms of immune evasion in cancer. Cancer Immunol Immunother *55*, 237-245.

Kusmartsev, S., Nagaraj, S., and Gabrilovich, D. I. (2005). Tumor-associated CD8+ T cell tolerance induced by bone marrow-derived immature myeloid cells. J Immunol *175*, 4583-4592.

Kusmartsev, S., Nefedova, Y., Yoder, D., and Gabrilovich, D. I. (2004). Antigen-specific inhibition of CD8+ T cell response by immature myeloid cells in cancer is mediated by reactive oxygen species. J Immunol *172*, 989-999.

Kusmartsev, S., Su, Z., Heiser, A., Dannull, J., Eruslanov, E., Kubler, H., Yancey, D., Dahm, P., and Vieweg, J. (2008). Reversal of myeloid cell-mediated immunosuppression in patients with metastatic renal cell carcinoma. Clin Cancer Res *14*, 8270-8278.

Kuwata, T., Wang, I. M., Tamura, T., Ponnamperuma, R. M., Levine, R., Holmes, K. L., Morse, H. C., De Luca, L. M., and Ozato, K. (2000). Vitamin A deficiency in mice causes a systemic expansion of myeloid cells. Blood *95*, 3349-3356.

Lathers, D. M., Clark, J. I., Achille, N. J., and Young, M. R. (2004). Phase 1B study to improve immune responses in head and neck cancer patients using escalating doses of 25-hydroxyvitamin D3. Cancer Immunol Immunother *53*, 422-430.

Lejeune, P., Lagadec, P., Onier, N., Pinard, D., Ohshima, H., and Jeannin, J. F. (1994). Nitric oxide involvement in tumor-induced immunosuppression. J Immunol *152*, 5077-5083.

Lengagne, R., Graff-Dubois, S., Garcette, M., Renia, L., Kato, M., Guillet, J. G., Engelhard, V. H., Avril, M. F., Abastado, J. P., and Prevost-Blondel, A. (2008). Distinct role for CD8 T cells toward cutaneous tumors and visceral metastases. J Immunol *180*, 130-137.

Lengagne, R., Pommier, A., Caron, J., Douguet, L., Garcette, M., Kato, M., Avril, M. F., Abastado, J. P., Bercovici, N., Lucas, B., and Prevost-Blondel, A. (2011). T cells contribute to tumor progression by favoring pro-tumoral properties of intra-tumoral myeloid cells in a mouse model for spontaneous melanoma. PLoS One *6*, e20235.

Li, H., Han, Y., Guo, Q., Zhang, M., and Cao, X. (2009). Cancer-expanded myeloid-derived suppressor cells induce anergy of NK cells through membrane-bound TGF-beta 1. J Immunol *182*, 240-249.

Linette, G. P., Zhang, D., Hodi, F. S., Jonasch, E. P., Longerich, S., Stowell, C. P., Webb, I. J., Daley, H., Soiffer, R. J., Cheung, A. M., *et al.* (2005). Immunization using autologous dendritic cells pulsed with the melanoma-associated antigen gp100-derived G280-9V peptide elicits CD8+ immunity. Clin Cancer Res *11*, 7692-7699.

Liu, C., Yu, S., Kappes, J., Wang, J., Grizzle, W. E., Zinn, K. R., and Zhang, H. G. (2007). Expansion of spleen myeloid suppressor cells represses NK cell cytotoxicity in tumor-bearing host. Blood *109*, 4336-4342.

Makarenkova, V. P., Bansal, V., Matta, B. M., Perez, L. A., and Ochoa, J. B. (2006). CD11b+/Gr-1+ myeloid suppressor cells cause T cell dysfunction after traumatic stress. J Immunol *176*, 2085-2094.

Mansoor, M. A., Svardal, A. M., and Ueland, P. M. (1992). Determination of the in vivo redox status of cysteine, cysteinylglycine, homocysteine, and glutathione in human plasma. Anal Biochem *200*, 218-229.

Markiewski, M. M., DeAngelis, R. A., Benencia, F., Ricklin-Lichtsteiner, S. K., Koutoulaki, A., Gerard, C., Coukos, G., and Lambris, J. D. (2008). Modulation of the antitumor immune response by complement. Nat Immunol *9*, 1225-1235.

Mazzoni, A., Bronte, V., Visintin, A., Spitzer, J. H., Apolloni, E., Serafini, P., Zanovello, P., and Segal, D. M. (2002). Myeloid suppressor lines inhibit T cell responses by an NO-dependent mechanism. J Immunol *168*, 689-695.

Medot-Pirenne, M., Heilman, M. J., Saxena, M., McDermott, P. E., and Mills, C. D. (1999). Augmentation of an antitumor CTL response In vivo by inhibition of suppressor macrophage nitric oxide. J Immunol *163*, 5877-5882.

Melani, C., Sangaletti, S., Barazzetta, F. M., Werb, Z., and Colombo, M. P. (2007). Amino-biphosphonate-mediated MMP-9 inhibition breaks the tumor-bone marrow axis responsible for myeloid-derived suppressor cell expansion and macrophage infiltration in tumor stroma. Cancer Res *67*, 11438-11446.

Mirza, N., Fishman, M., Fricke, I., Dunn, M., Neuger, A. M., Frost, T. J., Lush, R. M., Antonia, S., and Gabrilovich, D. I. (2006). All-trans-retinoic acid improves differentiation of myeloid cells and immune response in cancer patients. Cancer Res *66*, 9299-9307.

Moline-Velazquez, V., Cuervo, H., Vila-Del Sol, V., Ortega, M. C., Clemente, D., and de Castro, F. (2011). Myeloid-derived suppressor cells limit the inflammation by promoting T lymphocyte apoptosis in the spinal cord of a murine model of multiple sclerosis. Brain Pathol.

Morris, S. M., Jr. (2002). Regulation of enzymes of the urea cycle and arginine metabolism. Annu Rev Nutr *22*, 87-105.

Movahedi, K., Guilliams, M., Van den Bossche, J., Van den Bergh, R., Gysemans, C., Beschin, A., De Baetselier, P., and Van Ginderachter, J. A. (2008). Identification of discrete tumor-induced myeloid-derived suppressor cell subpopulations with distinct T cell-suppressive activity. Blood *111*, 4233-4244.

Movahedi, K., Laoui, D., Gysemans, C., Baeten, M., Stange, G., Van den Bossche, J., Mack, M., Pipeleers, D., In't Veld, P., De Baetselier, P., and Van Ginderachter, J. A. (2010). Different tumor microenvironments contain functionally distinct subsets of macrophages derived from Ly6C(high) monocytes. Cancer Res *70*, 5728-5739.

Nagaraj, S., Gupta, K., Pisarev, V., Kinarsky, L., Sherman, S., Kang, L., Herber, D. L., Schneck, J., and Gabrilovich, D. I. (2007). Altered recognition of antigen is a mechanism of CD8+ T cell tolerance in cancer. Nat Med *13*, 828-835.

Nakamura, Y., Yasuoka, H., Tsujimoto, M., Yoshidome, K., Nakahara, M., Nakao, K., Nakamura, M., and Kakudo, K. (2006). Nitric oxide in breast cancer: induction of vascular endothelial growth factor-C and correlation with metastasis and poor prognosis. Clin Cancer Res *12*, 1201-1207.

Nausch, N., Galani, I. E., Schlecker, E., and Cerwenka, A. (2008). Mononuclear myeloid-derived "suppressor" cells express RAE-1 and activate natural killer cells. Blood *112*, 4080-4089.

Nefedova, Y., Nagaraj, S., Rosenbauer, A., Muro-Cacho, C., Sebti, S. M., and Gabrilovich, D. I. (2005). Regulation of dendritic cell differentiation and antitumor immune response in cancer by pharmacologic-selective inhibition of the janus-activated kinase 2/signal transducers and activators of transcription 3 pathway. Cancer Res *65*, 9525-9535.

Oble, D. A., Loewe, R., Yu, P., and Mihm, M. C., Jr. (2009). Focus on TILs: prognostic significance of tumor infiltrating lymphocytes in human melanoma. Cancer Immun *9*, 3.

Ostrand-Rosenberg, S., and Sinha, P. (2009). Myeloid-derived suppressor cells: linking inflammation and cancer. J Immunol *182*, 4499-4506.

Otsuji, M., Kimura, Y., Aoe, T., Okamoto, Y., and Saito, T. (1996). Oxidative stress by tumor-derived macrophages suppresses the expression of CD3 zeta chain of T-cell receptor complex and antigen-specific T-cell responses. Proc Natl Acad Sci U S A *93*, 13119-13124.

Ozao-Choy, J., Ma, G., Kao, J., Wang, G. X., Meseck, M., Sung, M., Schwartz, M., Divino, C. M., Pan, P. Y., and Chen, S. H. (2009). The novel role of tyrosine kinase inhibitor in the reversal of immune suppression and modulation of tumor microenvironment for immune-based cancer therapies. Cancer Res *69*, 2514-2522.

Pan, P. Y., Ma, G., Weber, K. J., Ozao-Choy, J., Wang, G., Yin, B., Divino, C. M., and Chen, S. H. (2010). Immune stimulatory receptor CD40 is required for T-cell suppression and T regulatory cell activation mediated by myeloid-derived suppressor cells in cancer. Cancer Res *70*, 99-108.

Pan, P. Y., Wang, G. X., Yin, B., Ozao, J., Ku, T., Divino, C. M., and Chen, S. H. (2008). Reversion of immune tolerance in advanced malignancy: modulation of myeloid-derived suppressor cell development by blockade of stem-cell factor function. Blood *111*, 219-228.

Pekarek, L. A., Starr, B. A., Toledano, A. Y., and Schreiber, H. (1995). Inhibition of tumor growth by elimination of granulocytes. J Exp Med *181*, 435-440.

Peranzoni, E., Zilio, S., Marigo, I., Dolcetti, L., Zanovello, P., Mandruzzato, S., and Bronte, V. (2010). Myeloid-derived suppressor cell heterogeneity and subset definition. Curr Opin Immunol *22*, 238-244.

Pitcher, L. A., and van Oers, N. S. (2003). T-cell receptor signal transmission: who gives an ITAM? Trends Immunol *24*, 554-560.

Priceman, S. J., Sung, J. L., Shaposhnik, Z., Burton, J. B., Torres-Collado, A. X., Moughon, D. L., Johnson, M., Lusis, A. J., Cohen, D. A., Iruela-Arispe, M. L., and Wu, L. (2010).

Targeting distinct tumor-infiltrating myeloid cells by inhibiting CSF-1 receptor: combating tumor evasion of antiangiogenic therapy. Blood *115*, 1461-1471.

Raychaudhuri, B., Rayman, P., Ireland, J., Ko, J., Rini, B., Borden, E. C., Garcia, J., Vogelbaum, M. A., and Finke, J. (2011). Myeloid-derived suppressor cell accumulation and function in patients with newly diagnosed glioblastoma. Neuro Oncol *13*, 591-599.

Ribechini, E., Greifenberg, V., Sandwick, S., and Lutz, M. B. (2010). Subsets, expansion and activation of myeloid-derived suppressor cells. Med Microbiol Immunol *199*, 273-281.

Rivoltini, L., Carrabba, M., Huber, V., Castelli, C., Novellino, L., Dalerba, P., Mortarini, R., Arancia, G., Anichini, A., Fais, S., and Parmiani, G. (2002). Immunity to cancer: attack and escape in T lymphocyte-tumor cell interaction. Immunol Rev *188*, 97-113.

Rodriguez, P. C., Hernandez, C. P., Quiceno, D., Dubinett, S. M., Zabaleta, J., Ochoa, J. B., Gilbert, J., and Ochoa, A. C. (2005). Arginase I in myeloid suppressor cells is induced by COX-2 in lung carcinoma. J Exp Med *202*, 931-939.

Rodriguez, P. C., and Ochoa, A. C. (2008). Arginine regulation by myeloid derived suppressor cells and tolerance in cancer: mechanisms and therapeutic perspectives. Immunol Rev *222*, 180-191.

Rodriguez, P. C., Quiceno, D. G., and Ochoa, A. C. (2007). L-arginine availability regulates T-lymphocyte cell-cycle progression. Blood *109*, 1568-1573.

Rodriguez, P. C., Quiceno, D. G., Zabaleta, J., Ortiz, B., Zea, A. H., Piazuelo, M. B., Delgado, A., Correa, P., Brayer, J., Sotomayor, E. M., *et al.* (2004). Arginase I production in the tumor microenvironment by mature myeloid cells inhibits T-cell receptor expression and antigen-specific T-cell responses. Cancer Res *64*, 5839-5849.

Rodriguez, P. C., Zea, A. H., Culotta, K. S., Zabaleta, J., Ochoa, J. B., and Ochoa, A. C. (2002). Regulation of T cell receptor CD3zeta chain expression by L-arginine. J Biol Chem *277*, 21123-21129.

Rodriguez, P. C., Zea, A. H., DeSalvo, J., Culotta, K. S., Zabaleta, J., Quiceno, D. G., Ochoa, J. B., and Ochoa, A. C. (2003a). L-arginine consumption by macrophages modulates the expression of CD3 zeta chain in T lymphocytes. J Immunol *171*, 1232-1239.

Rodriguez, P. C., Zea, A. H., and Ochoa, A. C. (2003b). Mechanisms of tumor evasion from the immune response. Cancer Chemother Biol Response Modif *21*, 351-364.

Salcedo, M., Bercovici, N., Taylor, R., Vereecken, P., Massicard, S., Duriau, D., Vernel-Pauillac, F., Boyer, A., Baron-Bodo, V., Mallard, E., *et al.* (2006). Vaccination of melanoma patients using dendritic cells loaded with an allogeneic tumor cell lysate. Cancer Immunol Immunother *55*, 819-829.

Sato, H., Watanabe, H., Ishii, T., and Bannai, S. (1987). Neutral amino acid transport in mouse peritoneal macrophages. J Biol Chem *262*, 13015-13019.

Sato, K., Ozaki, K., Oh, I., Meguro, A., Hatanaka, K., Nagai, T., Muroi, K., and Ozawa, K. (2007). Nitric oxide plays a critical role in suppression of T-cell proliferation by mesenchymal stem cells. Blood *109*, 228-234.

Schmielau, J., and Finn, O. J. (2001). Activated granulocytes and granulocyte-derived hydrogen peroxide are the underlying mechanism of suppression of t-cell function in advanced cancer patients. Cancer Res *61*, 4756-4760.

Serafini, P., Carbley, R., Noonan, K. A., Tan, G., Bronte, V., and Borrello, I. (2004). High-dose granulocyte-macrophage colony-stimulating factor-producing vaccines impair the immune response through the recruitment of myeloid suppressor cells. Cancer Res *64*, 6337-6343.

Serafini, P., Meckel, K., Kelso, M., Noonan, K., Califano, J., Koch, W., Dolcetti, L., Bronte, V., and Borrello, I. (2006). Phosphodiesterase-5 inhibition augments endogenous antitumor immunity by reducing myeloid-derived suppressor cell function. J Exp Med *203*, 2691-2702.

Serafini, P., Mgebroff, S., Noonan, K., and Borrello, I. (2008). Myeloid-derived suppressor cells promote cross-tolerance in B-cell lymphoma by expanding regulatory T cells. Cancer Res *68*, 5439-5449.

Shojaei, F., Wu, X., Qu, X., Kowanetz, M., Yu, L., Tan, M., Meng, Y. G., and Ferrara, N. (2009). G-CSF-initiated myeloid cell mobilization and angiogenesis mediate tumor refractoriness to anti-VEGF therapy in mouse models. Proc Natl Acad Sci U S A *106*, 6742-6747.

Shojaei, F., Wu, X., Zhong, C., Yu, L., Liang, X. H., Yao, J., Blanchard, D., Bais, C., Peale, F. V., van Bruggen, N., *et al.* (2007). Bv8 regulates myeloid-cell-dependent tumour angiogenesis. Nature *450*, 825-831.

Sinha, P., Clements, V. K., Bunt, S. K., Albelda, S. M., and Ostrand-Rosenberg, S. (2007). Cross-talk between myeloid-derived suppressor cells and macrophages subverts tumor immunity toward a type 2 response. J Immunol *179*, 977-983.

Sinha, P., Clements, V. K., and Ostrand-Rosenberg, S. (2005). Reduction of myeloid-derived suppressor cells and induction of M1 macrophages facilitate the rejection of established metastatic disease. J Immunol *174*, 636-645.

Sinha, P., Okoro, C., Foell, D., Freeze, H. H., Ostrand-Rosenberg, S., and Srikrishna, G. (2008). Proinflammatory S100 proteins regulate the accumulation of myeloid-derived suppressor cells. J Immunol *181*, 4666-4675.

Smyth, M. J. (1991). Glutathione modulates activation-dependent proliferation of human peripheral blood lymphocyte populations without regulating their activated function. J Immunol *146*, 1921-1927.

Sosroseno, W., Bird, P. S., and Seymour, G. J. (2009). Effect of exogenous nitric oxide on murine splenic immune response induced by Aggregatibacter actinomycetemcomitans lipopolysaccharide. Anaerobe *15*, 95-98.

Squadrito, G. L., and Pryor, W. A. (1995). The formation of peroxynitrite in vivo from nitric oxide and superoxide. Chem Biol Interact *96*, 203-206.

Srivastava, M. K., Sinha, P., Clements, V. K., Rodriguez, P., and Ostrand-Rosenberg, S. (2010). Myeloid-derived suppressor cells inhibit T-cell activation by depleting cystine and cysteine. Cancer Res *70*, 68-77.

Sunderkotter, C., Nikolic, T., Dillon, M. J., Van Rooijen, N., Stehling, M., Drevets, D. A., and Leenen, P. J. (2004). Subpopulations of mouse blood monocytes differ in maturation stage and inflammatory response. J Immunol *172*, 4410-4417.

Suzuki, E., Kapoor, V., Jassar, A. S., Kaiser, L. R., and Albelda, S. M. (2005). Gemcitabine selectively eliminates splenic Gr-1+/CD11b+ myeloid suppressor cells in tumor-bearing animals and enhances antitumor immune activity. Clin Cancer Res *11*, 6713-6721.

Talmadge, J. E., Hood, K. C., Zobel, L. C., Shafer, L. R., Coles, M., and Toth, B. (2007). Chemoprevention by cyclooxygenase-2 inhibition reduces immature myeloid suppressor cell expansion. Int Immunopharmacol *7*, 140-151.

Terabe, M., Matsui, S., Park, J. M., Mamura, M., Noben-Trauth, N., Donaldson, D. D., Chen, W., Wahl, S. M., Ledbetter, S., Pratt, B., *et al.* (2003). Transforming growth factor-beta production and myeloid cells are an effector mechanism through which CD1d-restricted T cells block cytotoxic T lymphocyte-mediated tumor immunosurveillance: abrogation prevents tumor recurrence. J Exp Med *198*, 1741-1752.

Terabe, M., Swann, J., Ambrosino, E., Sinha, P., Takaku, S., Hayakawa, Y., Godfrey, D. I., Ostrand-Rosenberg, S., Smyth, M. J., and Berzofsky, J. A. (2005). A nonclassical non-Valpha14Jalpha18 CD1d-restricted (type II) NKT cell is sufficient for down-regulation of tumor immunosurveillance. J Exp Med *202*, 1627-1633.

Testa, U., Masciulli, R., Tritarelli, E., Pustorino, R., Mariani, G., Martucci, R., Barberi, T., Camagna, A., Valtieri, M., and Peschle, C. (1993). Transforming growth factor-beta potentiates vitamin D3-induced terminal monocytic differentiation of human leukemic cell lines. J Immunol *150*, 2418-2430.

Toh, B., Wang, X., Keeble, J., Sim, W. J., Khoo, K., Wong, W. C., Kato, M., Prevost-Blondel, A., Thiery, J. P., and Abastado, J. P. (2011). Mesenchymal transition and dissemination of cancer cells is driven by myeloid-derived suppressor cells infiltrating the primary tumor. PLoS Biol *9*, e1001162.

Umansky, V., Abschuetz, O., Osen, W., Ramacher, M., Zhao, F., Kato, M., and Schadendorf, D. (2008). Melanoma-specific memory T cells are functionally active in Ret transgenic mice without macroscopic tumors. Cancer Res *68*, 9451-9458.

van Deventer, H. W., Burgents, J. E., Wu, Q. P., Woodford, R. M., Brickey, W. J., Allen, I. C., McElvania-Tekippe, E., Serody, J. S., and Ting, J. P. (2010). The inflammasome component NLRP3 impairs antitumor vaccine by enhancing the accumulation of tumor-associated myeloid-derived suppressor cells. Cancer Res *70*, 10161-10169.

Vincent, J., Mignot, G., Chalmin, F., Ladoire, S., Bruchard, M., Chevriaux, A., Martin, F., Apetoh, L., Rebe, C., and Ghiringhelli, F. (2010). 5-Fluorouracil selectively kills tumor-associated myeloid-derived suppressor cells resulting in enhanced T cell-dependent antitumor immunity. Cancer Res *70*, 3052-3061.

von Felbert, V., Cordoba, F., Weissenberger, J., Vallan, C., Kato, M., Nakashima, I., Braathen, L. R., and Weis, J. (2005). Interleukin-6 gene ablation in a transgenic mouse model of malignant skin melanoma. Am J Pathol *166*, 831-841.

Wu, G., and Morris, S. M., Jr. (1998). Arginine metabolism: nitric oxide and beyond. Biochem J *336 (Pt 1)*, 1-17.

Xia, S., Sha, H., Yang, L., Ji, Y., Ostrand-Rosenberg, S., and Qi, L. (2011). Gr-1+ CD11b+ myeloid-derived suppressor cells suppress inflammation and promote insulin sensitivity in obesity. J Biol Chem.

Xia, Y., Roman, L. J., Masters, B. S., and Zweier, J. L. (1998). Inducible nitric-oxide synthase generates superoxide from the reductase domain. J Biol Chem *273*, 22635-22639.

Yan, H. H., Pickup, M., Pang, Y., Gorska, A. E., Li, Z., Chytil, A., Geng, Y., Gray, J. W., Moses, H. L., and Yang, L. (2010). Gr-1+CD11b+ myeloid cells tip the balance of immune protection to tumor promotion in the premetastatic lung. Cancer Res *70*, 6139-6149.

Yang, L., DeBusk, L. M., Fukuda, K., Fingleton, B., Green-Jarvis, B., Shyr, Y., Matrisian, L. M., Carbone, D. P., and Lin, P. C. (2004). Expansion of myeloid immune suppressor Gr+CD11b+ cells in tumor-bearing host directly promotes tumor angiogenesis. Cancer Cell *6*, 409-421.

Yang, L., Huang, J., Ren, X., Gorska, A. E., Chytil, A., Aakre, M., Carbone, D. P., Matrisian, L. M., Richmond, A., Lin, P. C., and Moses, H. L. (2008). Abrogation of TGF beta signaling in mammary carcinomas recruits Gr-1+CD11b+ myeloid cells that promote metastasis. Cancer Cell *13*, 23-35.

Yang, R., Cai, Z., Zhang, Y., Yutzy, W. H. t., Roby, K. F., and Roden, R. B. (2006). CD80 in immune suppression by mouse ovarian carcinoma-associated Gr-1+CD11b+ myeloid cells. Cancer Res *66*, 6807-6815.

Youn, J. I., Nagaraj, S., Collazo, M., and Gabrilovich, D. I. (2008). Subsets of myeloid-derived suppressor cells in tumor-bearing mice. J Immunol *181*, 5791-5802.

Zea, A. H., Rodriguez, P. C., Atkins, M. B., Hernandez, C., Signoretti, S., Zabaleta, J., McDermott, D., Quiceno, D., Youmans, A., O'Neill, A., *et al.* (2005). Arginase-producing myeloid suppressor cells in renal cell carcinoma patients: a mechanism of tumor evasion. Cancer Res *65*, 3044-3048.

Zhang, Y., Liu, Q., Zhang, M., Yu, Y., Liu, X., and Cao, X. (2009). Fas signal promotes lung cancer growth by recruiting myeloid-derived suppressor cells via cancer cell-derived PGE2. J Immunol *182*, 3801-3808.

Zhao, F., Falk, C., Osen, W., Kato, M., Schadendorf, D., and Umansky, V. (2009). Activation of p38 mitogen-activated protein kinase drives dendritic cells to become tolerogenic in ret transgenic mice spontaneously developing melanoma. Clin Cancer Res *15*, 4382-4390.

Zhu, B., Bando, Y., Xiao, S., Yang, K., Anderson, A. C., Kuchroo, V. K., and Khoury, S. J. (2007). CD11b+Ly-6C(hi) suppressive monocytes in experimental autoimmune encephalomyelitis. J Immunol *179*, 5228-5237.

Zippelius, A., Batard, P., Rubio-Godoy, V., Bioley, G., Lienard, D., Lejeune, F., Rimoldi, D., Guillaume, P., Meidenbauer, N., Mackensen, A., *et al.* (2004). Effector function of human tumor-specific CD8 T cells in melanoma lesions: a state of local functional tolerance. Cancer Res *64*, 2865-2873.

5

The Role of Hypoxia in Re-Educating Macrophages in the Tumour Environment

Reuben J. Harwood[1,2], Claire E. Lewis[1] and Subhra K. Biswas[2]
[1]*Academic Unit of Inflammation and Tumour Targeting, Faculty of Medicine, University of Sheffield, Sheffield,*
[2]*Singapore Immunology Network, BMSI, A*STAR,*
[1]*UK*
[2]*Singapore*

1. Introduction

Monocytes and macrophages are myeloid cells which originate in the bone marrow and are essential in the primary defence against infection by bacteria, viruses and other pathogens. These cells circulate as monocytes in the bloodstream before undergoing extravasation and migration into adjacent tissues, where they differentiate into resident macrophages. Considerable monocyte extravasation occurs at the initial stages of inflammation, wound healing, tumour onset and various other diseases in response to chemotactic signals. In many instances these inflamed and/or diseased tissues have been shown to include areas of extremely low oxygen tension, termed hypoxia, by the measurement of oxygen concentrations using microelectrodes, use of hypoxic cell markers and/or expression of specific hypoxia-upregulated proteins. Such hypoxic areas are evident in the majority of malignant human cancers, including those of the breast, brain, cervix, head/neck, and soft tissue sarcomas (Raleigh et al., 2001; Vaupel et al., 1989), and are caused by an inability of the supporting vasculature to keep up with the oxygen demands of the rapidly increasing tumour mass (Shannon et al., 2003; Vaupel et al., 2005).

As with inflammation, extensive monocyte extravasation is also an early event in cancer development. Infiltrated monocytes differentiate into tumour-associated macrophages (TAMs), a process which is driven by tumour-secreted chemoattractants (Murdoch et al., 2004). Moreover, TAMs accumulate in high numbers within hypoxic areas, which drives a change in their gene expression through the modulation of such transcription factors as hypoxia-inducible factors (HIFs) 1 and 2 (Burke et al., 2003; Talks et al., 2000), activating transcription factor-4 (ATF-4), and early growth response-1 (egr-1) (Elbarghati et al., 2008). Subsequently, a wide panel of protumour genes are upregulated by hypoxic macrophages which could support tumour growth, survival and metastasis (Fang et al., 2009). This is thought to explain the correlation between high numbers of TAMs and poor patient prognosis in many types of human tumours (Fujimoto et al., 2000; Hamada et al., 2002; Hanada et al., 2000; Heidl et al., 1987; Leek et al., 1996; Lissbrant et al., 2000; Salvesen and Akslen, 1999).

2. Hypoxia as an important microenvironmental signal for 'educating' macrophages in tumours

2.1 Monocyte infiltration into tumours

The mechanisms by which immune cells are recruited into tumours have been well studied, revealing crucial roles for several chemokines and cytokines in the extravasation and infiltration of these cells, including monocytes, from the blood vessels and into the tumour. The chemokine-driven migration of leukocytes is followed by regulation of tumour growth, angiogenesis and metastasis, through alterations in the tumour environment (Balkwill, 2003; Strieter et al., 2004; Vicari and Caux, 2002).

Perhaps the most important monocyte chemoattractants upregulated by tumours are the chemokines, CCL2 and CCL5 (also known as MCP-1 and RANTES, respectively), which are synthesised by several cell types including tumour cells, fibroblasts, endothelial cells and TAMs themselves. Correlation between the expression of CCL2 and the accumulation of TAMs within breast (Ueno et al., 2000), ovarian (Negus et al., 1997), esophageal and squamous cell (Ohta et al., 2002), non-small cell lung cancer (Arenberg et al., 2000), and also glioblastoma (Leung et al., 1997), underscore the importance of this chemokine in monocyte recruitment into tumours. In addition, Bottazzi et al. (1992) demonstrated that when the CCL2 gene was transferred to a murine melanoma and subsequently grown *in vivo*, infiltration of monocytes increased, as evidenced by a doubling of TAM numbers. However, the phenotype of these TAMs may have been anti-tumoural since these CCL2-producing tumours exhibited reduced tumour growth and increased overall survival.

The effects of CCL2 and CCL5 on human monocytes are not just limited to their direct chemotactic capabilities; both ligands are also known to support monocytes in the production of additional chemoattractants and tumour-promoting molecules – for example, analysis of CCL5-induced monocyte gene expression by oligonucleotide array revealed that CCL2, CCL3, CCL4, CXCL8, and CCR1 were consistently induced, suggesting a role for CCL5 in leukocyte recruitment into the tumour. This correlates with the finding that CCL3 and CCL4 are expressed in certain human tumours (Scotton et al., 2001), and that CXCL8 drives adhesion of monocytes to vascular endothelium as part of monocyte recruitment (Gerszten et al., 1999).

The cytokines CSF-1 (colony-stimulating factor-1) and VEGF (vascular endothelial growth factor) are also known to be monocyte chemotactic proteins, and are produced by a variety of cell types, including monocytes and macrophages. By crossing CSF-1 knock-out mice with mice which form spontaneous mammary tumours, Lin et al. (2001) demonstrated the importance of this cytokine in the recruitment of monocytes into tumours, since tumours in the daughter mice showed reduced TAM numbers and slower tumour progression. These features could be reversed by the introduction of CSF-1 by targeted gene expression, confirming that this cytokine is important for TAM infiltration and tumour progression.

The growth factor, VEGF, is best characterised as an angiogenic factor which functions as a potent and specific mitogen for endothelial cells. In the majority of tumour types tested, VEGF mRNA expression is upregulated within the tumour (Ferrara and Davis-Smyth, 1997), primarily by tumour cells and TAMs (Lewis et al., 2000), rather than endothelial cells. The inverse is true for mRNA expression of VEGF receptors, VEGF-R1 and -R2 (Brown et al., 1993; Plate et al., 1994; Plate et al., 1992), consistent with the hypothesis that VEGF predominantly acts as a paracrine factor to induce angiogenesis. Further studies suggested the expression of this growth factor by infiltrating lymphocytes (Freeman et al., 1995), and its role as a chemoattractant for monocytes and macrophages through VEGF-R1 was discovered (Barleon et al., 1996; Sawano et al., 2001), verified by the fact that murine macrophages lacking VEGF-R1 (from a model of embryonic angiogenesis) exhibited reduced migration in Boyden chambers in response to VEGF (Hiratsuka et al., 1998). Immunohistochemistry in surgically resected breast tumour samples showed that increased VEGF within tumours was associated with higher numbers of TAMs (Leek et al., 2000). These findings suggest that VEGF is not only important for angiogenesis, but also for the recruitment of monocytes (Figure 1a) (Toi et al., 1994).

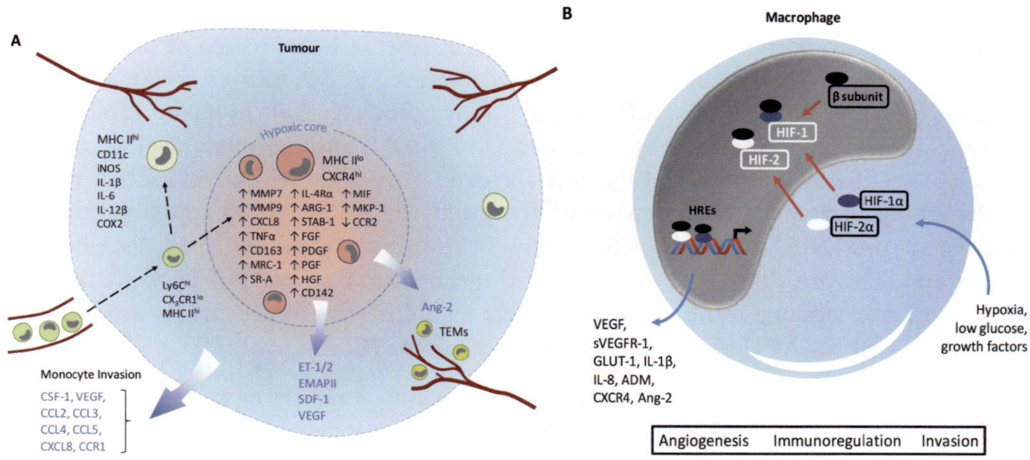

Fig. 1. Tumour hypoxia drives monocyte infiltration, polarization and transcription of hypoxia-regulated genes. a. Tumours and infiltrated macrophages secrete chemoattractants, resulting in the recruitment of monocytes from the blood. Hypoxic conditions commonly found within tumours enhance the polarisation of macrophages toward a protumour phenotype, which leads to the upregulation of a wide array of tumour-supporting genes (such as those shown in the figure) and the downregulation of MHC II. Almost all murine TAMs derive from a population of monocytes defined by Ly6C^{hi}CX$_3$CR1^{lo} expression, which continuously seed tumours. Two types of murine TAMs, MHC II^{hi} and MHC II^{lo}, have been shown to be located in normoxic and hypoxic areas of tumours, displaying M1 and M2 characteristics, respectively. TIE2-expressing macrophages (TEM) are recruited in response to release of Ang2 (as well as upregulation of Tie-2) by the hypoxic core. TEMs associate with blood vessels and promote tumour angiogenesis. Monocyte/macrophage-derived factors in black, tumour-derived factors in blue. b. Hypoxic conditions result in the stabilisation of HIF-1α and -2α in macrophages, which are then able to bind to a constitutively expressed common β subunit, located in the nucleus. The active transcription factors then bind to HREs in a variety of genes (shown at bottom left) which regulate the immunosuppressive and protumoural functions of macrophages.

2.2 Monocyte infiltration into areas of hypoxia

Following their infiltration into tumours, macrophages have been shown to accumulate specifically in hypoxic areas, a phenomenon which is thought to be guided by hypoxia-induced chemoattractants and maintained by the suppression of TAM motility in these areas by hypoxia (reviewed by Murdoch et al. (2004)). As would be expected, these oxygen-deprived regions of tumours have been found to have elevated levels of VEGF, produced by both tumour cells and macrophages (Brown et al., 1995; Lee et al., 1998; Lewis et al., 2000). In addition, VEGF expression in a murine model of Lewis lung carcinoma was shown by immunohistochemistry to correlate with pimonidazole stained areas, a marker for hypoxia (Kim et al., 2001). As mentioned previously, this factor is a chemoattractant for monocytes and macrophages and therefore is likely to play a major role in the accumulation of TAM at these sites (Lewis et al., 2000). However, it is worth noting that there is not always a correlation between hypoxia and VEGF expression in human tumours (Janssen et al., 2002; Raleigh et al., 1998). Matschurat and colleagues (2003) found that another monocyte chemotactic, EMAP II, is expressed at high levels in perinecrotic areas of methylcholanthrene fibrosarcomas and B16 murine melanomas in an inactive form, pro-EMAP II. Additionally, they showed that hypoxic tumour cell supernatants *in vitro* demonstrated an increase in EMAP II at the protein level, which was not supported by an induction at the mRNA level. This suggests that the active protein can be induced under hypoxia without the need for transcription, possibly through cleavage of pre-EMAP II to its active form by proteases released from necrotic cells (Zhang and Schwarz, 2002), providing a rapid mechanism for EMAP II upregulation and subsequent macrophage infiltration. This effect explains why macrophages are found at sites positive for EMAP II expression in uveal melanoma (Clarijs et al., 2003).

Also known to be regulated by hypoxia are endothelins, a family of secretory vasoactive peptides involved in vasoconstriction. They also have co-mitogenic functions, enhancing the effects of other such growth factors as PDGF by initiating intracellular signalling through endothelin receptors, ET-RA and ET-RB. Studies of endothelin regulation under hypoxic conditions demonstrated a co-localisation of hypoxia and endothelin ET-2 expression in murine mammary tumours (Grimshaw et al., 2002a). This is significant since ET-2 is thought to bind to ET-RB on macrophages and act as a chemoattractant, explaining the correlation seen between ET-2 expression and ET-RB-positive macrophages in breast tumours (Grimshaw et al., 2004; Grimshaw et al., 2002b). Furthermore, ET-1 (which acts through endothelin-1 receptor A) was recently shown to enhance the invasion and migration of both tumour cells and macrophages. The contribution of these factors to metastasis was supported by the finding that tumour expression of ET-1 and activity of its receptor are required for the development of lung metastases, through a process which is dependent on macrophage infiltration of the lung (Said et al., 2011).

More recently, Wang et al. (2012) identified stromal-derived factor-1 (SDF-1/CXCL12) as a tumour-derived chemoattractant and survival factor for TAMs. In a murine glioma model they showed that SDF-1^{kd} tumours have a different association of TAMs with hypoxia, implying that the secretion of this factor by tumour cells is critical for the accumulation of TAM in hypoxic areas of murine glioma. This factor is known to bind to its receptor, CXC receptor 4 (CXCR4), which is upregulated through a HIF-1-dependent mechanism in monocytes and macrophages (as well as endothelial cells and tumour cells). Therefore, SDF-1 and its receptor, CXCR4, are very important for the chemotaxis of TAMs to hypoxic tumour sites (Schioppa et al., 2003).

It has been suggested that the accumulation of infiltrating macrophages in tumours, primarily in hypoxic regions, is not just due to chemoattraction, but also to their retention in these areas. Downregulation of chemokine release by tumour cells, and of chemokine receptors by TAMs in hypoxia, effectively dampens TAM motility, thus causing large numbers of macrophages to be trapped in these sites. For example, the expression of CCR2 (the receptor for CCL2/MCP-1) and chemotactic responses to CCL2 in vitro were markedly higher for TAMs isolated from ovarian carcinomas than monocyte-derived macrophages in culture (Negus et al., 1998; Sica et al., 2000).

When cultured with human tumour ascites, the chemotactic response of fresh monocytes to CCL2 was greatly diminished, accompanied by a reduction in CCR2 mRNA levels. Furthermore, inhibition of TNF-α restored CCR2 mRNA expression in monocytes cultured in the presence of ascitic fluid, demonstrating that defective CCR2 expression in TAM may be regulated, at least in part, by this cytokine in tumours (Sica et al., 2000). Therefore, it is possible that macrophage TNF-α production within hypoxic areas of tumours (Guida and Stewart, 1998; Hempel et al., 1996; Scannell et al., 1993) may lead to a downregulation of CCR2 expression on TAMs, decreasing their responsiveness to chemotactic ligands.

An increase in TNF-α expression is also believed to induce mitogen-activated protein kinase phosphatase 1 (MKP-1) (Grimshaw and Balkwill, 2001), a molecule which dephosphorylates extracellular signal-regulated kinase (ERK) 1/2, and p38 mitogen activated protein kinase (p38 MAPK) (Franklin and Kraft, 1997; Sun et al., 1993). Intracellular signalling via p38 MAPK and ERK1/2 is required for the chemotactic response of monocytes and monocytic cell lines to hypoxia-regulated chemokines (Ashida et al., 2001; Wain et al., 2002). Therefore, TNF-α may be an important factor in the hypoxic tumour environment for the suppression of macrophage migration, via a downregulation of CCR2 and an upregulation of MKP-1 (Figure 1a).

3. Hypoxia and its impact on macrophage function

For a long time it has been known that macrophages can be stimulated by environmental signals to exhibit a wide array of phenotypes (Nibbering et al., 1987; Ogle et al., 1994; van Furth, 1980). Two main polarization phenotypes of macrophages have been recognized. These include the classically activated (M1) and alternatively activated (M2) macrophage phenotypes. M1 macrophages are induced by interferon gamma (IFN-γ) and lipopolysaccharide (LPS). These macrophages upregulate pro-inflammatory cytokines (e.g. IL-12, IL-23, TNF, CXCL10), co-stimulatory molecules, produce reactive nitrogen and oxygen intermediates (RNI/ROI), and very little anti-inflammatory cytokines (e.g. IL-10). These cells promote inflammation, apoptosis, and microbicidal activity. Conversely, M2 macrophages are induced by IL-4 and IL-13, promote angiogenesis, cell proliferation and other tissue remodelling and protumoral functions. These cells are characterized in general by an $IL\text{-}12^{lo}IL\text{-}10^{hi}$ phenotype, upregulate chemokines like CCL17, CCL18 and CCL22, various scavenging receptors and the production of Arginase I. Although the M1-M2 nomenclature is a useful one when assessing the phenotype of macrophages, it is however, an over-simplification. Not all macrophage fit into these two distinct populations, and so further sub-populations have been defined (Mantovani et al., 2004).

Recently, subsets of differentially polarized TAMs with distinct functions were described by Movahedi et al. (2010) in murine mammary tumours. Their findings showed that almost all TAMs from these tumours were derived from $Ly6C^{hi}CX_3CR1^{lo}$ monocytes, where Ly6C is a monocyte/macrophage differentiation antigen regulated by IFN-γ, and CX_3CR1 is a receptor for CX_3CL1, a chemokine involved in the adhesion and migration of leukocytes. Notably, they found that hypoxic areas had higher numbers of M2-like TAMs, which increased as the tumour progressed (in certain tumours), and were shown to have potent proangiogenic effects *in vivo*. This also correlated with the expression of major histocompatibility complex II (MHC II), whereby MHC II^{hi} macrophages resided in normoxic areas and displayed an M1-like phenotype, and MHC II^{lo} macrophages resided in hypoxic areas and displayed a more M2-like phenotype (Figure 1a). Expression of M1 molecules like Nos2 (iNOS), interleukin (Il)-1β, Il-6, Il-12β and Ptgs2 (or cycloxygenase 2, COX2) were reported in MHC II^{hi} monocytes at the RNA or protein level. By comparison, MHC II^{lo} monocytes expressed such M2-related molecules such as macrophage mannose receptor (MR), scavenger receptor 1 (SR-A), arginase-1 (ARG-1), CD163, stabilin-1 (STAB-1), and interleukin-4Rα (IL-4Rα) (Movahedi et al., 2010). Fitting with their M2-like phenotype and localisation in areas of hypoxia, MHC II^{lo} TAMs were found to have significantly elevated proangiogenic activity *in vivo*. The phenotypic similarity between MHC II^{hi} TAMs and IKKβ-deficient macrophages implies that differences in these MHC II^{hi} and MHC II^{lo} TAM subsets may be driven by NF-κβ activity (Movahedi et al., 2010).

Another monocyte population, thought to be distinct from MHC II^{lo} TAMs, are the Tie2-expressing monocytes (TEMs) (Figure 1a). Originally identified in tumour-bearing mice, these monocytes circulate in the mouse blood as $Tie2^+CD11b^+CD45^+$ cells. They comprise a small monocyte subset which migrate towards angiopoietin-2 (Ang-2), a TIE2 ligand that is primarily released by vascular endothelial cells; this is thought to be a possible mechanism by which TEMs are recruited to tumours (Venneri et al., 2007), and more specifically, to highly vascularised areas (De Palma et al., 2003) (Figure 1a). Their role in the promotion of angiogenesis was confirmed by De Palma et al. (2005), who found that selective depletion of TEMs in a murine cancer model resulted in the inhibition of tumour angiogenesis and growth. Furthermore, TEM depletion was found to increase the efficacy of vascular-disrupting agent (VDA) therapy of tumours, suggesting that the action of these cells counteracts the antitumour effects of VDAs (Welford et al., 2011). Understanding more about monocyte subsets uncovers new possibilities for targeting specific subpopulations, which could alter the overall balance of TAM phenotypes. Repolarisation of TAM from an M2- to an M1-like phenotype could restore their antitumour effects, leading to a better patient prognosis.

The implications of macrophage plasticity in cancer biology have gathered increasing interest, both in terms of the phenotypes driven by the tumour microenvironment, and more specifically, by the hypoxic tumour environment. Biswas and colleagues (2008) reviewed the experimental evidence demonstrating that TAMs initially have an M1-like phenotype in areas of chronic inflammation where tumours commonly develop. These, however, respond to secreted cytokines, chemokines, growth factors and stress signals in the (hypoxic) tumour microenvironment, to express more of an M2-like phenotype in established tumours. This suggests a "re-education" of macrophages, which are recruited by the tumour, initially expressing an M1-like phenotype (thus promoting an inflammatory response); however, their residency within tumours leads to their polarisation and differentiation into M2-skewed TAMs, where their re-educated phenotype is one which promotes angiogenesis, tissue remodelling, immunosuppression and cell proliferation (Biswas et al., 2008).

One important feature of the tumour environment which brings about this phenotypic change in macrophages is hypoxia. Hypoxic regions of tumours commonly form due to the leaky and disorganised nature of tumour blood vessels, meaning that the rapid tumour cell proliferation often surpasses the ability of the poorly-formed vasculature to deliver required oxygen and nutrients (Shannon et al., 2003; Vaupel et al., 2001). Studies with human breast carcinomas (Leek et al., 1999) or animal tumours (Collingridge et al., 2001) have shown that hypoxic tumours contain higher numbers of TAMs. A positive correlation that is also seen between hypoxia and TAM numbers in secondary liver tumours that form as metastases from breast and colorectal tumours (Stessels et al., 2004). There is an inverse relationship between TAM infiltration and patient prognosis seen in many human cancers (Fujimoto et al., 2000; Hamada et al., 2002; Hanada et al., 2000; Heidl et al., 1987; Leek et al., 1996; Lissbrant et al., 2000; Salvesen and Akslen, 1999), which implies that these macrophages adopt a pro-tumoural phenotype, contrasting with their more classic role as pathogen and tumour killing cells and with their ability to initiate an immune response.

4. Molecular pathways mediating the effects of hypoxia on macrophages

4.1 Transcription factors HIFs 1 and 2

The best understood transcription factors mediating the response of macrophages to hypoxia are the hypoxia-inducible factors (HIFs) 1 and 2 (Burke et al., 2003; Fang et al., 2009; Talks et al., 2000) (Figure 1b). Both HIFs are heterodimers consisting of an individual α subunit and a common β subunit which is constitutively expressed. HIF-1α and HIF-2α are tightly controlled, such that, in the presence of oxygen they are quickly degraded by the ubiquitin-proteasome pathway within the cytoplasm. However, hypoxic stress causes an increase in production and stabilisation of these subunits, which are then able to complex with the β subunit within the nucleus and bind to hypoxic response elements (HREs) of certain oxygen-sensitive genes to drive transcription (Jiang et al., 1996; Semenza, 2002). The hypoxia-responsive genes regulated by HIFs are known to be involved in tumour proliferation, metabolism, angiogenesis, apoptosis and metastasis (reviewed by (Harris, 2002)). The data supporting the expression of HIFs by macrophages, especially TAMs, is currently unclear. Talks et al. (2000) showed that hypoxia predominantly upregulates HIF-2α in the pro-monocytic cell line, U937, and the HIF over-expression studies by White et al. (2004), suggested that HIF-2 might be more important for macrophage pro-angiogenic responses to hypoxia. In contrast, human macrophages exposed to tumour-specific levels of hypoxia *in vitro*, as well as those in hypoxic areas of several human tumours *in vivo*, were shown to be capable of inducing high levels of HIF-1 as well as HIF-2 (Burke et al., 2002). Recently, Fang et al. (2009) demonstrated that 18 hour exposure of human macrophages to hypoxia induces expression of VEGF, IL-1β, IL-8, adrenomedullin, CXCR4, and angiopoietin-2. Induction of these genes suggests a potent, pro-tumoural macrophage phenotype. Using small interfering RNA (siRNA), this gene expression was shown to be mediated via HIF-1 and 2 signalling, thus implicating these transcription factors in the generation of the hypoxia-driven, tumour-promoting macrophage phenotype.

Both HIF-1 and 2 bind to the HRE sequence contained in the promoter region of the VEGF gene and cause its upregulation (Ema et al., 1997; Flamme et al., 1997; Tian et al., 1997). Evidence that TAMs themselves upregulate VEGF in poorly vascularised tumour areas (Lewis et al., 2000) suggests that hypoxia, at least in part, causes TAMs to align with tumour cells in their pro-angiogenic function to increase the supply of oxygen to these areas. Interestingly, the binding of HIF-1 and 2 to the promoter region of *VEGF* in GM-CSF-cultured macrophages is thought to have antagonistic effects on angiogenesis, whereby HIF-1 induces VEGF production and HIF-2 induces the production of the soluble VEGF receptor, sVEGFR-1, in low oxygen conditions. The secretion of sVEGFR-1 is able to neutralise VEGF biologic activity, inhibiting its angiogenic effect; this indicates that the binding of these two transcription factors may have opposing effects on the regulation of angiogenesis (Eubank et al., 2011).

Less is known about the third member of the HIF family, HIF-3α, which shows high similarity to HIFs 1 and 2 and also forms heterodimers with the same β subunit. However, experiments so far show that this factor lacks the C-terminal transactivation domain (CTAD) (Gu et al., 1998), and acts as a dominant-negative regulator of the HIF pathway by antagonising the effects of HIFs 1 and 2 (Makino et al., 2001). HIF-3 was found to be constitutively expressed in monocyte-derived macrophages (MDMs), and was not responsive to hypoxic conditions in either monocytes or MDMs (Elbarghati et al., 2008). However, it was found to be hypoxia-responsive in lung epithelial cells (A549) at both the mRNA and protein level (Li et al., 2006), and so it is clear that further investigation into this transcription factor, with regards to its expression and importance, is needed.

HIFs are not the only hypoxia-responsive transcription factors. Both activating transcription factor-4 (ATF-4) and early growth response-1 (Egr-1) are upregulated in response to hypoxia in several murine and human tumour cell types (Ameri et al., 2004; Yan et al., 1999) and macrophages (Elbarghati et al., 2008), respectively. Both ATF-4 and Egr-1 proteins were found to be transiently upregulated in macrophages following a short hypoxic incubation, but there was no induction seen in monocytes. Interestingly, hypoxic treatment caused Egr-1 protein accumulation in macrophages in both the nucleus and the cytoplasm, in contrast to HIFs 1 and 2, and ATF-4 (Elbarghati et al., 2008), and is thought to play a role in monocyte differentiation into macrophages. Kharbanda et al. (1991) showed that M-CSF-stimulated monocytes demonstrate a dose-dependent increase in EGR-1 mRNA levels, and that inhibition of monocyte differentiation with dexamethasone also abolishes this EGR-1 induction. Therefore, since hypoxia increases the levels of Egr-1 protein, it is possible that hypoxia accelerates the differentiation of monocytes into TAMs (Elbarghati et al., 2008). This is also supported by the work of Oda and colleagues (2006), who demonstrated an increase in the expression of HIF-1α and HIF-1β in differentiating THP-1 cells and human monocytes from peripheral blood. RNA interference studies determined that, although HIF-1α is not essential for macrophage differentiation, it is, however, required for macrophage functional maturation. These findings further suggest that macrophage differentiation may be facilitated by hypoxia.

Various experimental methods have been used to identify HIF targets, including loss of expression in HIF-null cells (Fang et al., 2009; Semenza, 2003), targeting transcribed HIF using siRNA treatment (Fang et al., 2009; Kamlah et al., 2009; Krishnamachary et al., 2003), overexpression of HIFs using expression vectors or induced gene expression in von Hippel-Lindau (*VHL*)-null cells (Wykoff et al., 2000), or by the identification of HREs and HIF binding sites within gene promoter regions (Benita et al., 2009; Hirani et al., 2001; Semenza and Wang, 1992; Zhang et al., 2006). Both HIF1 and 2 were shown to regulate hypoxic MDM induction of VEGFA, GLUT-1, CXCR4, IL-1β, IL-8, and ADM (Fang et al., 2009) (Figure 1b), validating other reports of these as HIF target genes (Benita et al., 2009; Hirani et al., 2001; Semenza, 2003; Zhang et al., 2006).

Evidence that hypoxia induces a protumour phenotype in TAMs is not just limited to observed changes in RNA and protein expression; functional studies with hypoxic or HIF-expressing TAMs have also confirmed this phenotypic shift in macrophages. TAM-induced endothelial cell migration and tubule formation, reported by Chen et al. (2011), confirms the angiogenesis-promoting actions of TAM suggested by RNA and protein expression. More specifically, HIF-1α has been implicated in these protumour functional effects of TAMs. Doedens et al. (2010) report a dose-dependent suppression of T-cell proliferation by macrophages, demonstrating this immunosuppressive effect to be enhanced under hypoxia in a HIF-1α-dependent manner.

4.2 HIF relation with other pathways

It is clear that hypoxia drives a tumour-promoting phenotype in macrophages - it does this through the activation of hypoxia-responsive transcription factors, predominantly HIF-1 and 2, and their crosstalk with other signalling pathways. One such example is Toll-like receptor (TLR) signalling; TLR receptors are known to activate the innate immune system upon recognition of various pathogen-associated molecular patterns (PAMPs), including Lipopolysaccharide (LPS), bacterial DNA, and double-stranded RNA (Kaisho and Akira, 2006). In humans there are 10 functional members of the TLR family (TLR1-TLR10), of which, TLR4 is possibly the most involved in macrophage hypoxic response. This particular receptor recognises LPS, but has more recently been shown to be a receptor for certain endogenous molecules associated with damaged cells and tissues (Zhang and Mosser, 2008).

In their study of the relationship between hypoxic stress and TLR activity of macrophages, Kim et al. (2010) showed that hypoxia (and the hypoxia mimetic, $CoCl_2$) increased TLR4 messenger RNA and protein expression in the murine macrophage cell line, RAW264.7. This was unique to TLR4 and not seen with any of the other TLRs. Through the manipulation of macrophage HIF-1α gene expression, they demonstrated that hypoxic upregulation of TLR4 was dependent upon HIF-1 signalling, as well as showing that overexpression of HIF-1α enhanced TLR4 expression. Using chromatin immunoprecipitation (ChIP) they discovered that HIF-1α binds to the TLR4 promoter under hypoxic conditions, and the resultant induction of TLR4 in these macrophages increased the expression of interleukin-6 (IL-6), cyclooxygenase-2 (COX-2) and interferon-inducible protein-10 (IP-10) (Kim et al., 2010). Therefore, it is likely that, at sites which are challenged by hypoxic stress, macrophages upregulate TLR4 and become more sensitive to infection and inflammatory signals.

In addition to HIF-1α regulating TLR4, Sumbayev (2008) demonstrated that the inverse is also true. In human myeloid cells, TLR4 signalling (induced by the gram-negative bacterial ligand, LPS), activates crosstalk of HIF-1α and apoptosis signal-regulating kinase 1 (ASK1) pathways. Through the activation of p38 mitogen-activated protein kinase (p38 MAPK), ASK1 was found to stabilise HIF-1α, and knockdown of HIF-1α led to a reduced TLR4-dependent induction of pro-inflammatory cytokines. Similarly, TLR7 and 8 (involved in the recognition of viral single-stranded RNA) were also found to induce HIF-1α, although ASK1 was not found to be involved (Nicholas and Sumbayev, 2009).

Evidence has been given for the role of HIFs 1 and 2 in these pro-tumour actions of TAM in hypoxic areas, but more recently it has emerged that HIF-1 may also be responsive under normoxic conditions. Such stimuli as LPS, cytokines (e.g. TNFα), growth factors, insulin, thrombin and vasoactive peptides cause HIF-1α stabilisation in normoxia, via nuclear factor-kappa B (NF-κB) signalling. This key transcription factor was shown by Rius et al. (2008) to be upregulated following a 2-4h exposure of murine bone marrow-derived macrophages (BMDMs) to low oxygen. They also demonstrated that basal levels of NF-κB were required for the accumulation of HIF-1α protein in hypoxic cells, using macrophages from an IKK-beta knock-out (IKKβ$^{-/-}$) mouse. This implies that IKKβ, an important activator of NF-κB through phosphorylation-induced degradation of IkB inhibitors, has important contributions to macrophage response to hypoxia. Since NF-κB has a crucial and well characterised role in inflammation, IKKβ represents a significant molecule which may link the hypoxic response to innate immunity and infection (Rius et al., 2008).

5. Hypoxia, macrophage function and tumour progression

By contributing to angiogenesis, metastasis, invasion, immunosuppression, chemo- and radio-resistance, and altering metabolism, macrophages are known to greatly influence the survival and progression of cancer (see Biswas et al. (2008)). This phenotype of TAMs is also known to be influenced by hypoxia, which induces a distinct protumour phenotype. Expression of various growth factors, including fibroblast growth factor 2 (FGF2), platelet-derived growth factor (PDGF), placental growth factor (PGF), and hepatocyte growth factor (HGF), have been found to be upregulated *in vitro* by macrophages under hypoxia (White et al., 2004). These factors, in addition to VEGF, function as tumour cell mitogens and support tumour growth in hypoxic regions (Fang et al., 2009; Lewis et al., 2000).

Another key process in tumour progression is angiogenesis. The expression of VEGF (a potent mitogen and well characterised pro-angiogenic factor) by hypoxic macrophages has been discussed previously. However, other key proteins reported by White and colleagues (2004) include CXCL8, angiopoietin, cyclooxygenase-2 (COX-2) and inducible nitric oxide synthase (iNOS), all of which were identified in cDNA arrays as genes that are transcriptionally upregulated in primary macrophages under hypoxia. Induction of these genes by macrophages is likely to be crucial for tumour angiogenesis.

Additionally, hypoxic TAMs also release tissue factor (CD142) (Compeau et al., 1994) and macrophage inhibitory factor (MIF) (Schmeisser et al., 2005), which are thought to be involved in invasion and metastasis. Tissue factor expression by hypoxic TAMs (as well as tumour cells, endothelial cells and fibroblasts), induces the production of thrombin, which in turn promotes tumour cell metastasis (Versteeg et al., 2004). Furthermore, MIF has been shown to promote tumour cell motility in a murine colon cancer cell line *in vitro* and *in vivo* (Sun et al., 2005). These factors may act indirectly through matrix metalloproteases (MMPs), such as MMP-9, which is stimulated by MIF and degrades the basement membrane and extracellular matrix (ECM) (Hagemann et al., 2004). This weakens the attachment of tumour cells to these structural supports and enables their subsequent invasion and metastasis. Further evidence of MMP induction comes from a co-culture of macrophages with tumour cells in hypoxia, which revealed an upregulation of macrophage MMP-7 production in low oxygen conditions *in vitro* and human tumours (Burke et al., 2003).

Finally, the hypoxic phenotype of TAMs also includes various immunosuppressive functions which are achieved through several mechanisms; these include the expression of immunosuppressive factors prostaglandin E_2 (PGE2) and IL-10 (Ertel et al., 1993; Murata et al., 2002), whose presence within the tumour microenvironment can downregulate the tumouricidal abilities of TAMs. In addition, PGE2 and IL-10 inhibit the functions of T cells and other effector cells of the immune system (Elgert et al., 1998), which combined with hypoxic inhibition of macrophage phagocytosis and presentation of antigens (Leeper-Woodford and Mills, 1992; Murata et al., 2002), suppresses the triggering of an adaptive immune response directed toward the tumour. Doedens et al. (2010) recently reported hypoxia- and HIF-1α-dependent suppression of T-cell proliferation by macrophages. Hypoxia, therefore, drives the macrophage towards a protumour phenotype which regulates tumour growth, angiogenesis, invasion, metastasis and immunosuppression.

6. Targeting tumour hypoxia for therapy

Under the stresses associated with hypoxia in areas of tumour ischemia (predominantly low oxygen and low glucose concentrations), tumour cells are forced to respire anaerobically and reduce their proliferation. This challenges many conventional cancer therapies such as chemotherapy, since their mechanism of action relies on the rapidly replication of tumour cells. In addition to this, the poorly developed tumour vasculature, which contributes to the development of hypoxia in the first place, also impedes the delivery of drugs to these areas of the tumour.

In light of this, antiangiogenic "vessel normalizing" strategies are being developed which aim to improve tumour vasculature for better anticancer treatment and reduced metastasis. Rolny and colleagues (2011) demonstrated that histidine-rich glycoprotein (HRG), a host-derived factor, is able to significantly reduce hypoxia and to polarise TAMs away from a protumour phenotype.

The concept of delivering a prodrug systemically - for subsequent activation in specific areas of the body - has been applied to cancer biology, but is most often limited by the level of expression of the activating enzyme at the target site. Rather than hypoxia inhibiting cancer therapy, some recent therapeutic strategies have focussed on utilising cellular responses to these harsh conditions, twinned with the prodrug therapeutic design, to creatively activate cytotoxic agents within the hypoxic tumour microenvironment. Griffiths et al. (2000) made use of macrophage accumulation in areas of low oxygen to deliver gene therapy to pathological hypoxia. They genetically modified macrophages to express the enzyme cytochrome p450 under hypoxic conditions, which when expressed, converts the systemically administered pro-drug cyclophosphamide into its active form exclusively in these areas and causes tumour cell death. This system was then adapted further to deliver an oncolytic adenovirus to these areas by co-transducing macrophages with a hypoxia-regulated E1A/B construct, as well as an E1A-dependent virus which can only proliferate within a prostate-tumour (using a prostate-specific promoter) (Muthana et al., 2011). E1A/B proteins were only synthesised once the host cell (the macrophage) had infiltrated into areas of extreme hypoxia in tumours. This then subsequently activated the proliferation of the oncolytic adenovirus and its release. The virus then infected and killed surrounding prostate tumour cells – in both hypoxic and non-hypoxic areas of tumours. This three-step process (the homing of macrophages to hypoxic sites, hypoxia-responsive proliferation of the adenovirus, and the limiting of viral replication to within prostate tumour cells), makes this system very specific for killing tumour cells within the hypoxic areas prostate tumours (Muthana et al., 2011). This hypoxia-based therapy was seen to eradicate both primary and secondary tumours in mice.

It has been suggested that the best use of this therapy would be in combination with conventional therapies, since this could potentially eliminate both the slower proliferating (hypoxic) and the highly proliferating areas of the tumour. Using a mathematical model, Owen et al. (2011) predict that the use of a macrophage-based, hypoxia-responsive therapy immediately before or during conventional chemotherapy would produce significant antitumour effects.

7. Concluding remarks

Macrophage accumulation in tumours is known to correlate with poor patient prognosis in the majority of cancer types (Fujimoto et al., 2000; Hamada et al., 2002; Hanada et al., 2000; Heidl et al., 1987; Leek et al., 1996; Lissbrant et al., 2000; Salvesen and Akslen, 1999). This can be explained by the tumour-promoting phenotype of TAMs, induced by the tumour microenvironment. Here we have reviewed how hypoxia, a key component of many malignant tumours (Raleigh et al., 2001; Vaupel et al., 1989), is centrally involved in the polarisation of TAMs. The shift in TAM phenotype under hypoxia has been shown not just at the expression level, but also at a functional level as well. In many of these reports, the HIF-1 transcription factor was found to be crucially important. Studies with HIF-1α knockout mice have revealed its role, not just in regulating responses to pathological hypoxia, but also to physiological low oxygen conditions as part of normal oxygen homeostasis. It is possible that HIF-1 signalling (including its activation of other pathways), is a major factor in determining the polarisation and function of macrophages in different environments (Dehne and Brune, 2009).

With considerable assistance from hypoxic, M2-like TAMs, tumour cells in hypoxic areas have the necessary support and drive to migrate and invade into adjacent tissues, evade the immune system and prevent a targeted adaptive immune response, and travel through the vasculature to form metastases at secondary sites. This has large implications in cancer therapy, especially since hypoxic tumour cells are less affected by most conventional therapeutic strategies. Inefficient targeting of such tumour cells is likely to contribute to the well-documented relapse in many chemotherapy- and radiotherapy-treated cancer patients; therefore, more creative and innovative therapeutic methodologies need to be developed based on our continually growing understanding of tumour hypoxia, to enhance patient long-term survival.

8. Acknowledgement

SKB is grateful to funding support from Biomedical Research Council, A*STAR, Singapore. RH is supported by an ARAP fellowship (A*STAR, Singapore).

9. References

Ameri, K., Lewis, C. E., Raida, M., Sowter, H., Hai, T., and Harris, A. L. (2004). Anoxic induction of ATF-4 through HIF-1-independent pathways of protein stabilization in human cancer cells. Blood *103*, 1876-1882.

Arenberg, D. A., Keane, M. P., DiGiovine, B., Kunkel, S. L., Strom, S. R., Burdick, M. D., Iannettoni, M. D., and Strieter, R. M. (2000). Macrophage infiltration in human non-small-cell lung cancer: the role of CC chemokines. Cancer Immunol Immunother *49*, 63-70.

Ashida, N., Arai, H., Yamasaki, M., and Kita, T. (2001). Differential signaling for MCP-1-dependent integrin activation and chemotaxis. Ann N Y Acad Sci *947*, 387-389.

Balkwill, F. (2003). Chemokine biology in cancer. Semin Immunol *15*, 49-55.

Barleon, B., Sozzani, S., Zhou, D., Weich, H. A., Mantovani, A., and Marme, D. (1996). Migration of human monocytes in response to vascular endothelial growth factor (VEGF) is mediated via the VEGF receptor flt-1. Blood *87*, 3336-3343.

Benita, Y., Kikuchi, H., Smith, A. D., Zhang, M. Q., Chung, D. C., and Xavier, R. J. (2009). An integrative genomics approach identifies Hypoxia Inducible Factor-1 (HIF-1)-target genes that form the core response to hypoxia. Nucleic Acids Res *37*, 4587-4602.

Biswas, S. K., Sica, A., and Lewis, C. E. (2008). Plasticity of macrophage function during tumor progression: regulation by distinct molecular mechanisms. J Immunol *180*, 2011-2017.

Bottazzi, B., Walter, S., Govoni, D., Colotta, F., and Mantovani, A. (1992). Monocyte chemotactic cytokine gene transfer modulates macrophage infiltration, growth, and susceptibility to IL-2 therapy of a murine melanoma. J Immunol *148*, 1280-1285.

Brown, L. F., Berse, B., Jackman, R. W., Tognazzi, K., Guidi, A. J., Dvorak, H. F., Senger, D. R., Connolly, J. L., and Schnitt, S. J. (1995). Expression of vascular permeability factor (vascular endothelial growth factor) and its receptors in breast cancer. Hum Pathol *26*, 86-91.

Brown, L. F., Berse, B., Jackman, R. W., Tognazzi, K., Manseau, E. J., Senger, D. R., and Dvorak, H. F. (1993). Expression of vascular permeability factor (vascular endothelial growth factor) and its receptors in adenocarcinomas of the gastrointestinal tract. Cancer Res *53*, 4727-4735.

Burke, B., Giannoudis, A., Corke, K. P., Gill, D., Wells, M., Ziegler-Heitbrock, L., and Lewis, C. E. (2003). Hypoxia-induced gene expression in human macrophages: implications for ischemic tissues and hypoxia-regulated gene therapy. Am J Pathol *163*, 1233-1243.

Burke, B., Tang, N., Corke, K. P., Tazzyman, D., Ameri, K., Wells, M., and Lewis, C. E. (2002). Expression of HIF-1alpha by human macrophages: implications for the use of macrophages in hypoxia-regulated cancer gene therapy. J Pathol *196*, 204-212.

Chen, P., Huang, Y., Bong, R., Ding, Y., Song, N., Wang, X., Song, X., and Luo, Y. (2011). Tumor-associated macrophages promote angiogenesis and melanoma growth via adrenomedullin in a paracrine and autocrine manner. Clin Cancer Res *17*, 7230-7239.

Clarijs, R., Schalkwijk, L., Ruiter, D. J., and de Waal, R. M. (2003). EMAP-II expression is associated with macrophage accumulation in primary uveal melanoma. Invest Ophthalmol Vis Sci *44*, 1801-1806.

Collingridge, D. R., Hill, S. A., and Chaplin, D. J. (2001). Proportion of infiltrating IgG-binding immune cells predict for tumour hypoxia. Br J Cancer *84*, 626-630.

Compeau, C. G., Ma, J., DeCampos, K. N., Waddell, T. K., Brisseau, G. F., Slutsky, A. S., and Rotstein, O. D. (1994). In situ ischemia and hypoxia enhance alveolar macrophage tissue factor expression. Am J Respir Cell Mol Biol *11*, 446-455.

De Palma, M., Venneri, M. A., Galli, R., Sergi Sergi, L., Politi, L. S., Sampaolesi, M., and Naldini, L. (2005). Tie2 identifies a hematopoietic lineage of proangiogenic monocytes required for tumor vessel formation and a mesenchymal population of pericyte progenitors. Cancer Cell *8*, 211-226.

De Palma, M., Venneri, M. A., Roca, C., and Naldini, L. (2003). Targeting exogenous genes to tumor angiogenesis by transplantation of genetically modified hematopoietic stem cells. Nat Med *9*, 789-795.

Dehne, N., and Brune, B. (2009). HIF-1 in the inflammatory microenvironment. Exp Cell Res *315*, 1791-1797.

Doedens, A. L., Stockmann, C., Rubinstein, M. P., Liao, D., Zhang, N., DeNardo, D. G., Coussens, L. M., Karin, M., Goldrath, A. W., and Johnson, R. S. (2010). Macrophage expression of hypoxia-inducible factor-1 alpha suppresses T-cell function and promotes tumor progression. Cancer Res *70*, 7465-7475.

Elbarghati, L., Murdoch, C., and Lewis, C. E. (2008). Effects of hypoxia on transcription factor expression in human monocytes and macrophages. Immunobiology *213*, 899-908.

Elgert, K. D., Alleva, D. G., and Mullins, D. W. (1998). Tumor-induced immune dysfunction: the macrophage connection. J Leukoc Biol *64*, 275-290.

Ema, M., Taya, S., Yokotani, N., Sogawa, K., Matsuda, Y., and Fujii-Kuriyama, Y. (1997). A novel bHLH-PAS factor with close sequence similarity to hypoxia-inducible factor 1alpha regulates the VEGF expression and is potentially involved in lung and vascular development. Proc Natl Acad Sci U S A *94*, 4273-4278.

Ertel, W., Singh, G., Morrison, M. H., Ayala, A., and Chaudry, I. H. (1993). Chemically induced hypotension increases PGE2 release and depresses macrophage antigen presentation. Am J Physiol *264*, R655-660.

Eubank, T. D., Roda, J. M., Liu, H., O'Neil, T., and Marsh, C. B. (2011). Opposing roles for HIF-1alpha and HIF-2alpha in the regulation of angiogenesis by mononuclear phagocytes. Blood *117*, 323-332.

Fang, H. Y., Hughes, R., Murdoch, C., Coffelt, S. B., Biswas, S. K., Harris, A. L., Johnson, R. S., Imityaz, H. Z., Simon, M. C., Fredlund, E., *et al.* (2009). Hypoxia-inducible factors 1 and 2 are important transcriptional effectors in primary macrophages experiencing hypoxia. Blood *114*, 844-859.

Ferrara, N., and Davis-Smyth, T. (1997). The biology of vascular endothelial growth factor. Endocr Rev *18*, 4-25.

Flamme, I., Frohlich, T., von Reutern, M., Kappel, A., Damert, A., and Risau, W. (1997). HRF, a putative basic helix-loop-helix-PAS-domain transcription factor is closely related to hypoxia-inducible factor-1 alpha and developmentally expressed in blood vessels. Mech Dev *63*, 51-60.

Franklin, C. C., and Kraft, A. S. (1997). Conditional expression of the mitogen-activated protein kinase (MAPK) phosphatase MKP-1 preferentially inhibits p38 MAPK and stress-activated protein kinase in U937 cells. J Biol Chem *272*, 16917-16923.

Freeman, M. R., Schneck, F. X., Gagnon, M. L., Corless, C., Soker, S., Niknejad, K., Peoples, G. E., and Klagsbrun, M. (1995). Peripheral blood T lymphocytes and lymphocytes infiltrating human cancers express vascular endothelial growth factor: a potential role for T cells in angiogenesis. Cancer Res *55*, 4140-4145.

Fujimoto, J., Sakaguchi, H., Aoki, I., and Tamaya, T. (2000). Clinical implications of expression of interleukin 8 related to angiogenesis in uterine cervical cancers. Cancer Res *60*, 2632-2635.

Gerszten, R. E., Garcia-Zepeda, E. A., Lim, Y. C., Yoshida, M., Ding, H. A., Gimbrone, M. A., Jr., Luster, A. D., Luscinskas, F. W., and Rosenzweig, A. (1999). MCP-1 and IL-8 trigger firm adhesion of monocytes to vascular endothelium under flow conditions. Nature *398*, 718-723.

Griffiths, L., Binley, K., Iqball, S., Kan, O., Maxwell, P., Ratcliffe, P., Lewis, C., Harris, A., Kingsman, S., and Naylor, S. (2000). The macrophage - a novel system to deliver gene therapy to pathological hypoxia. Gene Ther *7*, 255-262.

Grimshaw, M. J., and Balkwill, F. R. (2001). Inhibition of monocyte and macrophage chemotaxis by hypoxia and inflammation--a potential mechanism. Eur J Immunol *31*, 480-489.

Grimshaw, M. J., Hagemann, T., Ayhan, A., Gillett, C. E., Binder, C., and Balkwill, F. R. (2004). A role for endothelin-2 and its receptors in breast tumor cell invasion. Cancer Res *64*, 2461-2468.

Grimshaw, M. J., Naylor, S., and Balkwill, F. R. (2002a). Endothelin-2 is a hypoxia-induced autocrine survival factor for breast tumor cells. Mol Cancer Ther *1*, 1273-1281.

Grimshaw, M. J., Wilson, J. L., and Balkwill, F. R. (2002b). Endothelin-2 is a macrophage chemoattractant: implications for macrophage distribution in tumors. Eur J Immunol *32*, 2393-2400.

Gu, Y. Z., Moran, S. M., Hogenesch, J. B., Wartman, L., and Bradfield, C. A. (1998). Molecular characterization and chromosomal localization of a third alpha-class hypoxia inducible factor subunit, HIF3alpha. Gene Expr *7*, 205-213.

Guida, E., and Stewart, A. (1998). Influence of hypoxia and glucose deprivation on tumour necrosis factor-alpha and granulocyte-macrophage colony-stimulating factor expression in human cultured monocytes. Cell Physiol Biochem *8*, 75-88.

Hagemann, T., Robinson, S. C., Schulz, M., Trumper, L., Balkwill, F. R., and Binder, C. (2004). Enhanced invasiveness of breast cancer cell lines upon co-cultivation with macrophages is due to TNF-alpha dependent up-regulation of matrix metalloproteases. Carcinogenesis *25*, 1543-1549.

Hamada, I., Kato, M., Yamasaki, T., Iwabuchi, K., Watanabe, T., Yamada, T., Itoyama, S., Ito, H., and Okada, K. (2002). Clinical effects of tumor-associated macrophages and dendritic cells on renal cell carcinoma. Anticancer Res *22*, 4281-4284.

Hanada, T., Nakagawa, M., Emoto, A., Nomura, T., Nasu, N., and Nomura, Y. (2000). Prognostic value of tumor-associated macrophage count in human bladder cancer. Int J Urol *7*, 263-269.

Harris, A. L. (2002). Hypoxia--a key regulatory factor in tumour growth. Nat Rev Cancer *2*, 38-47.

Heidl, G., Davaris, P., Zwadlo, G., Jagoda, M. S., Duchting, S., Bierhoff, E., Gruter, T., Krieg, V., and Sorg, C. (1987). Association of macrophages detected with monoclonal antibody 25 F 9 with progression and pathobiological classification of gastric carcinoma. J Cancer Res Clin Oncol *113*, 567-572.

Hempel, S. L., Monick, M. M., and Hunninghake, G. W. (1996). Effect of hypoxia on release of IL-1 and TNF by human alveolar macrophages. Am J Respir Cell Mol Biol *14*, 170-176.

Hirani, N., Antonicelli, F., Strieter, R. M., Wiesener, M. S., Ratcliffe, P. J., Haslett, C., and Donnelly, S. C. (2001). The regulation of interleukin-8 by hypoxia in human macrophages--a potential role in the pathogenesis of the acute respiratory distress syndrome (ARDS). Mol Med *7*, 685-697.

Hiratsuka, S., Minowa, O., Kuno, J., Noda, T., and Shibuya, M. (1998). Flt-1 lacking the tyrosine kinase domain is sufficient for normal development and angiogenesis in mice. Proc Natl Acad Sci U S A *95*, 9349-9354.

Janssen, H. L., Haustermans, K. M., Sprong, D., Blommestijn, G., Hofland, I., Hoebers, F. J., Blijweert, E., Raleigh, J. A., Semenza, G. L., Varia, M. A., *et al.* (2002). HIF-1A, pimonidazole, and iododeoxyuridine to estimate hypoxia and perfusion in human head-and-neck tumors. Int J Radiat Oncol Biol Phys *54*, 1537-1549.

Jiang, B. H., Semenza, G. L., Bauer, C., and Marti, H. H. (1996). Hypoxia-inducible factor 1 levels vary exponentially over a physiologically relevant range of O2 tension. Am J Physiol *271*, C1172-1180.

Kaisho, T., and Akira, S. (2006). Toll-like receptor function and signaling. J Allergy Clin Immunol *117*, 979-987; quiz 988.

Kamlah, F., Eul, B. G., Li, S., Lang, N., Marsh, L. M., Seeger, W., Grimminger, F., Rose, F., and Hanze, J. (2009). Intravenous injection of siRNA directed against hypoxia-inducible factors prolongs survival in a Lewis lung carcinoma cancer model. Cancer Gene Ther *16*, 195-205.

Kharbanda, S., Nakamura, T., Stone, R., Hass, R., Bernstein, S., Datta, R., Sukhatme, V. P., and Kufe, D. (1991). Expression of the early growth response 1 and 2 zinc finger genes during induction of monocytic differentiation. J Clin Invest *88*, 571-577.

Kim, M. S., Kwon, H. J., Lee, Y. M., Baek, J. H., Jang, J. E., Lee, S. W., Moon, E. J., Kim, H. S., Lee, S. K., Chung, H. Y., *et al.* (2001). Histone deacetylases induce angiogenesis by negative regulation of tumor suppressor genes. Nat Med *7*, 437-443.

Kim, S. Y., Choi, Y. J., Joung, S. M., Lee, B. H., Jung, Y. S., and Lee, J. Y. (2010). Hypoxic stress up-regulates the expression of Toll-like receptor 4 in macrophages via hypoxia-inducible factor. Immunology *129*, 516-524.

Krishnamachary, B., Berg-Dixon, S., Kelly, B., Agani, F., Feldser, D., Ferreira, G., Iyer, N., LaRusch, J., Pak, B., Taghavi, P., and Semenza, G. L. (2003). Regulation of colon carcinoma cell invasion by hypoxia-inducible factor 1. Cancer Res *63*, 1138-1143.

Lee, A. H., Dublin, E. A., Bobrow, L. G., and Poulsom, R. (1998). Invasive lobular and invasive ductal carcinoma of the breast show distinct patterns of vascular endothelial growth factor expression and angiogenesis. J Pathol *185*, 394-401.

Leek, R. D., Hunt, N. C., Landers, R. J., Lewis, C. E., Royds, J. A., and Harris, A. L. (2000). Macrophage infiltration is associated with VEGF and EGFR expression in breast cancer. J Pathol *190*, 430-436.

Leek, R. D., Landers, R. J., Harris, A. L., and Lewis, C. E. (1999). Necrosis correlates with high vascular density and focal macrophage infiltration in invasive carcinoma of the breast. Br J Cancer *79*, 991-995.

Leek, R. D., Lewis, C. E., Whitehouse, R., Greenall, M., Clarke, J., and Harris, A. L. (1996). Association of macrophage infiltration with angiogenesis and prognosis in invasive breast carcinoma. Cancer Res *56*, 4625-4629.

Leeper-Woodford, S. K., and Mills, J. W. (1992). Phagocytosis and ATP levels in alveolar macrophages during acute hypoxia. Am J Respir Cell Mol Biol *6*, 326-334.

Leung, S. Y., Wong, M. P., Chung, L. P., Chan, A. S., and Yuen, S. T. (1997). Monocyte chemoattractant protein-1 expression and macrophage infiltration in gliomas. Acta Neuropathol *93*, 518-527.

Lewis, J. S., Landers, R. J., Underwood, J. C., Harris, A. L., and Lewis, C. E. (2000). Expression of vascular endothelial growth factor by macrophages is up-regulated in poorly vascularized areas of breast carcinomas. J Pathol *192*, 150-158.

Li, Q. F., Wang, X. R., Yang, Y. W., and Lin, H. (2006). Hypoxia upregulates hypoxia inducible factor (HIF)-3alpha expression in lung epithelial cells: characterization and comparison with HIF-1alpha. Cell Res *16*, 548-558.

Lin, E. Y., Nguyen, A. V., Russell, R. G., and Pollard, J. W. (2001). Colony-stimulating factor 1 promotes progression of mammary tumors to malignancy. J Exp Med *193*, 727-740.

Lissbrant, I. F., Stattin, P., Wikstrom, P., Damber, J. E., Egevad, L., and Bergh, A. (2000). Tumor associated macrophages in human prostate cancer: relation to clinicopathological variables and survival. Int J Oncol *17*, 445-451.

Makino, Y., Cao, R., Svensson, K., Bertilsson, G., Asman, M., Tanaka, H., Cao, Y., Berkenstam, A., and Poellinger, L. (2001). Inhibitory PAS domain protein is a negative regulator of hypoxia-inducible gene expression. Nature *414*, 550-554.

Mantovani, A., Sica, A., Sozzani, S., Allavena, P., Vecchi, A., and Locati, M. (2004). The chemokine system in diverse forms of macrophage activation and polarization. Trends Immunol *25*, 677-686.

Matschurat, S., Knies, U. E., Person, V., Fink, L., Stoelcker, B., Ebenebe, C., Behrensdorf, H. A., Schaper, J., and Clauss, M. (2003). Regulation of EMAP II by hypoxia. Am J Pathol *162*, 93-103.

Movahedi, K., Laoui, D., Gysemans, C., Baeten, M., Stange, G., Van den Bossche, J., Mack, M., Pipeleers, D., In't Veld, P., De Baetselier, P., and Van Ginderachter, J. A. (2010). Different tumor microenvironments contain functionally distinct subsets of macrophages derived from Ly6C(high) monocytes. Cancer Res *70*, 5728-5739.

Murata, Y., Ohteki, T., Koyasu, S., and Hamuro, J. (2002). IFN-gamma and pro-inflammatory cytokine production by antigen-presenting cells is dictated by intracellular thiol redox status regulated by oxygen tension. Eur J Immunol *32*, 2866-2873.

Murdoch, C., Giannoudis, A., and Lewis, C. E. (2004). Mechanisms regulating the recruitment of macrophages into hypoxic areas of tumors and other ischemic tissues. Blood *104*, 2224-2234.

Muthana, M., Giannoudis, A., Scott, S. D., Fang, H. Y., Coffelt, S. B., Morrow, F. J., Murdoch, C., Burton, J., Cross, N., Burke, B., *et al.* (2011). Use of macrophages to target therapeutic adenovirus to human prostate tumors. Cancer Res *71*, 1805-1815.

Negus, R. P., Stamp, G. W., Hadley, J., and Balkwill, F. R. (1997). Quantitative assessment of the leukocyte infiltrate in ovarian cancer and its relationship to the expression of C-C chemokines. Am J Pathol *150*, 1723-1734.

Negus, R. P., Turner, L., Burke, F., and Balkwill, F. R. (1998). Hypoxia down-regulates MCP-1 expression: implications for macrophage distribution in tumors. J Leukoc Biol *63*, 758-765.

Nibbering, P. H., Leijh, P. C., and van Furth, R. (1987). Quantitative immunocytochemical characterization of mononuclear phagocytes. II. Monocytes and tissue macrophages. Immunology *62*, 171-176.

Nicholas, S. A., and Sumbayev, V. V. (2009). The involvement of hypoxia-inducible factor 1 alpha in Toll-like receptor 7/8-mediated inflammatory response. Cell Res *19*, 973-983.

Oda, T., Hirota, K., Nishi, K., Takabuchi, S., Oda, S., Yamada, H., Arai, T., Fukuda, K., Kita, T., Adachi, T., *et al.* (2006). Activation of hypoxia-inducible factor 1 during macrophage differentiation. Am J Physiol Cell Physiol *291*, C104-113.

Ogle, C. K., Wu, J. Z., Mao, X., Szczur, K., Alexander, J. W., and Ogle, J. D. (1994). Heterogeneity of Kupffer cells and splenic, alveolar, and peritoneal macrophages for the production of TNF, IL-1, and IL-6. Inflammation *18*, 511-523.

Ohta, M., Kitadai, Y., Tanaka, S., Yoshihara, M., Yasui, W., Mukaida, N., Haruma, K., and Chayama, K. (2002). Monocyte chemoattractant protein-1 expression correlates with macrophage infiltration and tumor vascularity in human esophageal squamous cell carcinomas. Int J Cancer *102*, 220-224.

Owen, M. R., Stamper, I. J., Muthana, M., Richardson, G. W., Dobson, J., Lewis, C. E., and Byrne, H. M. (2011). Mathematical modeling predicts synergistic antitumor effects of combining a macrophage-based, hypoxia-targeted gene therapy with chemotherapy. Cancer Res *71*, 2826-2837.

Plate, K. H., Breier, G., Weich, H. A., Mennel, H. D., and Risau, W. (1994). Vascular endothelial growth factor and glioma angiogenesis: coordinate induction of VEGF receptors, distribution of VEGF protein and possible in vivo regulatory mechanisms. Int J Cancer *59*, 520-529.

Plate, K. H., Breier, G., Weich, H. A., and Risau, W. (1992). Vascular endothelial growth factor is a potential tumour angiogenesis factor in human gliomas in vivo. Nature *359*, 845-848.

Raleigh, J. A., Calkins-Adams, D. P., Rinker, L. H., Ballenger, C. A., Weissler, M. C., Fowler, W. C., Jr., Novotny, D. B., and Varia, M. A. (1998). Hypoxia and vascular endothelial growth factor expression in human squamous cell carcinomas using pimonidazole as a hypoxia marker. Cancer Res *58*, 3765-3768.

Raleigh, J. A., Chou, S. C., Bono, E. L., Thrall, D. E., and Varia, M. A. (2001). Semiquantitative immunohistochemical analysis for hypoxia in human tumors. Int J Radiat Oncol Biol Phys *49*, 569-574.

Rius, J., Guma, M., Schachtrup, C., Akassoglou, K., Zinkernagel, A. S., Nizet, V., Johnson, R. S., Haddad, G. G., and Karin, M. (2008). NF-kappaB links innate immunity to the hypoxic response through transcriptional regulation of HIF-1alpha. Nature *453*, 807-811.

Rolny, C., Mazzone, M., Tugues, S., Laoui, D., Johansson, I., Coulon, C., Squadrito, M. L., Segura, I., Li, X., Knevels, E., *et al.* (2011). HRG inhibits tumor growth and metastasis by inducing macrophage polarization and vessel normalization through downregulation of PlGF. Cancer Cell *19*, 31-44.

Said, N., Smith, S., Sanchez-Carbayo, M., and Theodorescu, D. (2011). Tumor endothelin-1 enhances metastatic colonization of the lung in mouse xenograft models of bladder cancer. J Clin Invest *121*, 132-147.

Salvesen, H. B., and Akslen, L. A. (1999). Significance of tumour-associated macrophages, vascular endothelial growth factor and thrombospondin-1 expression for tumour angiogenesis and prognosis in endometrial carcinomas. Int J Cancer *84*, 538-543.

Sawano, A., Iwai, S., Sakurai, Y., Ito, M., Shitara, K., Nakahata, T., and Shibuya, M. (2001). Flt-1, vascular endothelial growth factor receptor 1, is a novel cell surface marker for the lineage of monocyte-macrophages in humans. Blood *97*, 785-791.

Scannell, G., Waxman, K., Kaml, G. J., Ioli, G., Gatanaga, T., Yamamoto, R., and Granger, G. A. (1993). Hypoxia induces a human macrophage cell line to release tumor necrosis factor-alpha and its soluble receptors in vitro. J Surg Res *54*, 281-285.

Schioppa, T., Uranchimeg, B., Saccani, A., Biswas, S. K., Doni, A., Rapisarda, A., Bernasconi, S., Saccani, S., Nebuloni, M., Vago, L., *et al.* (2003). Regulation of the chemokine receptor CXCR4 by hypoxia. J Exp Med *198*, 1391-1402.

Schmeisser, A., Marquetant, R., Illmer, T., Graffy, C., Garlichs, C. D., Bockler, D., Menschikowski, D., Braun-Dullaeus, R., Daniel, W. G., and Strasser, R. H. (2005). The expression of macrophage migration inhibitory factor 1alpha (MIF 1alpha) in human atherosclerotic plaques is induced by different proatherogenic stimuli and associated with plaque instability. Atherosclerosis *178*, 83-94.

Scotton, C., Milliken, D., Wilson, J., Raju, S., and Balkwill, F. (2001). Analysis of CC chemokine and chemokine receptor expression in solid ovarian tumours. Br J Cancer *85*, 891-897.

Semenza, G. (2002). Signal transduction to hypoxia-inducible factor 1. Biochem Pharmacol *64*, 993-998.

Semenza, G. L. (2003). Targeting HIF-1 for cancer therapy. Nat Rev Cancer *3*, 721-732.

Semenza, G. L., and Wang, G. L. (1992). A nuclear factor induced by hypoxia via de novo protein synthesis binds to the human erythropoietin gene enhancer at a site required for transcriptional activation. Mol Cell Biol *12*, 5447-5454.

Shannon, A. M., Bouchier-Hayes, D. J., Condron, C. M., and Toomey, D. (2003). Tumour hypoxia, chemotherapeutic resistance and hypoxia-related therapies. Cancer Treat Rev *29*, 297-307.

Sica, A., Saccani, A., Bottazzi, B., Bernasconi, S., Allavena, P., Gaetano, B., Fei, F., LaRosa, G., Scotton, C., Balkwill, F., and Mantovani, A. (2000). Defective expression of the monocyte chemotactic protein-1 receptor CCR2 in macrophages associated with human ovarian carcinoma. J Immunol *164*, 733-738.

Stessels, F., Van den Eynden, G., Van der Auwera, I., Salgado, R., Van den Heuvel, E., Harris, A. L., Jackson, D. G., Colpaert, C. G., van Marck, E. A., Dirix, L. Y., and Vermeulen, P. B. (2004). Breast adenocarcinoma liver metastases, in contrast to colorectal cancer liver metastases, display a non-angiogenic growth pattern that preserves the stroma and lacks hypoxia. Br J Cancer *90*, 1429-1436.

Strieter, R. M., Belperio, J. A., Phillips, R. J., and Keane, M. P. (2004). Chemokines: angiogenesis and metastases in lung cancer. Novartis Found Symp *256*, 173-184; discussion 184-178, 259-169.

Sumbayev, V. V. (2008). LPS-induced Toll-like receptor 4 signalling triggers cross-talk of apoptosis signal-regulating kinase 1 (ASK1) and HIF-1alpha protein. FEBS Lett *582*, 319-326.

Sun, B., Nishihira, J., Yoshiki, T., Kondo, M., Sato, Y., Sasaki, F., and Todo, S. (2005). Macrophage migration inhibitory factor promotes tumor invasion and metastasis via the Rho-dependent pathway. Clin Cancer Res *11*, 1050-1058.

Sun, H., Charles, C. H., Lau, L. F., and Tonks, N. K. (1993). MKP-1 (3CH134), an immediate early gene product, is a dual specificity phosphatase that dephosphorylates MAP kinase in vivo. Cell *75*, 487-493.

Talks, K. L., Turley, H., Gatter, K. C., Maxwell, P. H., Pugh, C. W., Ratcliffe, P. J., and Harris, A. L. (2000). The expression and distribution of the hypoxia-inducible factors HIF-1alpha and HIF-2alpha in normal human tissues, cancers, and tumor-associated macrophages. Am J Pathol *157*, 411-421.

Tian, H., McKnight, S. L., and Russell, D. W. (1997). Endothelial PAS domain protein 1 (EPAS1), a transcription factor selectively expressed in endothelial cells. Genes Dev *11*, 72-82.

Toi, M., Hoshina, S., Takayanagi, T., and Tominaga, T. (1994). Association of vascular endothelial growth factor expression with tumor angiogenesis and with early relapse in primary breast cancer. Jpn J Cancer Res *85*, 1045-1049.

Ueno, T., Toi, M., Saji, H., Muta, M., Bando, H., Kuroi, K., Koike, M., Inadera, H., and Matsushima, K. (2000). Significance of macrophage chemoattractant protein-1 in macrophage recruitment, angiogenesis, and survival in human breast cancer. Clin Cancer Res *6*, 3282-3289.

van Furth, R. (1980). Monocyte origin of Kupffer cells. Blood Cells *6*, 87-92.

Vaupel, P., Kallinowski, F., and Okunieff, P. (1989). Blood flow, oxygen and nutrient supply, and metabolic microenvironment of human tumors: a review. Cancer Res *49*, 6449-6465.

Vaupel, P., Kelleher, D. K., and Hockel, M. (2001). Oxygen status of malignant tumors: pathogenesis of hypoxia and significance for tumor therapy. Semin Oncol *28*, 29-35.

Vaupel, P., Mayer, A., Briest, S., and Hockel, M. (2005). Hypoxia in breast cancer: role of blood flow, oxygen diffusion distances, and anemia in the development of oxygen depletion. Adv Exp Med Biol *566*, 333-342.

Venneri, M. A., De Palma, M., Ponzoni, M., Pucci, F., Scielzo, C., Zonari, E., Mazzieri, R., Doglioni, C., and Naldini, L. (2007). Identification of proangiogenic TIE2-expressing monocytes (TEMs) in human peripheral blood and cancer. Blood *109*, 5276-5285.

Versteeg, H. H., Spek, C. A., Peppelenbosch, M. P., and Richel, D. J. (2004). Tissue factor and cancer metastasis: the role of intracellular and extracellular signaling pathways. Mol Med *10*, 6-11.

Vicari, A. P., and Caux, C. (2002). Chemokines in cancer. Cytokine Growth Factor Rev *13*, 143-154.

Wain, J. H., Kirby, J. A., and Ali, S. (2002). Leucocyte chemotaxis: Examination of mitogen-activated protein kinase and phosphoinositide 3-kinase activation by Monocyte Chemoattractant Proteins-1, -2, -3 and -4. Clin Exp Immunol *127*, 436-444.

Wang, S. C., Hong, J. H., Hsueh, C., and Chiang, C. S. (2012). Tumor-secreted SDF-1 promotes glioma invasiveness and TAM tropism toward hypoxia in a murine astrocytoma model. Lab Invest *92*, 151-162.

Welford, A. F., Biziato, D., Coffelt, S. B., Nucera, S., Fisher, M., Pucci, F., Di Serio, C., Naldini, L., De Palma, M., Tozer, G. M., and Lewis, C. E. (2011). TIE2-expressing macrophages limit the therapeutic efficacy of the vascular-disrupting agent combretastatin A4 phosphate in mice. J Clin Invest *121*, 1969-1973.

White, J. R., Harris, R. A., Lee, S. R., Craigon, M. H., Binley, K., Price, T., Beard, G. L., Mundy, C. R., and Naylor, S. (2004). Genetic amplification of the transcriptional response to hypoxia as a novel means of identifying regulators of angiogenesis. Genomics *83*, 1-8.

Wykoff, C. C., Pugh, C. W., Maxwell, P. H., Harris, A. L., and Ratcliffe, P. J. (2000). Identification of novel hypoxia dependent and independent target genes of the von Hippel-Lindau (VHL) tumour suppressor by mRNA differential expression profiling. Oncogene *19*, 6297-6305.

Yan, S. F., Lu, J., Zou, Y. S., Soh-Won, J., Cohen, D. M., Buttrick, P. M., Cooper, D. R., Steinberg, S. F., Mackman, N., Pinsky, D. J., and Stern, D. M. (1999). Hypoxia-associated induction of early growth response-1 gene expression. J Biol Chem *274*, 15030-15040.

Zhang, A., Meng, L., Wang, Q., Xi, L., Chen, G., Wang, S., Zhou, J., Lu, Y., and Ma, D. (2006). Enhanced in vitro invasiveness of ovarian cancer cells through up-regulation of VEGF and induction of MMP-2. Oncol Rep *15*, 831-836.

Zhang, F. R., and Schwarz, M. A. (2002). Pro-EMAP II is not primarily cleaved by caspase-3 and -7. Am J Physiol Lung Cell Mol Physiol *282*, L1239-1244.

Zhang, X., and Mosser, D. M. (2008). Macrophage activation by endogenous danger signals. J Pathol *214*, 161-178.

6

Tumor Inflammatory Microenvironment in EMT and Metastasis

Tingting Yuan[1,3], Yadi Wu[2,3] and Binhua P. Zhou[1,3]
[1]Departments of Molecular and Cellular Biochemistry,
[2]Molecular and Biomedical Pharmacology,
[3]Markey Cancer Center, University of Kentucky School of Medicine, Lexington, KY, USA

1. Introduction

Approximately 90% of cancer-related death is caused by metastasis. The increased motility and invasiveness of metastatic tumor cells is reminiscent of events that occur at the epithelial-mesenchymal transition (EMT), which is a characteristic that occurs during embryonic development, tissue remodeling, wound healing and metastasis. Interestingly, EMT is a dynamic process and mainly occurs at the edges of wounds during healing and at the invasive fronts of metastatic tumors, which suggest that EMT is influenced by stimuli that emanate from the inflammatory microenvironment. The tumor microenvironment consists of many kinds of cells including infiltrated inflammatory cells, such as neutrophils, lymphocytes, macrophages and myeloid derived suppressor cells (MDSC). These infiltrated immune cells secrete cytokines, chemokines and growth factors, such as TNF-α, TGF-β, IL-6, fibroblast growth factor (FGF) and epidermal growth factor (EGF). These growth factors contribute significantly to the invasive and metastatic traits of cancer cells by inducing EMT. Here, we discuss new insights into the molecular pathways and key regulators that link inflammatory tumor microenvironment to EMT and metastasis.

2. Cancer and immunity: Immunity's roles in tumor suppression and promotion

One of the most challenging questions in immunology is to understand how the immune system affects cancer development and progression. In recent years, after a long eclipse, different lines of work have lead to a renaissance of the inflammation-cancer connection (Balkwill and Mantovani 2001; Coussens and Werb 2002; Mantovani, Allavena et al. 2008). It is now believed that the immune system plays a dual role in cancer: on one hand , it can function as an extrinsic tumor suppressor (Dighe, Richards et al. 1994; Kaplan, Shankaran et al. 1998; Smyth, Thia et al. 2000; Girardi, Oppenheim et al. 2001; Shankaran, Ikeda et al. 2001; Street, Trapani et al. 2002) by destroying cancer cells or inhibiting their outgrowth; on the other hand, the immune system can also promote tumor progression by establishing conditions within the tumor microenvironment that facilitate tumor outgrowth (Schreiber, Old et al.). Inflammatory responses play decisive roles at different stages of tumor development, including initiation, promotion, malignant conversion, invasion, and metastasis (de Visser, Eichten et al. 2006; Grivennikov, Greten et al. 2010).

3. EMT and metastasis

Epithelial-mesenchymal transition (EMT) is a phenotypic conversion during embryonic development when tissue remodeling and cell migration shape the future organism, such as in embryonic development and wound healing. During EMT, epithelial cells lose the adherent junctions that keep them in contact with their neighbors. They gain a mesenchymal cell phenotype that enables them to break through the basal membrane and migrate over a long distance, a result of profound changes in their cytoskeleton architecture and gene expression profile (Kalluri and Neilson 2003). This concept was pioneered by the seminal study from Elizabeth Hay using chick primitive streak formation as a model in 1967 (Hay 1995). Hay realized that an epithelial phenotypic conversion was of crucial importance during gastrulation and cell migration in the early vertebrate embryo. She proposed that differentiated epithelial cells could undergo a dramatic "transformation" into mesenchymal cells (Greenburg and Hay 1988; Hay 1995). However, this "transformation" is reversible: mesenchymal cells can revert back to epithelial cells through a reverse process called mesenchymal-epithelial transition (MET). As a result, the term "transition" is now used.

EMT does not only occur during embryonic development or as a physiological response to injury. It is also an important element in cancer progression and other pathologies that involve organ degeneration, such as fibrosis. At the cellular level, pathological EMTs are very similar to physiological EMTs in that they are governed by similar signaling pathways, regulators, and effective molecules.

From a clinical perspective, metastasis is the most critical aspect of tumorigenesis: we have already addressed that more than 90% of cancer mortality is caused by metastasis. Aberrant control of epithelial proliferation and angiogenesis underlie the initiation and growth of primary carcinomas (Hanahan and Weinberg 2011). However, additional steps must be completed before a metastatic tumor is successfully established. The spread of malignant cells consists of a series of steps, all of which are thought to be important for metastatic outgrowth in different organs. Basically, these steps include local invasion toward and entry into blood vasculature (intravasation), survival within the circulation system, arrest in distant capillary beds or "homing" to distal organs, exit from blood vasculature (extravasation), and eventual outgrowth and re-establishment of malignant growths in secondary locations (Woodhouse, Chuaqui et al. 1997; Chambers, Naumov et al. 2001; Fidler 2003; Hanahan and Weinberg 2011).

3.1 Classification of EMT into three different subtypes

Based on recent intensive study in this field, EMT can be divided into three subtypes, which have different biological functional consequences (Kalluri 2009; Kalluri and Weinberg 2009; Zeisberg and Neilson 2009). Type 1 EMT occurs during implantation, embryo formation, gastrulation, and neural crest migration, which describes the transition of epithelial cells to generate diverse mesenchymal cell types. These primary mesenchymal cells can revert back to form secondary epithelia in mesodermal and endodermal organs through MET. Type 2 EMT occurs during wound healing, tissue regeneration and organ fibrosis, which is usually associated with injury and chronic inflammation. Type 2 EMT ceases once inflammation is attenuated, but if inflammation persists, this type of EMT will eventually lead to tissue fibrosis and organ destruction. Unlike Type 1 EMT, these mesenchymal cells have no potential to undergo MET and turn back to epithelial cells. Type 3 EMT occurs during tumor progression, which describes how neoplastic cells at the invasive front of primary tumors undergo a transition to acquire increased motility and invasive ability, enabling them to invade and metastasize through the blood stream or lymph node system, eventually generating life-threatening metastatic lesions at distant organs.

Because studies of EMT often involve various model systems ranging from different epithelial cell types to assorted stimulations, it is important to use validated biomarkers to examine the phenotypic conversion during all three classes of EMT. Common biomarkers include cell-surface and extracellular molecules, cytoskeletal proteins and specific transcription factors. For example, down-regulation of E-cadherin is a hallmark of EMT, and loss of E-cadherin expression facilitates the induction of EMT (Huber, Kraut et al. 2005). E-cadherin is a cell-cell adhesion molecule that participates in homotypic, calcium-dependent interactions to form epithelial adherent junctions (Cowin, Rowlands et al. 2005; Junghans, Haas et al. 2005). In addition, E-cadherin repressors, such as Snail, Slug, Twist and ZEB1/2, are commonly used as EMT markers. Snail is the first described E-cadherin repressor and is also the common downstream target of various signaling pathways that lead to EMT. Vimentin, an intermediate filament mainly expressed in fibroblasts, endothelial cells and hematopoietic cells, is also commonly used as an indicator for Type 3 EMT, since expression of vimentin in tumor cells correlates with their invasiveness and metastatic potential. Furthermore, differential expression of integrin is also used as a biomarker of EMT, since integrins modulate the interaction of cells with extracellular matrix (ECM). For example, increased expression of α5 integrin is commonly found in Type 2 and Type 3 EMT (Qian, Zhang et al. 2005; Davidson, Marsden et al. 2006; White, Blanchette et al. 2007).

3.2 Type1 EMT in the formation of mesoderm and neural crest

EMT is crucially important to tissue morphogenetic events during embryonic development, such as the mesoderm formation, neural crest formation, heart valve development, and secondary palate formation. Without EMT, development cannot proceed through the blastula stage. Mesoderm formation and neural crest development represent the major EMT programs that occur during early embryonic development; the resulting mesenchymal and neural crest cells act as progenitors and further differentiate into various cell types via MET. For example, gastrulation EMT produces the mesoderm, giving rise to muscle, bone and connective tissues, whereas neural crest delamination EMT gives rise to glial and neuronal cells, adrenal glandular tissues, pigment-containing cells of the epidermis and skeletal and connective tissues. The heart valve development and secondary palate formation occur in relatively well-differentiated epithelial cells that are destined to become defined mesenchymal cells types.

The formation of mesoderm from the primitive ectoderm during gastrulation is the classic example of EMT. Gastrulation, observed in all metazoans, is accompanied by drastic morphogenic changes from a single epithelial layer (the epiblast) into three embryonic germ layers, the ectoderm, mesoderm, and endoderm, to form a complex three-dimensional multilayered embryo (Shook and Keller 2003). In chicken and mouse embryo, Wnt and TGF-β signaling provide the initial induction signals for EMT, while the FGF signal is necessary to maintain the EMT regulatory network during mesoderm formation. All these signaling events activate the expression of Snail, which represses the expression of E-cadherin and other tight junction components (such as claudins, occludins, and Crumbs) and promotes cell migration. In Snail knock-out mice the cells that form are unable to migrate, although mesoderm specification is not affected.

Neural crest formation is another example of Type 1 EMT in embryogenesis where premigratory neural crest cells form at the border of the neural plate and non-neural ectoderm as a result of signals emanating from these two tissues. Interestingly, similar signaling pathways operating during EMT at gastrulation are used in the neural crest formation. Indeed, a combination of Wnt, FGF, and TGF-β (mainly BMP) induce the expression of Snail, Sox and forkhead box D3 transcription factors (Villanueva, Glavic et al. 2002). In addition, experimental evidence shows that Notch signalling pathway plays an important role in neural crest formation through induction of Slug in frog and chick embryo (Nieto 2002). The combination of these transcription factors generates the full spectrum of phenotypic changes associated with EMT and primes the precursor cells to become migratory neural crest cells. These neural crest cells are equipped with the ability to migrate over extraordinarily long distances in the embryo, prior to their reaggregation via MET for further differentiation.

3.3 Type 2 EMT in tissue and organ fibrosis

3.3.1 Implications of EMT in fibrosis

Re-epithelization, tissue regeneration and organ fibrosis constitute Type 2 EMT. Organ fibrosis is mediated by inflammatory cells and fibroblasts, which deposit collagens, elastin, tenacin and other matrix molecules. Fibrosis-associated Type 2 EMT specifically occurs in kidney, liver, lung and intestine (Zeisberg, Tarnavski et al. 2007). A series of typical experiments has shown that EMT is an important process during tissue injury that leads to organ fibrosis. In terms of EMT proteomes, fibroblast-specific protein 1 (FSP1, also known S100A4 and MTS-1), α-SMA (smooth muscle actin) and collagen I are reliable markers to characterize the mesenchymal products generated by EMTs in the development of fibrosis in various organs. TGF-β1, as the major pro-fibrotic cytokine, induces many of the central processes involved in fibrosis, including differentiation of fibroblast to myfibroblasat, ECM deposition and EMT. TGF-β not only contributes to pulmonary and hepatic fibrosis, but also plays a key role in cardiac fibrosis (Gressner, Weiskirchen et al. 2002; Willis and Borok 2007; Zeisberg, Tarnavski et al. 2007). TGF-β induces EMT via both a Smad2/3-dependent pathway and a MAPK-dependent pathway. The relevance of TGF-β-induced EMT for progression of organ fibrosis was recently further elucidated using BMP-7 as an intracellular competitor of TGF-β signaling in mouse models of kidney, liver, billiard tract, lung and intestinal fibrosis (Zeisberg, Bottiglio et al. 2003; Zeisberg, Hanai et al. 2003). The function of TGF-β in fibrosis is highlighted by the finding that Smad3-/- mice are resistant to the induction of several fibrotic diseases (Flanders 2004). TGF-β levels are also over-produced and are associated with functional impairment in patients with fibrotic pulmonary diseases such as idiopathic pulmonary fibrosis (Salez, Gosset et al. 1998). Clinical studies have also demonstrated the correlation between fibrosis and EMT (Rastaldi, Ferrario et al. 2002). Using immunohistochemistry and in situ hybridization, an EMT was demonstrated with the expression of several markers of tubular phenotype transition, such as cytokeratin, vimentin, α-SMA and zona occludens (ZO-1) in 133 kidney biopsies (Rastaldi, Ferrario et al. 2002). Similarly, an expression pattern of EMT was found in areas of fibrosis in the colon in patients with Crohn's disease (Bataille, Rohrmeier et al. 2008).

3.3.2 Re-epithelialization of wounded skin

Re-epithelialization recapitulates several aspects of EMT. Re-epithelialization requires epithelial cells at the edge of wounded tissue to loosen their cell--cell and cell--ECM contacts and assume a migratory phenotype, reminiscent of EMT. Slug has a crucial role in wound-healing, which is expressed in keratinocytes at the boundary of wounds. Importantly, epithelial cell outgrowth from skin explants was markedly reduced in Slug knockout mice, whereas overexpression of Slug in cultured human keratinocytes result in increased cell spreading and desmosomal disruption (Savagner, Kusewitt et al. 2005). Arnoux et al further found that EGF can activate Erk5, which specifically enhances Slug promoter activity and controls wound healing in keratinocyte-derived HacaT cells in vitro (Arnoux, Nassour et al. 2008). However, it should be noted that not all features of EMT are seen. First, the migrating keratinocytes remain part of a cohesive cell sheet since they retain some intercellular junction. Second, the epithelial cells do not actually become mesenchymal (i.e., interstitial) cells. They retain epithelial characteristics. Once wound closure is complete, the involved epithelial cells revert to their tissue-specific, differentiated state.

3.4 Type 3 EMT in cancer metastasis

Cancer metastasis is believed to consist of four distinct steps: invasion, intravasation, extravasation and metastatic colonization (Chambers, Groom et al. 2002; Pantel and Brakenhoff 2004). During invasion, tumor cells lose cell-cell adhesion, gain mobility and leave the site of the primary tumor to invade adjacent tissues. In intravasation, tumor cells penetrate through the endothelial barrier and enter systemic circulation through blood and lymphatic vessels. In extravasation, cells that survive anchorage-independent growth conditions in the bloodstream attach to vessels at distant sites and leave the bloodstream. Finally, in metastatic colonization, tumor cells form macrometastases in the new host environment (Chambers, Groom et al. 2002; Pantel and Brakenhoff 2004). All of these steps, from initial breakdown of tissue structure through increased invasiveness, and ultimately distribution and colonization throughout the body, are characteristics of the developmental process at EMT/MET. The similarity of genetic controls and biochemical mechanisms underlying the acquisition of the invasive phenotype, and the subsequent systemic spread of the cancer cells, highlights that tumor cells usurp this developmental pathway for their metastatic dissemination. We will further discuss this type of EMT, with more detail on how it is regulated by different signaling pathways and molecular in various tumor microenvironments.

3.5 Molecular regulation of EMT

The hallmark of EMT is the loss of E-cadherin expression, an important caretaker of the epithelial phenotype. Loss of E-cadherin expression is often correlated with the tumor grade and stage, because it results in disruption of the cell-cell adhesion and an increase in nuclear β-catenin (Cowin, Rowlands et al. 2005; Junghans, Haas et al. 2005). Several transcription factors have been implicated in the regulation of EMT, including zinc finger proteins of the Snail/Slug family, the basic helix-loop-helix factor Twist, E12/E47, Goosecoid, δEF1/ZEB1 and SIP1 (Nieto 2002; Yang, Mani et al. 2004; Hartwell, Muir et al. 2006). These factors act as a molecular switch of EMT program by repressing a subset of common genes that encode cadherins, claudins, integrins, mucins, plakophilin, occludin and ZO1 to induce EMT. For example, Snail expression is associated with E-cadherin repression in metastasis; it also correlates with tumor recurrence and poor prognosis in various cancers (Elloul, Elstrand et al. 2005; Moody, Perez et al. 2005; Bruyere, Namdarian et al. 2009). In addition, extensive crosstalk among these transcription factors forms a signaling network that is responsible for establishing and maintaining mesenchymal cell phenotypes. Furthermore, some of these transcription factors, including Snail, play an important part in overcoming oncogene-induced senescence (Ansieau, Bastid et al. 2008), inhibiting tumor immunosuppression (Kudo-Saito, Shirako et al. 2009) and generating tumorigenic cancer stem cells (Mani, Guo et al. 2008). These transcription factors communicate and respond to extracellular signals such as growth factors, cytokines and hypoxia from their microenvironment to induce EMT.

Many signaling pathways trigger EMT in both embryonic development and in normal and transformed cell lines. The signaling pathways include those triggered by different members of the TGF-β superfamily, Wnts, Notch, EGF, FGF and many others (Fig.1).

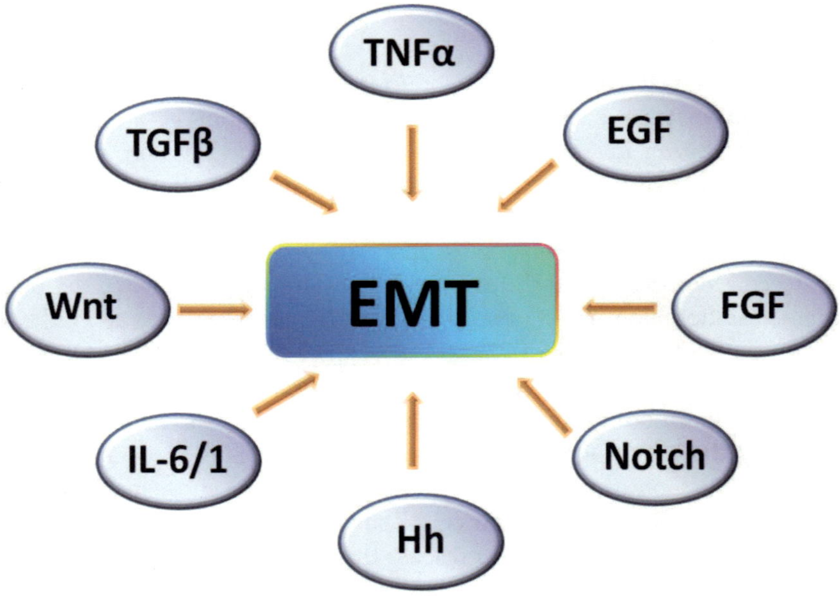

Fig. 1. Overview of the Molecular regulation of EMT.

TGF-β is a primary inducer of EMT. It not only contributes to EMT during embryonic development, but also induces EMT during tumor progression in vivo (Zavadil and Bottinger 2005). Overexpression of Smad2 and Smad3 result in increased EMT in a mammary epithelial model (Valcourt, Kowanetz et al. 2005). Knockout of Smad3 blocks TGF-β-induced EMT in primary tubular epithelial cells; the reduction of Smad2 and Smad3 function is associated with the decreased metastatic potential of breast cancer cell lines in a xenograft model (Zavadil, Cermak et al. 2004). It is interesting that SMAD3 and SMAD4 interact and form a complex with Snail, targeting the promoters of CAR (a tight-junction protein) and E-cadherin during TGF-β-inducing EMT in breast epithelial cells (Vincent, Neve et al. 2009). Bos et al identified that TGF-β primed cancer cells for lung metastasis through angiopoietin-like 4 via Smad signaling pathway (Bos, Zhang et al. 2009). In contrast, inhibition of TGF-β or TGF-β receptor reduces the invasive and metastatic activities of cancer cells. TGF-β can also downregulate various epithelial molecules, including E-cadherin, ZO-1 and several specific keratins; it also upregulates certain mesenchymal proteins such as fibronectin, fibroblast specific protein 1, α-smooth muscle actin and vimentin. In addition, TGF-β cooperates with numerous kinases such as RAS, MAPK, and p38MAP, to promote EMT (Zavadil and Bottinger 2005; Buijs, Henriquez et al. 2007). More specifically, p38 MAPK and RhoA mediate an autocrine TGF-β-induced EMT in NMuMG mouse mammary epithelial cells (Bhowmick, Ghiassi et al. 2001). ECM molecules, such as integrin β1 and Fibulin-5, augment TGF-β-induced EMT in a MAPK-dependent mechanism (Bhowmick, Ghiassi et al. 2001; Lee, Albig et al. 2008). Constitutive activation of Raf enhances the function of TGF-β in inducing EMT via MAPK in MDCK cells (Janda, Lehmann et al. 2002). TGF-β also induces EMT through changes in the expression of certain cell polarity molecules. For example, TGF-β can induce phosphorylation of Par6, which in turn stimulates binding of Par6 to E3 ligase Smurf1. The Par6-Smurf1 complex then mediates the localized ubiquitination of RhoA to disrupt tight junctions during EMT (Ozdamar, Bose et al. 2005). TGF-β can also downregulate Par3 expression to destroy cell polarity (Wang, Nie et al. 2008). It is interesting to note that Abl can inhibit TGF-β-mediated EMT in normal and metastatic mammary epithelial cells (MECs) (Allington, Galliher-Beckley et al. 2009). Furthermore, TGF-β can cooperate with other oncogenic pathways, such as Notch, Wnt/β-catenin and NF-κB, to maintain the mesenchymal phenotype of invasive/metastatic tumor cells (Nawshad, Lagamba et al. 2005; Zavadil and Bottinger 2005; Neth, Ries et al. 2007).

The Wnt/β-catenin pathway has a particularly tight link with EMT (Li, Hively et al. 2000). On one hand, β-catenin is an essential component of adherent junctions, where it provides the link between E-cadherin and α-catenin and modulates cell-cell adhesion and cell migration. On the other hand, β-catenin also functions as a transcription cofactor with T cell factor (TCF). Nuclear translocation of β-catenin can activate expression of Slug, thus inducing EMT. Expression of β-catenin in oocyte induces a premature EMT in the epiblast, concomitant with Snail transcription. Interestingly, Snail is a highly unstable protein and is dually regulated by protein stability and cellular location. We showed that GSK-3β binds and phosphorylates Snail at two consensus motifs to dually regulate the function of this protein: phosphorylation at the first motif regulates its ubiquitination mediated by β-Trcp, and phosphorylation at the second motif controls its subcellular localization (Zhou, Deng et al. 2004). Thus, Wnt can suppress the activity of GSK-3β, and it stabilizes the protein level of Snail and β-catenin to induce EMT and cancer metastasis (Yook, Li et al. 2005; Yook, Li et al. 2006). Meanwhile, Snail can functionally interact with β-catenin to increase Wnt-dependent target gene expression, promoting EMT (Stemmer, de Craene et al. 2008). Increasing evidence indicates that Wnt signaling is strongly associated with human basal-like breast cancer. Inhibiting Wnt signaling through LRP6 reduces the capacity of cancer cells to self-renew and colonize in vivo. It also results in the re-expression of breast epithelial markers and repression of EMT transcription factors Slug and Twist (DiMeo, Anderson et al. 2009). How the synergistic activation of Snail and β-catenin by the Wnt signaling pathway, enhancing EMT and metastasis, remains to be further defined.

Notch is an evolutionarily conserved signaling pathway that regulates cell fate specification, self-renewal and differentiation in embryonic and postnatal tissues. Four Notch (Notch 1−4) and five ligands (Jagged1, 2 and Deltalike1, 3, 4) have been identified. Notch signaling is normally activated followed by ligand-receptor binding between two neighboring cells. Notch undergoes intramembrane cleavage by γ-secretase, and its intracellular domain (NICD) is released and translocates to the nucleus to activate gene transcription by associating with Mastermind-like 1 (MAM) and histone acetyltransferase p300/CBP. Alteration of Notch signaling has been associated with various types of cancer in which Notch can act as an oncogene or as a tumor suppressor, depending on the cellular context. The first observation that Notch pathway is required for EMT was derived from cardiac valve and cushion formation at heart development (Timmerman, Grego-Bessa et al. 2004). This implies that Notch, acting through a similar mechanism, induces EMT during tumor progression and converts polarized epithelial cells into motile and invasive ones (Grego-Bessa, Diez et al. 2004). Indeed, overexpression of Jagged1 and Notch1 induces the expression of Slug and correlates with poor prognosis in various human cancers (Leong, Niessen et al. 2007). Slug is essential for Notch-mediated EMT by repressing E-cadherin expression, which results in β-catenin activation and resistance to anoikis. Inhibition of Notch signaling in xenografted, Slug-positive/E-cadherin-negative breast tumors promotes apoptosis and inhibits tumor growth and metastasis (Leong, Niessen et al. 2007). In addition, Notch signaling deploys two distinct mechanisms that act in synergy to control the expression of Snail (Sahlgren, Gustafsson et al. 2008). First, Notch directly upregulates Snail expression by recruiting the Notch intracellular domain to the Snail promoter. Second, Notch potentiates hypoxia-inducible factor 1α (HIF-1α) recruitment to the lysyl oxidase (LOX) promoter and elevates the hypoxia-induced upregulation of LOX, which stabilizes the Snail protein. Thus, Notch signaling is required to convert the hypoxic stimulus into EMT, and it increases the invasiveness of tumor cells. In addition, the Notch signaling pathway is involved in the acquisition of EMT phenotype of gemcitabine-resistant (GR) cells in pancreatic cancer (Wang, Li et al. 2009). Down-regulation of Notch signaling is associated with decreased invasive behavior of GR cells. Moreover, Notch signaling leads to the increased expression of vimentin, ZEB1, Slug, Snail, and NF-κB, and it results in EMT. Thus, inhibition of Notch signaling by novel therapeutic strategies can be clinically important in overcoming drug resistance and EMT phenotype of tumor cells.

The Hedgehog (Hh) signaling pathway was first identified in a large screen for Drosophila genes required for patterning of the early embryo (Hooper and Scott 2005; Jacob and Lum 2007). The Hh ligands, Sonic-, Desert-, and Indian Hh in vertebrates and Hh in Drosophila, are secreted proteins that undergo several posttranslational modifications to gain full activity. Key effectors of Hh signaling include zinc-finger proteins of the Gli1-3 transcription factors. Hh signaling can initiate cell growth, cell division, lineage specification and axon guidance and can also function as a survival factor. Activation of Hh signaling also leads to EMT. In mouse epidermal cells or in rat kidney epithelial cells immortalized with adenovirus E1A, Gli1 rapidly induces transcription of Snail and promotes EMT (Li, Deng et al. 2006; Li, Deng et al. 2007). Targeted expression of Gli1 in the epithelial cells of mammary gland of mice induces the expression of Snail, resulting in the disruption of the mammary epithelial network and alveologenesis during pregnancy (Fiaschi, Rozell et al. 2007). In addition, Hedgehog signals induce JAG2 up-regulation for Notch-CSL-mediated Snail expression; on the other hand, Hedgehog induces TGF-β1 secretion to induce ZEB1 and ZEB2 expression through TGF-β and NF-κB pathways. Conversely, blocking Hedgehog signaling by inhibitor cyclopamine suppresses pancreatic cancer invasion and metastasis by inhibiting EMT (Feldmann, Dhara et al. 2007). The crosstalk between the Hh and EMT also presents in human esophageal squamous cell carcinoma (ESCC) (Isohata, Aoyagi et al. 2009). Hh and EMT signaling genes are co-expressed on the undifferentiated esophageal epithelial cells and in most ESCCs. These findings suggest that mesenchymal gene expression is maintained or strengthened through Hh signaling in cancer cells.

3.6 Microenvironmental regulation of EMT/metastasis

Metastasis is a multi-step process that requires cancer cells to escape from the primary tumor, survive in circulation, seed at distant sites and grow. Each of these processes involves rate-limiting steps influenced by non-malignant cells of the tumor microenvironment (Joyce and Pollard 2009), composed of multiple cell types, such as stroma fibroblasts, epithelial cells, and a variety of bone marrow-derived cells (BMDCs) including macrophages, myeloid-derived suppressor cells (MDSCs), and so on. In this surrounding environment, a variety of stromal cells are recruited to tumors, not only enhance growth of the primary tumor, but also to facilitate its metastatic dissemination to distant organs (Tse and Kalluri 2007; Lunt, Chaudary et al. 2009).

Recent work has indicated that EMT is a dynamic process controlled by signals that cells receive from their microenvironment. By adopting a mesenchymal phenotype through EMT, individual carcinoma cells can infiltrate adjacent tissues, cross endothelial barriers, and enter the circulation through blood and lymphatic vessels. Once the tumor cells reach their secondary tissues or organs, they no longer encounter the signals they experienced in the primary tumor, and they can revert to an epithelial state via a mesenchymal-epithelial transition (MET). Consistent with this notion, EMT commonly occurs at the invasive front (tumor-stromal boundary) of many invasive carcinomas (Christofori 2006; Franci, Takkunen et al. 2006). These observations indicate that EMT is triggered by cellular signals from microenvironment. These immune and inflammatory cells secrete cytokines, chemokines, and growth factors, which play essential roles for supporting tumor progression and metastasis. Because it is analogous with the role of inflammation in mediating wound healing, we hypothesize that the migratory and invasive ability of tumor cells at the invasive front is initiated and propelled by an inflammatory microenvironment through the induction of EMT.

4. The role of inflammatory cells and cytokines in EMT/metastasis

4.1 Tumor-Associated Macrophages (TAMs)

Consistent with our hypothesis, a high content of inflammatory cells, particularly tumor-associated macrophages, is commonly found at the invasive fronts of advanced carcinoma (Condeelis and Pollard 2006). Macrophages are key cells in chronic inflammation. M1 macrophages are involved in Type 1 reactions and are classically activated by microbial products, killing microorganisms and producing reactive oxygen and nitrogen intermediates. In contrast, M2 cells (tumor associated macrophage; TAM) are important components of infiltrated leukocytes in most malignant tumors. They are involved in Type 2 reactions, tune inflammation and adaptive immunity, promote cell proliferation by producing growth factors and enhance angiogenesis, tissue remodeling, and repair. Macrophage directly influences the behavior and function of tumor cells and has been regarded as an "obligate partner for tumor-cell migration, invasion and metastasis" (Condeelis and Pollard 2006). Clinical studies indicate a correlation between TAM density and poor prognosis (Pollard 2004). For example, in PyMT-induced mammary tumors, macrophages are present in the areas of basement membrane breakdown during the development of "early-stage" metastatic lesions and systemic depletion of macrophages results in reduced formation of lung metastasis (Lin, Nguyen et al. 2001). TAMs produce a wide variety of growth factors (such as FGF, HGF, EGF, PDGF and TGF-β and cytokines [such as TNFα, interleukin-6, interleukin-1, and interferons]) to stimulate the growth, motility, and invasiveness of tumor cells. TAMs also produce many proteases, ranging from uPA to a variety of matrix metalloproteinases, to degrade the basement membrane in order to create a channel for tumor cell invasion. In our recent study, we found that the EMT/invasiveness of tumor cells was dramatically enhanced when they were co-cultured with macrophages or macrophage-conditioned medium (Wu, Deng et al. 2009). We showed that this effect, mainly mediated by the secretion of TNFα from macrophages as neutralization of TNFα by TNFα antibody, greatly suppressed macrophage-mediated tumor cell invasion and metastasis(Wu, Deng et al. 2009). Consistent with our finding, Hagemann et al found that co-culturing macrophages with tumor cells enhanced their invasive ability in a manner dependent on TNFα and matrix metalloproteinases (MMP)(Hagemann, Wilson et al. 2005). Interestingly, expression of Snail in the non-metastatic breast cancer cell lines MCF7 and T47D, which contain little endogenous Snail, greatly increased the invasiveness of these cells by inflammation, indicating that Snail, through the induction of EMT, is critical for mediating inflammation-induced invasion/metastasis of breast cancer cells. Knockdown Snail expression significantly inhibited cell migration and invasion induced by inflammatory cytokines; it also suppressed inflammation-mediated breast cancer metastasis in animal model. Thus, macrophages, the major inflammatory component of the stroma in malignancies, facilitate angiogenesis, extracellular matrix breakdown, invasion, and metastasis through multiple mechanisms.

4.2 T-reg cells

Regulatory T cells (Treg), which include many populations that differ in phenotype, cytokine secretion profile and suppressive mechanism (Maloy and Powrie 2001; Shevach 2002; Wood and Sakaguchi 2003), were reported to interact with tumor cells, promoting rather than inhibiting cancer development and progression. High Treg levels have been found in peripheral blood, lymph nodes, and tumor specimens from patients with different types of cancer (Wang 2008). Treg have been characterized by the constitutive expression of Forkhead box P3 (FoxP3), glucocorticoid-induecd THFR family-related receptor (GITR), cytotoxic T lymphocyte associated antigen 4 (CTLA-4), and high levels of the alpha chain of the IL-2 receptor (CD25). It was found that Treg numbers were significantly higher in patients with metastatic cancer compared to healthy donors (Audia, Nicolas et al. 2007; Watanabe, Oda et al. 2010).

The level of FoxP3, an indicator of Treg activity, might also be an indicator of breast tumorigenesis (Gupta, Joshi et al. 2007). It has been demonstrated that high numbers of FoxP3-positive Tregs were present in high-grade tumors, increasing the risk of relapse/metastasis (Bates, Fox et al. 2006). Interestingly, the FoxP3 transcription factor, recently found to be expressed in tumor cells, can regulate a large number of genes. Besides, FoxP3 binds to the gene region upstream of the transcriptional start site of CCR7 and CXCR4 (Zheng and Rudensky 2007), two chemokine receptors recently reported to play an important role in cancer invasion and metastasis (Kodama, Hasengaowa et al. 2007; Pitkin, Luangdilok et al. 2007). Thus, FoxP3 expressed in breast cancer cells might influence metastasis by modulating the expression of these chemokine receptors or other genes, which encode cell surface or secrete molecules that regulate the response of tumor cells to the microenvironment (Merlo, Casalini et al. 2009).

Recently, it has been demonstrated that pulmonary metastasis of breast cancer requires recruitment and expansion of Treg that promote escape from host protective immune cells. Arya Biragyn's group reported that the primary role of tBregs (tumor-evoked Bregs) in lung metastases of breast cancer in the mouse 4T1 model is to induce TGF-β–dependent conversion of FoxP3+ Tregs from resting CD4+ T cells. In the absence of tBregs, 4T1 tumors cannot metastasize into the lungs efficiently due to poor Treg conversion, which suggest that tBregs must be controlled to interrupt the initiation of a key cancer-induced-immunosuppressive event that is critical to support cancer metastasis.(Olkhanud, Damdinsuren et al. 2011)

Tregs were selectively recruited within lymphoid infiltrates and activated by mature dendritic cells likely through the recognition of tumor-associated antigen presentation, which result in the prevention of effector T cell activation, immune escape, and ultimately, tumor progression (Gobert, Treilleux et al. 2009). Treg depletion may become a successful anticancer strategy, and Treg manipulation in terms of frequency and functional activity should be added to the therapeutic regimen to enhance tumor immunity in humans (Wolf, Wolf et al. 2003).

4.3 Myeloid-Drived Suppressor Cells (MDSC) and others

Myeloid-derived suppressor cells (MDSC) are present in many cancer patients and mice with transplanted or spontaneous tumors (Young and Lathers 1999; Almand, Clark et al. 2001). MDSC, characterized as CD11b+ Gr-1+ in mice, can be recruited and activated by multiple factors, such as VEGF, IL-1β and IL-6, many of which are associated with chronic inflammation (Gabrilovich and Nagaraj 2009). Recent studies indicated that these cells also have a crucial role in tumor progression. MDSCs can directly incorporate into tumor endothelium. They secret many pro-angiogenic factors as well. In addition, they play an essential role in cancer invasion and metastasis through inducing the production of matrix metalloproteinases (MMPs), chemoattractants and creating a pre-metastatic environment. Recruitment of MDSCs further produces pro-inflammatory factors, resulting in the amplification of the pro-inflammatory response. MDSCs not only suppress the adaptive immune responses but also regulate innate immune responses by modulating the cytokine production of macrophages (Sinha, Clements et al. 2007), thus directly facilitating metastasis. Recent studies have shown a close correlation between the level of MDSCs and cancer stage, metastatic tumor burden, and responsiveness to chemotherapy (Diaz-Montero,

Salem et al. 2009). MDSCs from mammary carcinoma can promote tumor invasion and metastasis (Bunt, Yang et al. 2007). In Tgfbr2-decificent mice, MDSCs are concentrated at the invasive tumor front and facilitate tumor cell invasion and metastasis through chemokine receptors CXCR2 and CXCR4 (Yang, Huang et al. 2008). It has been recently found that MDSCs accumulated in pregnant mice and exerted an inhibitory effect on NK cell activity, and decreased NK cell activity is responsible for the observed increase in metastasis during murine gestation, providing a candidate mechanism for the enhanced metastatic tumor growth observed in gestant mice.(Mauti, Le Bitoux et al. 2011)

In addition to macrophages and MDSC, fibroblasts/myofibroblasts comprise another major component of tumor stroma. These cancer-associated fibroblasts (CAF) share a lot of characteristics with activated fibroblasts in wound healing and promote tumor progression. Recent studies have demonstrated that CAF are important in tumor cell migration and metastasis. CAF isolated from metastatic breast cancer produce elevated levels of IL-6 and enhance cancer cell invasiveness (Studebaker, Storci et al. 2008). Similarly, De Wever et al found that the invasive growth of breast and colon cancer cells could be stimulated using myofibroblasts isolated from surgical colon cancer specimens (De Wever, Westbroek et al. 2004). In addition, CAF in pancreatic ductal adenocarcinoma are responsible for a poorly vascularized architecture that imposes a barrier for drug delivery and spurs metastasis (Olive, Jacobetz et al. 2009). Furthermore, fibroblasts promote tumor cell proliferation and metastasis through the production of several growth factors, cytokines, chemokines, and matrix metalloproteinases (MMPs). MMPs derived from tumor cells and stromal components are regarded as major players in assisting the metastasis of tumor cells. For example, transgenic expression of MMP3 stimulates expression of Snail through the increased cellular reactive oxygen species, inducing down-regulation of E-cadherin and increased tumor progression (Radisky, Levy et al. 2005). Besides, Reisfeld's group demonstrated recently that CAF are key modulators of immune polarization in the tumor microenvironment of a 4T1 murine model of metastatic breast cancer. Elimination of CAF in vivo by a DNA vaccine targeted to fibroblast activation protein results in a shift of the immune microenvironment from a Th2 to Th1 polarization. This shift is characterized by increased protein expression of IL-2 and IL-7, suppressed recruitment of tumor-associated macrophages, myeloid derived suppressor cells, T regulatory cells, and decreased tumor angiogenesis and lymphangiogenesis. (Liao, Luo et al. 2009)

Neutrophils are also noted as important cells in the tumor inflammatory microenvironment. CXCR2 can induce the expression of matrix metalloproteinase 9 (MMP9) and vascular endothelial growth factor (VEGF) to recruit neutrophils (Albini, Mirisola et al. 2008). This subsequently leads to endothelial cell invasion and blood vessel formation. On the other hand, there are reports demonstrated that neutrophils accumulate in the lung prior to the arrival of metastatic cells in mouse models of breast cancer. Those tumor entrained neutrophils (TENs) inhibit metastatic seeding in the lungs by generating H2O2. TENs are present in the peripheral blood of breast cancer patients prior to surgical resection but not in healthy individuals. Thus, whereas tumor-secreted factors contribute to tumor progression at the primary site, they concomitantly induce a neutrophil-mediated inhibitory process at the metastatic site. These neutrophils acquire a cytotoxic phenotype and provide anti-metastatic protection by eliminating disseminated tumor cells. Although the neutrophils are eventually outcompeted by continued influx of metastatic cells, infusion of exogenous neutrophils effectively blocks metastasis and therefore represents a potential therapeutic strategy for management of micro-metastatic disease.(Granot, Henke et al. 2011)

Taken together, all of these infiltrated inflammatory cells secret different cytokines, chemokines, and other factors to influence the tumor cell migration and invasion and contribute to inflammation-mediated metastasis.

4.4 Cytokines

TNF-α, a key inflammatory cytokine, plays a central role in tumor progression. Constitutive expression of TNF-α from the tumor microenvironment is a characteristic of many malignant tumors and its presence is often associated with poor prognosis. Several lines of evidence point to the tumor-promoting effects of TNF-α in inflammation-driven tumorigenesis. First, overexpression of TNF-α confers migratory and invasive properties of many tumor cell lines (Rosen, Goldberg et al. 1991). Second, TNF-α and TNF-α receptor 1 (TNFR1) knock-out mice are resistant to chemical-induced-carcinogenesis in skin and liver metastasis in an experimental colon cancer model (Knight, Yeoh et al. 2000; Arnott, Scott et al. 2004). Third, various tumor-promoting effects of TNF-α are further confirmed in enhancing tumor cell motility, activating oncogenic pathways, and triggering EMT. TNF-α can also promote breast cancer cell migration through up-regulating LOX (Liang, Zhang et al. 2007). Endogenous TNFα contributes to the growth and invasiveness of primary pancreatic ductal adenocarcinoma, and anti-TNFα inhibit metastasis of these tumors (Egberts, Cloosters et al. 2008). Using RNA interference technology, Kulbe et al demonstrated that tumor growth and dissemination were significantly inhibited when TNFα production was blocked (Kulbe, Thompson et al. 2007). In addition, TNF-α can up-regulate SELECTIN and VCAM1 on endothelial cells that promote tumor cell adhesion and migration (Mannel, Orosz et al. 1994; Stoelcker, Hafner et al. 1995). Furthermore, TNF-α enhances the invasive property of cancer cells by inducing EMT through Snail or ZEB1/ZEB2 (Chua, Bhat-Nakshatri et al. 2007; Chuang, Sun et al. 2008). In our recent study, we found that inflammatory cytokine TNF-α is the major signal to induce Snail stabilization and EMT induction (Wu, Deng et al. 2009). We showed that TNF-α greatly enhanced the migration and invasion of tumor cells by inducing EMT program through NF-κB-mediated Snail stabilization. Knockdown of Snail expression not only inhibits TNF-α-induced cancer cell migration and invasion in vitro but also suppresses LPS-mediated metastasis in vivo. Furthermore, knockdown of Snail expression not only blocks metastasis that is intrinsic to the metastatic breast cancer cells but also greatly suppresses inflammation-accelerated metastasis. Collectively, our study indicates that Snail stabilization and EMT induction mediated by the inflammatory cytokine TNF-α are critical for metastasis. Our study provides a plausible molecular mechanism for tumor cell dissemination and invasion at the tumor invasive front.

In fact, under hypoxic and inflammatory conditions, the tumor microenvironment generates and sustains a tumor-promoting cytokine network for facilitating tumor growth and metastasis. For example, the production of TGF-β from myeloid cells, mesenchymal cells, and cancer cells is significantly enhanced in a hypoxic or inflammatory state. TGF-β is a multifunctional growth factor with a complicated dual role in tumorigenesis(Leivonen and Kahari 2007). At the early stages of tumor formation, TGF-β acts as a tumor suppressor by inhibiting proliferation and inducing apoptosis of tumor cells. At the later stages of tumorigenesis, TGF-β functions as a tumor promoter by increasing tumor growth, survival, motility, and invasion. TGF-β has also been shown to induce EMT in normal mammary epithelial cells and breast cancer cell lines (Miettinen, Ebner et al. 1994) (Forrester, Chytil et al. 2005). As we mentioned in part-2.5 (Molecular regulation of EMT), TGF-β plays an important role in the process of EMT.

IL-6 is another important inflammatory cytokine linking inflammation and cancer. IL-6 transmits its signal through a common signaling receptor, gp130, expressed in many cell types. IL-6 binds to the sIL-6R receptor (gp80, present either on the cell surface or in solution), which then induces dimerization of gp130 chains, resulting in activation of the associated Janus kinases (JAKs). JAKs phosphorylate gp130, leading to the recruitment and activation of the STAT3 and STAT1 transcription factors, as well as other molecules (SHP2, Ras-MAPK, and PI3K) (Mumm and Oft 2008). The role of IL-6 in accelerating tumorigenesis is becoming clear as exogenous administration of IL-6 to mice during tumor initiation results in an increase in tumor burden and multiplicity (Grivennikov, Karin et al. 2009). IL-6 also enhances tumor proliferation in tumor-initiating intestinal epithelial cells (IECs) through NF-κB-IL-6-STAT3 cascade (Bollrath, Phesse et al. 2009; Bromberg and Wang 2009; Grivennikov, Karin et al. 2009). IL-6 can also act as an inducer of EMT in breast cancer cells. Ectopic expression of IL-6 in breast adenocarcinoma cells exhibits an EMT phenotype characterized by suppressing E-cadherin expression and inducting vimentin, N-cadherin, Snail and Twist (Sullivan, Sasser et al. 2009). In addition, IL-6 also synergizes with EGF in inducing EMT through the activation JNK2/STAT3 in ovarian carcinomas (Colomiere, Ward et al. 2009).

The interleukin-1 (IL-1) also promotes inflammatory processes and augments metastasis. There are two forms of IL-1 protein, IL-1α and IL-1β, and one antagonistic protein IL-1 receptor antagonist (IL-1ra). IL-1β is active solely in its secreted form, whereas IL-1α is active mainly as an intracellular precursor. IL-1 is abundant at tumor sites, where it affects the process of carcinogenesis, tumor growth and invasiveness, and the patterns of tumor-host interactions (Apte, Krelin et al. 2006). Genetic ablation of IL-1β in mice results in the absence of metastatic tumors in vivo (Voronov, Shouval et al. 2003). Liver metastasis can be almost completely inhibited in mice with deletion of the interleukin-1β converting enzyme, which is required for the processing of IL-1β (Vidal-Vanaclocha, Fantuzzi et al. 2000). IL-1β also directly induces uPA expression and NF-κB activation, which results in the migration of A549 cells (Cheng, Hsieh et al. 2009).

Together with chemotaxis, chemokines, a family of inducible chemo-attractant cytokines that regulate the chemotaxis of tumor cells and other cell types, are thought to be involved in every crucial step of tumor cell dissemination (Roussos, Condeelis et al. 2011). Chemotaxis of carcinoma cells and tumor-associated inflammatory and stromal cells is mediated by chemokines, chemokine receptors, growth factors and growth factor receptors. Chemotaxis helps to shape the tumor microenvironment. Directional migration to a chemokine source is evident both in vitro and in vivo for most cells of the tumor microenvironment. The most common chemokine receptor detected in cancer cells is CXCR4; another common one is CCR7 (Muller, Homey et al. 2001; Lazennec and Richmond 2010). In standard chemotaxis assays in vitro, CXCR4-positive cancer cells can migrate in a directional manner toward CXCL12, whereas CCR7-expressing cancer cells can migrate towards CCL21 (Kodama, Hasengaowa et al. 2007; Pitkin, Luangdilok et al. 2007). Recently, it has been reported that the recruitment of inflammatory monocytes, which express CCR2, is dependent on CCL2 synthesized by both the tumor and the stroma, facilitating breast-tumor metastasis; the same is true for the subsequent recruitment of metastasis-associated macrophages and their interaction with metastasizing tumor cells (Qian, Li et al. 2011).

5. Summary

Every year about 500,000 people in the United States die as a result of cancer, among which 90% exhibit systemic disease with metastasis. That's why it is so important to understand the mechanism behind EMT and metastasis. Based on thousands of studies in this field in recent years, significant progress has been made regarding our understanding of EMT and metastasis, which point out that EMT is the most critical mechanism implicated in tumor metastasis and recurrence. It is now quite clearly that solid tumors are not simply clones of cancer cells. A variety of stromal cells in the surrounding environment are recruited to tumors, which including mesenchymal supporting cells (e.g. fibroblasts), cells of the vascular system, and cells from immune system, such as TAMs, Treg, MDSC, Neutrophils and so on. The dynamic interaction which exists between cancer cells and the inflammatory microenvironment not only enhances growth of the primary cancer but also facilitates its metastatic dissemination to distant organs. There are many evidences show that the induction of EMT is dependent on the signals that cells received from their microenvironment, and the crosstalk between inflammation and metastasis has an un-replaceable role in each step for the successful establishment of a metastatic tumor (Fig. 2).

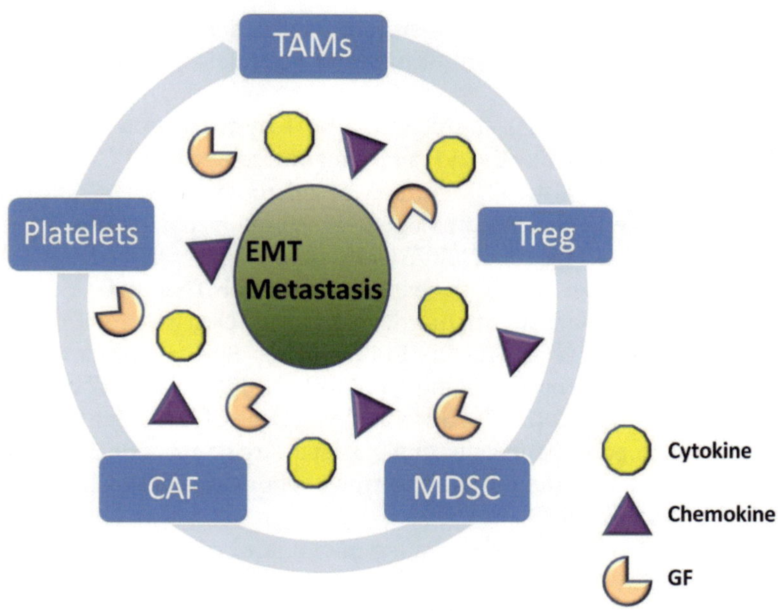

Fig. 2. Tumor Inflammatory Microenvironment in EMT and Metastasis.

Understanding how inflammatory microenvironment is maintained and how it contributes to the tumor progression and metastasis will be crucial for understanding tumor biology as well as the development of new effective cancer prevention and therapy. Hopefully, with recent research illuminating the involvement of infiltrated inflammatory cells and many kinds of cytokines in tumor progression and EMT/Metastasis, a more comprehensive view of how cancer cells spreads to different organs in a specific manner will emerge in the near future. However, we have to realize that several challenges still need to be addressed about how to translate these basic findings into clinical practice and find novel treatment strategies targeting the inflammatory microenvironment which could efficiently kill both primary and metastatic tumor cells.

6. Acknowledgement

We apologize to those whose work is important but that we are unable to cite here due to the limitation of space. We thank Dr. Nathan L. Vanderford for critical reading and editing of this manuscript. Our study is supported by the grants from NIH (RO1CA125454), the Susan G Komen Foundation (KG081310), and the Mary Kay Ash Foundation (to B.P. Zhou).

7. References

Albini, A., V. Mirisola, et al. (2008). "Metastasis signatures: genes regulating tumor-microenvironment interactions predict metastatic behavior." *Cancer Metastasis Rev* 27(1): 75-83.

Allington, T. M., A. J. Galliher-Beckley, et al. (2009). "Activated Abl kinase inhibits oncogenic transforming growth factor-{beta} signaling and tumorigenesis in mammary tumors." *FASEB J.*

Almand, B., J. I. Clark, et al. (2001). "Increased production of immature myeloid cells in cancer patients: a mechanism of immunosuppression in cancer." *J Immunol* 166(1): 678-689.

Ansieau, S., J. Bastid, et al. (2008). "Induction of EMT by twist proteins as a collateral effect of tumor-promoting inactivation of premature senescence." *Cancer Cell* 14(1): 79-89.

Apte, R. N., Y. Krelin, et al. (2006). "Effects of micro-environment- and malignant cell-derived interleukin-1 in carcinogenesis, tumour invasiveness and tumour-host interactions." *Eur J Cancer* 42(6): 751-759.

Arnott, C. H., K. A. Scott, et al. (2004). "Expression of both TNF-alpha receptor subtypes is essential for optimal skin tumour development." *Oncogene* 23(10): 1902-1910.

Arnoux, V., M. Nassour, et al. (2008). "Erk5 controls Slug expression and keratinocyte activation during wound healing." *Mol Biol Cell* 19(11): 4738-4749.

Audia, S., A. Nicolas, et al. (2007). "Increase of CD4+ CD25+ regulatory T cells in the peripheral blood of patients with metastatic carcinoma: a Phase I clinical trial using cyclophosphamide and immunotherapy to eliminate CD4+ CD25+ T lymphocytes." *Clin Exp Immunol* 150(3): 523-530.

Balkwill, F. and A. Mantovani (2001). "Inflammation and cancer: back to Virchow?" *Lancet* 357(9255): 539-545.

Bataille, F., C. Rohrmeier, et al. (2008). "Evidence for a role of epithelial mesenchymal transition during pathogenesis of fistulae in Crohn's disease." *Inflamm Bowel Dis* 14(11): 1514-1527.

Bates, G. J., S. B. Fox, et al. (2006). "Quantification of regulatory T cells enables the identification of high-risk breast cancer patients and those at risk of late relapse." *J Clin Oncol* 24(34): 5373-5380.

Bhowmick, N. A., M. Ghiassi, et al. (2001). "Transforming growth factor-beta1 mediates epithelial to mesenchymal transdifferentiation through a RhoA-dependent mechanism." *Mol Biol Cell* 12(1): 27-36.

Bollrath, J., T. J. Phesse, et al. (2009). "gp130-mediated Stat3 activation in enterocytes regulates cell survival and cell-cycle progression during colitis-associated tumorigenesis." *Cancer Cell* 15(2): 91-102.

Bos, P. D., X. H. Zhang, et al. (2009). "Genes that mediate breast cancer metastasis to the brain." *Nature* 459(7249): 1005-1009.

Bromberg, J. and T. C. Wang (2009). "Inflammation and cancer: IL-6 and STAT3 complete the link." *Cancer Cell* 15(2): 79-80.

Bruyere, F., B. Namdarian, et al. (2009). "Snail expression is an independent predictor of tumor recurrence in superficial bladder cancers." *Urol Oncol.*

Buijs, J. T., N. V. Henriquez, et al. (2007). "TGF-beta and BMP7 interactions in tumour progression and bone metastasis." *Clin Exp Metastasis* 24(8): 609-617.

Bunt, S. K., L. Yang, et al. (2007). "Reduced inflammation in the tumor microenvironment delays the accumulation of myeloid-derived suppressor cells and limits tumor progression." *Cancer Res* 67(20): 10019-10026.

Chambers, A. F., A. C. Groom, et al. (2002). "Dissemination and growth of cancer cells in metastatic sites." *Nat Rev Cancer* 2(8): 563-572.

Chambers, A. F., G. N. Naumov, et al. (2001). "Critical steps in hematogenous metastasis: an overview." *Surg Oncol Clin N Am* 10(2): 243-255, vii.

Cheng, C. Y., H. L. Hsieh, et al. (2009). "IL-1 beta induces urokinase-plasminogen activator expression and cell migration through PKC alpha, JNK1/2, and NF-kappaB in A549 cells." *J Cell Physiol* 219(1): 183-193.

Christofori, G. (2006). "New signals from the invasive front." *Nature* 441(7092): 444-450.

Chua, H. L., P. Bhat-Nakshatri, et al. (2007). "NF-kappaB represses E-cadherin expression and enhances epithelial to mesenchymal transition of mammary epithelial cells: potential involvement of ZEB-1 and ZEB-2." *Oncogene* 26(5): 711-724.

Chuang, M. J., K. H. Sun, et al. (2008). "Tumor-derived tumor necrosis factor-alpha promotes progression and epithelial-mesenchymal transition in renal cell carcinoma cells." *Cancer Sci* 99(5): 905-913.

Colomiere, M., A. C. Ward, et al. (2009). "Cross talk of signals between EGFR and IL-6R through JAK2/STAT3 mediate epithelial-mesenchymal transition in ovarian carcinomas." *Br J Cancer* 100(1): 134-144.

Condeelis, J. and J. W. Pollard (2006). "Macrophages: obligate partners for tumor cell migration, invasion, and metastasis." *Cell* 124(2): 263-266.

Coussens, L. M. and Z. Werb (2002). "Inflammation and cancer." *Nature* 420(6917): 860-867.

Cowin, P., T. M. Rowlands, et al. (2005). "Cadherins and catenins in breast cancer." *Curr Opin Cell Biol* 17(5): 499-508.

Davidson, L. A., M. Marsden, et al. (2006). "Integrin alpha5beta1 and fibronectin regulate polarized cell protrusions required for Xenopus convergence and extension." *Curr Biol* 16(9): 833-844.

de Visser, K. E., A. Eichten, et al. (2006). "Paradoxical roles of the immune system during cancer development." *Nat Rev Cancer* 6(1): 24-37.

De Wever, O., W. Westbroek, et al. (2004). "Critical role of N-cadherin in myofibroblast invasion and migration in vitro stimulated by colon-cancer-cell-derived TGF-beta or wounding." *J Cell Sci* 117(Pt 20): 4691-4703.

Diaz-Montero, C. M., M. L. Salem, et al. (2009). "Increased circulating myeloid-derived suppressor cells correlate with clinical cancer stage, metastatic tumor burden, and doxorubicin-cyclophosphamide chemotherapy." *Cancer Immunol Immunother* 58(1): 49-59.

Dighe, A. S., E. Richards, et al. (1994). "Enhanced in vivo growth and resistance to rejection of tumor cells expressing dominant negative IFN gamma receptors." *Immunity* 1(6): 447-456.

DiMeo, T. A., K. Anderson, et al. (2009). "A novel lung metastasis signature links Wnt signaling with cancer cell self-renewal and epithelial-mesenchymal transition in basal-like breast cancer." *Cancer Res* 69(13): 5364-5373.

Egberts, J. H., V. Cloosters, et al. (2008). "Anti-tumor necrosis factor therapy inhibits pancreatic tumor growth and metastasis." *Cancer Res* 68(5): 1443-1450.

Elloul, S., M. B. Elstrand, et al. (2005). "Snail, Slug, and Smad-interacting protein 1 as novel parameters of disease aggressiveness in metastatic ovarian and breast carcinoma." *Cancer* 103(8): 1631-1643.

Feldmann, G., S. Dhara, et al. (2007). "Blockade of hedgehog signaling inhibits pancreatic cancer invasion and metastases: a new paradigm for combination therapy in solid cancers." *Cancer Res* 67(5): 2187-2196.

Fiaschi, M., B. Rozell, et al. (2007). "Targeted expression of GLI1 in the mammary gland disrupts pregnancy-induced maturation and causes lactation failure." *J Biol Chem* 282(49): 36090-36101.

Fidler, I. J. (2003). "The pathogenesis of cancer metastasis: the 'seed and soil' hypothesis revisited." *Nat Rev Cancer* 3(6): 453-458.

Flanders, K. C. (2004). "Smad3 as a mediator of the fibrotic response." *Int J Exp Pathol* 85(2): 47-64.

Forrester, E., A. Chytil, et al. (2005). "Effect of conditional knockout of the type II TGF-beta receptor gene in mammary epithelia on mammary gland development and polyomavirus middle T antigen induced tumor formation and metastasis." *Cancer Res* 65(6): 2296-2302.

Franci, C., M. Takkunen, et al. (2006). "Expression of Snail protein in tumor-stroma interface." *Oncogene* 25(37): 5134-5144.

Gabrilovich, D. I. and S. Nagaraj (2009). "Myeloid-derived suppressor cells as regulators of the immune system." *Nat Rev Immunol* 9(3): 162-174.

Girardi, M., D. E. Oppenheim, et al. (2001). "Regulation of cutaneous malignancy by gammadelta T cells." *Science* 294(5542): 605-609.

Gobert, M., I. Treilleux, et al. (2009). "Regulatory T cells recruited through CCL22/CCR4 are selectively activated in lymphoid infiltrates surrounding primary breast tumors and lead to an adverse clinical outcome." *Cancer Res* 69(5): 2000-2009.

Granot, Z., E. Henke, et al. (2011). "Tumor entrained neutrophils inhibit seeding in the premetastatic lung." *Cancer Cell* 20(3): 300-314.

Greenburg, G. and E. D. Hay (1988). "Cytoskeleton and thyroglobulin expression change during transformation of thyroid epithelium to mesenchyme-like cells." *Development* 102(3): 605-622.

Grego-Bessa, J., J. Diez, et al. (2004). "Notch and epithelial-mesenchyme transition in development and tumor progression: another turn of the screw." *Cell Cycle* 3(6): 718-721.

Gressner, A. M., R. Weiskirchen, et al. (2002). "Roles of TGF-beta in hepatic fibrosis." *Front Biosci* 7: d793-807.

Grivennikov, S., E. Karin, et al. (2009). "IL-6 and Stat3 are required for survival of intestinal epithelial cells and development of colitis-associated cancer." *Cancer Cell* 15(2): 103-113.

Grivennikov, S. I., F. R. Greten, et al. (2010). "Immunity, inflammation, and cancer." *Cell* 140(6): 883-899.

Gupta, S., K. Joshi, et al. (2007). "Intratumoral FOXP3 expression in infiltrating breast carcinoma: Its association with clinicopathologic parameters and angiogenesis." *Acta Oncol* 46(6): 792-797.

Hagemann, T., J. Wilson, et al. (2005). "Macrophages induce invasiveness of epithelial cancer cells via NF-kappa B and JNK." *J Immunol* 175(2): 1197-1205.

Hanahan, D. and R. A. Weinberg (2011). "Hallmarks of cancer: the next generation." *Cell* 144(5): 646-674.

Hartwell, K. A., B. Muir, et al. (2006). "The Spemann organizer gene, Goosecoid, promotes tumor metastasis." *Proc Natl Acad Sci U S A* 103(50): 18969-18974.

Hay, E. D. (1995). "An overview of epithelio-mesenchymal transformation." *Acta Anat (Basel)* 154(1): 8-20.

Hooper, J. E. and M. P. Scott (2005). "Communicating with Hedgehogs." *Nat Rev Mol Cell Biol* 6(4): 306-317.

Huber, M. A., N. Kraut, et al. (2005). "Molecular requirements for epithelial-mesenchymal transition during tumor progression." *Curr Opin Cell Biol* 17(5): 548-558.

Isohata, N., K. Aoyagi, et al. (2009). "Hedgehog and epithelial-mesenchymal transition signaling in normal and malignant epithelial cells of the esophagus." *Int J Cancer* 125(5): 1212-1221.

Jacob, L. and L. Lum (2007). "Deconstructing the hedgehog pathway in development and disease." *Science* 318(5847): 66-68.

Janda, E., K. Lehmann, et al. (2002). "Ras and TGF[beta] cooperatively regulate epithelial cell plasticity and metastasis: dissection of Ras signaling pathways." *J Cell Biol* 156(2): 299-313.

Joyce, J. A. and J. W. Pollard (2009). "Microenvironmental regulation of metastasis." *Nat Rev Cancer* 9(4): 239-252.

Junghans, D., I. G. Haas, et al. (2005). "Mammalian cadherins and protocadherins: about cell death, synapses and processing." *Curr Opin Cell Biol* 17(5): 446-452.

Kalluri, R. (2009). "EMT: when epithelial cells decide to become mesenchymal-like cells." *J Clin Invest* 119(6): 1417-1419.

Kalluri, R. and E. G. Neilson (2003). "Epithelial-mesenchymal transition and its implications for fibrosis." *J Clin Invest* 112(12): 1776-1784.

Kalluri, R. and R. A. Weinberg (2009). "The basics of epithelial-mesenchymal transition." *J Clin Invest* 119(6): 1420-1428.

Kaplan, D. H., V. Shankaran, et al. (1998). "Demonstration of an interferon gamma-dependent tumor surveillance system in immunocompetent mice." *Proc Natl Acad Sci U S A* 95(13): 7556-7561.

Knight, B., G. C. Yeoh, et al. (2000). "Impaired preneoplastic changes and liver tumor formation in tumor necrosis factor receptor type 1 knockout mice." *J Exp Med* 192(12): 1809-1818.

Kodama, J., Hasengaowa, et al. (2007). "Association of CXCR4 and CCR7 chemokine receptor expression and lymph node metastasis in human cervical cancer." *Ann Oncol* 18(1): 70-76.

Kudo-Saito, C., H. Shirako, et al. (2009). "Cancer metastasis is accelerated through immunosuppression during Snail-induced EMT of cancer cells." *Cancer Cell* 15(3): 195-206.

Kulbe, H., R. Thompson, et al. (2007). "The inflammatory cytokine tumor necrosis factor-alpha generates an autocrine tumor-promoting network in epithelial ovarian cancer cells." *Cancer Res* 67(2): 585-592.

Lazennec, G. and A. Richmond (2010). "Chemokines and chemokine receptors: new insights into cancer-related inflammation." *Trends Mol Med* 16(3): 133-144.

Lee, Y. H., A. R. Albig, et al. (2008). "Fibulin-5 initiates epithelial-mesenchymal transition (EMT) and enhances EMT induced by TGF-beta in mammary epithelial cells via a MMP-dependent mechanism." *Carcinogenesis* 29(12): 2243-2251.

Leivonen, S. K. and V. M. Kahari (2007). "Transforming growth factor-beta signaling in cancer invasion and metastasis." *Int J Cancer* 121(10): 2119-2124.

Leong, K. G., K. Niessen, et al. (2007). "Jagged1-mediated Notch activation induces epithelial-to-mesenchymal transition through Slug-induced repression of E-cadherin." *J Exp Med* 204(12): 2935-2948.

Li, X., W. Deng, et al. (2007). "Gli1 acts through Snail and E-cadherin to promote nuclear signaling by beta-catenin." *Oncogene* 26(31): 4489-4498.

Li, X., W. Deng, et al. (2006). "Snail induction is an early response to Gli1 that determines the efficiency of epithelial transformation." *Oncogene* 25(4): 609-621.

Li, Y., W. P. Hively, et al. (2000). "Use of MMTV-Wnt-1 transgenic mice for studying the genetic basis of breast cancer." *Oncogene* 19(8): 1002-1009.

Liang, M., P. Zhang, et al. (2007). "Up-regulation of LOX-1 expression by TNF-alpha promotes trans-endothelial migration of MDA-MB-231 breast cancer cells." *Cancer Lett* 258(1): 31-37.

Liao, D., Y. Luo, et al. (2009). "Cancer associated fibroblasts promote tumor growth and metastasis by modulating the tumor immune microenvironment in a 4T1 murine breast cancer model." *PLoS One* 4(11): e7965.

Lin, E. Y., A. V. Nguyen, et al. (2001). "Colony-stimulating factor 1 promotes progression of mammary tumors to malignancy." *J Exp Med* 193(6): 727-740.

Lunt, S. J., N. Chaudary, et al. (2009). "The tumor microenvironment and metastatic disease." *Clin Exp Metastasis* 26(1): 19-34.

Maloy, K. J. and F. Powrie (2001). "Regulatory T cells in the control of immune pathology." *Nat Immunol* 2(9): 816-822.

Mani, S. A., W. Guo, et al. (2008). "The epithelial-mesenchymal transition generates cells with properties of stem cells." *Cell* 133(4): 704-715.

Mannel, D. N., P. Orosz, et al. (1994). "Mechanisms involved in metastasis enhanced by inflammatory mediators." *Circ Shock* 44(1): 9-13.

Mantovani, A., P. Allavena, et al. (2008). "Cancer-related inflammation." *Nature* 454(7203): 436-444.

Mauti, L. A., M. A. Le Bitoux, et al. (2011). "Myeloid-derived suppressor cells are implicated in regulating permissiveness for tumor metastasis during mouse gestation." *J Clin Invest* 121(7): 2794-2807.

Merlo, A., P. Casalini, et al. (2009). "FOXP3 expression and overall survival in breast cancer." *J Clin Oncol* 27(11): 1746-1752.

Miettinen, P. J., R. Ebner, et al. (1994). "TGF-beta induced transdifferentiation of mammary epithelial cells to mesenchymal cells: involvement of type I receptors." *J Cell Biol* 127(6 Pt 2): 2021-2036.

Moody, S. E., D. Perez, et al. (2005). "The transcriptional repressor Snail promotes mammary tumor recurrence." *Cancer Cell* 8(3): 197-209.

Muller, A., B. Homey, et al. (2001). "Involvement of chemokine receptors in breast cancer metastasis." *Nature* 410(6824): 50-56.

Mumm, J. B. and M. Oft (2008). "Cytokine-based transformation of immune surveillance into tumor-promoting inflammation." *Oncogene* 27(45): 5913-5919.

Nawshad, A., D. Lagamba, et al. (2005). "Transforming growth factor-beta signaling during epithelial-mesenchymal transformation: implications for embryogenesis and tumor metastasis." *Cells Tissues Organs* 179(1-2): 11-23.

Neth, P., C. Ries, et al. (2007). "The Wnt signal transduction pathway in stem cells and cancer cells: influence on cellular invasion." *Stem Cell Rev* 3(1): 18-29.

Nieto, M. A. (2002). "The snail superfamily of zinc-finger transcription factors." *Nat Rev Mol Cell Biol* 3(3): 155-166.

Olive, K. P., M. A. Jacobetz, et al. (2009). "Inhibition of Hedgehog signaling enhances delivery of chemotherapy in a mouse model of pancreatic cancer." *Science* 324(5933): 1457-1461.

Olkhanud, P. B., B. Damdinsuren, et al. (2011). "Tumor-evoked regulatory B cells promote breast cancer metastasis by converting resting CD4 T cells to T-regulatory cells." *Cancer Res* 71(10): 3505-3515.

Ozdamar, B., R. Bose, et al. (2005). "Regulation of the polarity protein Par6 by TGFbeta receptors controls epithelial cell plasticity." *Science* 307(5715): 1603-1609.

Pantel, K. and R. H. Brakenhoff (2004). "Dissecting the metastatic cascade." *Nat Rev Cancer* 4(6): 448-456.

Pitkin, L., S. Luangdilok, et al. (2007). "Expression of CC chemokine receptor 7 in tonsillar cancer predicts cervical nodal metastasis, systemic relapse and survival." *Br J Cancer* 97(5): 670-677.

Pollard, J. W. (2004). "Tumour-educated macrophages promote tumour progression and metastasis." *Nat Rev Cancer* 4(1): 71-78.

Qian, B. Z., J. Li, et al. (2011). "CCL2 recruits inflammatory monocytes to facilitate breast-tumour metastasis." *Nature* 475(7355): 222-225.

Qian, F., Z. C. Zhang, et al. (2005). "Interaction between integrin alpha(5) and fibronectin is required for metastasis of B16F10 melanoma cells." *Biochem Biophys Res Commun* 333(4): 1269-1275.

Radisky, D. C., D. D. Levy, et al. (2005). "Rac1b and reactive oxygen species mediate MMP-3-induced EMT and genomic instability." *Nature* 436(7047): 123-127.

Rastaldi, M. P., F. Ferrario, et al. (2002). "Epithelial-mesenchymal transition of tubular epithelial cells in human renal biopsies." *Kidney Int* 62(1): 137-146.

Rosen, E. M., I. D. Goldberg, et al. (1991). "Tumor necrosis factor stimulates epithelial tumor cell motility." *Cancer Res* 51(19): 5315-5321.

Roussos, E. T., J. S. Condeelis, et al. (2011). "Chemotaxis in cancer." *Nat Rev Cancer* 11(8): 573-587.

Sahlgren, C., M. V. Gustafsson, et al. (2008). "Notch signaling mediates hypoxia-induced tumor cell migration and invasion." *Proc Natl Acad Sci U S A* 105(17): 6392-6397.

Salez, F., P. Gosset, et al. (1998). "Transforming growth factor-beta1 in sarcoidosis." *Eur Respir J* 12(4): 913-919.

Savagner, P., D. F. Kusewitt, et al. (2005). "Developmental transcription factor slug is required for effective re-epithelialization by adult keratinocytes." *J Cell Physiol* 202(3): 858-866.

Schreiber, R. D., L. J. Old, et al. "Cancer immunoediting: integrating immunity's roles in cancer suppression and promotion." *Science* 331(6024): 1565-1570.

Shankaran, V., H. Ikeda, et al. (2001). "IFNgamma and lymphocytes prevent primary tumour development and shape tumour immunogenicity." *Nature* 410(6832): 1107-1111.

Shevach, E. M. (2002). "CD4+ CD25+ suppressor T cells: more questions than answers." *Nat Rev Immunol* 2(6): 389-400.

Shook, D. and R. Keller (2003). "Mechanisms, mechanics and function of epithelial-mesenchymal transitions in early development." *Mech Dev* 120(11): 1351-1383.

Sinha, P., V. K. Clements, et al. (2007). "Cross-talk between myeloid-derived suppressor cells and macrophages subverts tumor immunity toward a type 2 response." *J Immunol* 179(2): 977-983.

Smyth, M. J., K. Y. Thia, et al. (2000). "Perforin-mediated cytotoxicity is critical for surveillance of spontaneous lymphoma." *J Exp Med* 192(5): 755-760.

Stemmer, V., B. de Craene, et al. (2008). "Snail promotes Wnt target gene expression and interacts with beta-catenin." *Oncogene* 27(37): 5075-5080.

Stoelcker, B., M. Hafner, et al. (1995). "Role of adhesion molecules and platelets in TNF-induced adhesion of tumor cells to endothelial cells: implications for experimental metastasis." *J Inflamm* 46(3): 155-167.

Street, S. E., J. A. Trapani, et al. (2002). "Suppression of lymphoma and epithelial malignancies effected by interferon gamma." *J Exp Med* 196(1): 129-134.

Studebaker, A. W., G. Storci, et al. (2008). "Fibroblasts isolated from common sites of breast cancer metastasis enhance cancer cell growth rates and invasiveness in an interleukin-6-dependent manner." *Cancer Res* 68(21): 9087-9095.

Sullivan, N. J., A. K. Sasser, et al. (2009). "Interleukin-6 induces an epithelial-mesenchymal transition phenotype in human breast cancer cells." *Oncogene*.

Timmerman, L. A., J. Grego-Bessa, et al. (2004). "Notch promotes epithelial-mesenchymal transition during cardiac development and oncogenic transformation." *Genes Dev* 18(1): 99-115.

Tse, J. C. and R. Kalluri (2007). "Mechanisms of metastasis: epithelial-to-mesenchymal transition and contribution of tumor microenvironment." *J Cell Biochem* 101(4): 816-829.

Valcourt, U., M. Kowanetz, et al. (2005). "TGF-beta and the Smad signaling pathway support transcriptomic reprogramming during epithelial-mesenchymal cell transition." *Mol Biol Cell* 16(4): 1987-2002.

Vidal-Vanaclocha, F., G. Fantuzzi, et al. (2000). "IL-18 regulates IL-1beta-dependent hepatic melanoma metastasis via vascular cell adhesion molecule-1." *Proc Natl Acad Sci U S A* 97(2): 734-739.

Villanueva, S., A. Glavic, et al. (2002). "Posteriorization by FGF, Wnt, and retinoic acid is required for neural crest induction." *Dev Biol* 241(2): 289-301.

Vincent, T., E. P. Neve, et al. (2009). "A SNAIL1-SMAD3/4 transcriptional repressor complex promotes TGF-beta mediated epithelial-mesenchymal transition." *Nat Cell Biol*.

Voronov, E., D. S. Shouval, et al. (2003). "IL-1 is required for tumor invasiveness and angiogenesis." *Proc Natl Acad Sci U S A* 100(5): 2645-2650.

Wang, R. F. (2008). "CD8+ regulatory T cells, their suppressive mechanisms, and regulation in cancer." *Hum Immunol* 69(11): 811-814.

Wang, X., J. Nie, et al. (2008). "Downregulation of Par-3 expression and disruption of Par complex integrity by TGF-beta during the process of epithelial to mesenchymal transition in rat proximal epithelial cells." *Biochim Biophys Acta* 1782(1): 51-59.

Wang, Z., Y. Li, et al. (2009). "Acquisition of epithelial-mesenchymal transition phenotype of gemcitabine-resistant pancreatic cancer cells is linked with activation of the notch signaling pathway." *Cancer Res* 69(6): 2400-2407.

Watanabe, M. A., J. M. Oda, et al. (2010). "Regulatory T cells and breast cancer: implications for immunopathogenesis." *Cancer Metastasis Rev* 29(4): 569-579.

White, L. R., J. B. Blanchette, et al. (2007). "The characterization of alpha5-integrin expression on tubular epithelium during renal injury." *Am J Physiol Renal Physiol* 292(2): F567-576.

Willis, B. C. and Z. Borok (2007). "TGF-beta-induced EMT: mechanisms and implications for fibrotic lung disease." *Am J Physiol Lung Cell Mol Physiol* 293(3): L525-534.

Wolf, A. M., D. Wolf, et al. (2003). "Increase of regulatory T cells in the peripheral blood of cancer patients." *Clin Cancer Res* 9(2): 606-612.

Wood, K. J. and S. Sakaguchi (2003). "Regulatory T cells in transplantation tolerance." *Nat Rev Immunol* 3(3): 199-210.

Woodhouse, E. C., R. F. Chuaqui, et al. (1997). "General mechanisms of metastasis." *Cancer* 80(8 Suppl): 1529-1537.

Wu, Y., J. Deng, et al. (2009). "Stabilization of snail by NF-kappaB is required for inflammation-induced cell migration and invasion." *Cancer Cell* 15(5): 416-428.

Yang, J., S. A. Mani, et al. (2004). "Twist, a master regulator of morphogenesis, plays an essential role in tumor metastasis." *Cell* 117(7): 927-939.

Yang, L., J. Huang, et al. (2008). "Abrogation of TGF beta signaling in mammary carcinomas recruits Gr-1+CD11b+ myeloid cells that promote metastasis." *Cancer Cell* 13(1): 23-35.

Yook, J. I., X. Y. Li, et al. (2005). "Wnt-dependent regulation of the E-cadherin repressor snail." *J Biol Chem* 280(12): 11740-11748.

Yook, J. I., X. Y. Li, et al. (2006). "A Wnt-Axin2-GSK3beta cascade regulates Snail1 activity in breast cancer cells." *Nat Cell Biol* 8(12): 1398-1406.

Young, M. R. and D. M. Lathers (1999). "Myeloid progenitor cells mediate immune suppression in patients with head and neck cancers." *Int J Immunopharmacol* 21(4): 241-252.

Zavadil, J. and E. P. Bottinger (2005). "TGF-beta and epithelial-to-mesenchymal transitions." *Oncogene* 24(37): 5764-5774.

Zavadil, J., L. Cermak, et al. (2004). "Integration of TGF-beta/Smad and Jagged1/Notch signalling in epithelial-to-mesenchymal transition." *EMBO J* 23(5): 1155-1165.

Zeisberg, E. M., O. Tarnavski, et al. (2007). "Endothelial-to-mesenchymal transition contributes to cardiac fibrosis." *Nat Med* 13(8): 952-961.

Zeisberg, M., C. Bottiglio, et al. (2003). "Bone morphogenic protein-7 inhibits progression of chronic renal fibrosis associated with two genetic mouse models." *Am J Physiol Renal Physiol* 285(6): F1060-1067.

Zeisberg, M., J. Hanai, et al. (2003). "BMP-7 counteracts TGF-beta1-induced epithelial-to-mesenchymal transition and reverses chronic renal injury." *Nat Med* 9(7): 964-968.

Zeisberg, M. and E. G. Neilson (2009). "Biomarkers for epithelial-mesenchymal transitions." *J Clin Invest* 119(6): 1429-1437.

Zheng, Y. and A. Y. Rudensky (2007). "Foxp3 in control of the regulatory T cell lineage." *Nat Immunol* 8(5): 457-462.

Zhou, B. P., J. Deng, et al. (2004). "Dual regulation of Snail by GSK-3beta-mediated phosphorylation in control of epithelial-mesenchymal transition." *Nat Cell Biol* 6(10): 931-940.

Part 2

Tumor Microenvironment and Myelomonocytic Cell Interaction in Specific Cancer Subtypes

7

Lung Tumor Microenvironment and Myelomonocytic Cells

Minu K. Srivastava, Åsa Andersson, Li Zhu, Marni Harris-White, Jay M. Lee, Steven Dubinett and Sherven Sharma
University of California Los Angeles and Veterans Affairs Greater Los Angeles, USA

1. Introduction

The lung tumor microenvironment consists of tumor cells, stroma, blood vessels, immune infiltrates and the extracellular matrix. Genetic alterations in oncogenes and tumor suppressor genes or epigenetic changes in the tumor that modulate tumor growth and invasion into the surrounding tissue orchestrate the persistence of inflammatory infiltrates. These cellular infiltrates modulate tumor development and progression. The infiltrates vary by size and composition in diverse tumor types and at different stages of tumor development. The lung tumor programs the cellular infiltrates and dysregulates inflammation to sustain tumor growth, progression and hypo responsiveness of the tumor. Characterization of the complex interactions among the infiltrates and lung cancer will aid in defining their role in tumor progression. This understanding will be important for the development of novel anticancer therapies. Although this is not a trivial undertaking, the information garnered will take us a step closer to personalized medicine. If we know an individual's lung tumor inflammatory infiltrates, we will be able to predict the risk of tumor progression and then give specific treatment to reprogram the tumor microenvironment to control the disease.

Contributing to the inflammatory infiltrates are members of the innate system including natural killer cells (NK) and the cells of the myelomonocytic lineage consisting of immature macrophages, granulocytes, dendritic cells (DC) as well as myeloid cells at earlier stages of differentiation (Sica and Bronte 2007; Talmadge 2007; Gabrilovich and Nagaraj 2009; Peranzoni et al. 2010). The down regulation of MHC expression by tumors enables them to evade T cell immune responses. The presence of NK cells in the infiltrates can contribute to antitumor activity because NK effectors recognize tumor targets independent of MHC expression (Moretta et al. 2001). However, there is usually a paucity of NK cells in the tumor microenvironment suggesting evasion mechanisms preventing their recruitment. Macrophages in the tumor microenvironment play an important modulatory role in the generation of anti tumor responses. The production of chemotactic factors such as CCL2, VEGF and M-CSF (Condeelis and Pollard 2006; Sica et al. 2008) in the tumor microenvironment recruits macrophages. The type of macrophages infiltrating the tumor correlates with favorable or unfavorable prognoses (Lewis and Pollard 2006). The M1 macrophages have potent antigen presentation function and stimulate Type 1 immune responses that lead to tumor rejection, tissue destruction, and host defense. M1 macrophage density in the tumor islets is positively associated with extended survival of non-small cell lung cancer (NSCLC) patients (Ma et al. 2010). The M1 macrophages produce high levels of IL-12, CXCL10 and inducible nitric oxide synthase (iNOS) (Mantovani et al. 2007). In contrast, M2 macrophages are thought to promote tumor formation by enhancing wound healing and tissue remodeling via inhibition of Type1 immune responses by IL-10 and TGFβ secretion. The M2 macrophages express high levels of IL-10 and arginase that suppress antitumor immune responses (Mantovani et al. 2002; Mantovani et al. 2005; Mantovani et al. 2007; Sinha et al. 2007). These macrophages increase metastatic potential by increasing tumor cell migration, invasion and angiogenesis. The tumor microenvironment also consists of T and B lymphocytes of the adaptive immunity. The phenotypes of the T and B subsets evoked in chronic inflammatory state of the tumor microenvironment are regulatory in nature and dampen immune responses against the tumor. B cells and antibodies have a key role in orchestrating macrophage-driven, tumor-promoting inflammation (Andreu et al. 2011), suggesting that modulating the pathways involved might be of therapeutic benefit in cancers driven by chronic inflammation.

Lung cancers contain a significant population of tumor infiltrating myeloid cells that promote tumor growth by suppressing the immune system. In this review we will focus on the interaction between lung cancer and myeloid derived suppressor cells (MDSC) that suppress antitumor immune responses and contribute to tumor progression.

2. Immune modulation in the lung tumor microenvironment by myeloid derived suppressor cells

2.1 Myeloid mediated downregulation of immune responses in the tumor microenvironment

MDSC are a heterogeneous population of immature myeloid cells (IMC) that consists of myeloid progenitors and precursors of macrophages, granulocytes and DC. In tumors immature myeloid cells are partially blocked at the immature state and do not differentiate into mature myeloid cells that results in an expansion of this population. The activation of these cells in cancer results in the upregulated expression of immune suppressive factors such as arginase and iNOS and an increase in the production of nitric oxide (NO) and reactive oxygen species (ROS). These expanded IMC populations with immune suppressive activity; are collectively known as MDSC. Investigations on diverse tumor types have demonstrated that MDSC accrual in the tumor microenvironment is dependent on tumor derived soluble factors including growth factors, cytokines and chemokines. Granulocyte macrophage colony stimulating factor (GM-CSF) supports the survival and expansion of MDSC in the tumor microenvironment (Serafini et al. 2004). The sources of GM-CSF are tumors or activated immune effectors such as T, NK and DC. IL-1β has been demonstrated to accumulate MDSC in tumors of mice (Lu et al. 2011). Tumor derived PGE2 has also been shown to cause an accumulation of MDSC in lung cancer (Zhang et al. 2009). MDSC accumulation and immune suppression, provides one of the mechanisms through which inflammation can contribute to lung cancer development and progression.

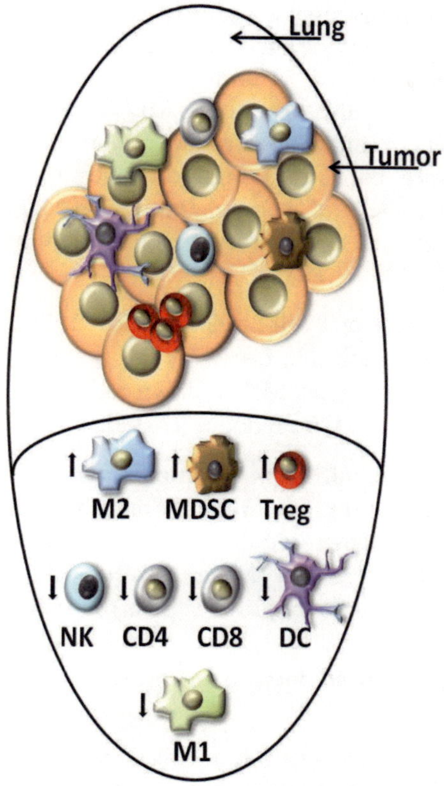

Fig. 1. Modulation in the balance of immune effectors and suppressors in the lung tumor microenvironment. The lung tumor microenvironment has increased myelomonocytic and T regulatory immune suppressors and decreased immune effectors (NK, DC, CD4T, CD8T and M1) that promote tumor growth kinetics and progression.

2.2 Molecular mechanisms of myeloid derived suppressor cell mediated T cell inactivation

MDSC suppress immune responses to newly displayed tumor antigens and promote tumor progression and the metastatic potential of the tumor. MDSC suppress T cell activation in tumor tissues and draining lymph nodes through several mechanisms. MDSC use two enzymes involved in L-arginine metabolism to control T-cell responses: Arginase which depletes the milieu of L-arginine and iNOS which generates NO. L-arginine is essential for T-cell function, including the optimal use of IL-2 and the development of a T-cell memory phenotype. MDSC arginase 1 gene (ARG1) is induced by cytokines such as TGFβ and IL-10 within the tumor microenvironment. The MDSC mediated depletion of arginine suppresses CD4 and CD8 T cell activation. IFNγ and TNFα in the tumor microenvironment induce iNOS in MDSC releasing NO which blocks the phosphorylation and activation of several targets in the IL-2 receptor signaling pathway and induces T-cell apoptosis (Mazzoni et al. 2002).

Cysteine another essential amino acid for T cell activation is depleted by MDSC. T cells lack the enzyme to convert methionine to cysteine and the membrane transporter to import cystine for intracellular reduction to cysteine. T cells obtain their cysteine from extracellular sources. During normal antigen processing and presentation activity, DC and macrophages synthesize cysteine from methionine and import extracellular cystine for cysteine conversion. Cysteine is then exported by antigen presenting cells (APC) during antigen presentation, and imported by T cells. Like T cells, MDSC are unable to convert methionine to cysteine and are dependent on importing cystine for conversion to cysteine. In the tumor microenvironment MDSC are present in high concentration and import most of the available cystine that deprive DC and macrophages. Since MDSC do not export cysteine, they deprive T cells of cysteine that is necessary for synthesizing proteins required for T cell activation (Srivastava et al. 2010).

MDSC mediated down regulation of T cell L-selectin (CD62L) further impairs T cell activity. CD62L is a plasma membrane molecule necessary for homing of naive T cells to lymph nodes for activation by tumor antigens. MDSC down-regulate CD62L on naive T cell that reduces T cell capacity to migrate to lymph nodes (Hanson et al. 2009).

MDSC-produced ROS and peroxynitrite in the tumor microenvironment inhibit CD8+ T cells by catalyzing the nitration of the T cell receptor and thereby preventing T cell-peptide-MHC interactions. MDSC also down-regulate the T cell receptor-associated ζ chain, a phenomenon common in cancer patients (Nagaraj et al. 2009). In the absence of the zeta chain, T cells are unable to transmit the required signals for activation.

2.3 Cellular mechanisms of myeloid derived suppressor cell mediated immune suppression

MDSC impair T cell activation by directly inducing T regulatory cells (Treg) through the production of IL-10 and TGFβ, or arginase that is independent of TGFβ. The Treg cells actively down regulate the activation and expansion of antitumor reactive T cells (Boon et al. 1994; Sakaguchi 2000; Li et al. 2007) and NK cells (Smyth et al. 2006). MDSC affect tumor immunity by polarizing T cells towards a tumor-promoting type 2 phenotype by producing IL-10 and down-regulating macrophage production of IL-12 (Sinha et al. 2007). The suppressive activity of MDSC on T cells can be antigen-specific or non-specific and can vary depending on the MDSC subpopulation. MDSC impair NK cells by inhibiting their cytotoxicity ability and IFNγ production (Liu et al. 2007; Li et al. 2009).

2.4 Lung cancer genetic signatures as drivers of immune suppression

Our laboratory has been evaluating tumor signatures that maintain tumor growth kinetics through the modulation of immune activity (Huang et al. 1996; Huang et al. 1998). Many tumors, including lung cancer, have the capacity to promote immune tolerance and escape host immune surveillance (Chouaib et al. 1997; Smyth and Trapani 2001). Tumors utilize numerous pathways to inhibit immune responses including the elaboration of immune inhibitory cytokines. In addition to directly secreting immunosuppressive cytokines, lung cancer cells may induce host cells to release immune inhibitors (Huang et al. 1996; Huang et al. 1998; Alleva et al. 1994; Maeda et al. 1996; Halak et al. 1999). In previous studies, we found an immune suppressive network in non-small cell lung cancer (NSCLC) that is due to over expression of tumor cyclooxygenase 2 (COX-2) (Huang et al. 1998; Stolina et al. 2000), which is constitutively expressed in a variety of malignancies. We and others have reported that COX-2 is constitutively elevated in human NSCLC frequently (Hida et al. 1998; Huang et al. 1998; Hida et al. 2000; Hosomi et al. 2000). Although multiple genetic alterations are necessary for lung cancer invasion and metastasis, COX-2 may be a central element in orchestrating this process (Hida et al. 1998; Huang et al. 1998; Wolff et al. 1998; Achiwa et al. 1999; Hosomi et al. 2000; Riedl et al. 2004). Over expression of COX-2 is associated with apoptosis resistance (Tsujii and Dubois 1995; Lin et al. 2001), angiogenesis promotion (Tsujii et al. 1998; Masferrer et al. 2000), enhanced tumor invasion and metastasis (Tsujii et al. 1998; Dohadwala et al. 2001; Dohadwala et al. 2002) and decreased host immunity (Huang et al. 1998; Stolina et al. 2000; Sharma et al. 2003). In murine lung cancer models, we found that specific genetic or pharmacological inhibition of COX-2 reduced tumor growth (Stolina et al. 2000). In other related studies, we documented that COX-2 inhibition prevented tumor-induced suppression of DC activities (Sharma et al. 2003). In recent studies, we have demonstrated that treatment of mice with a COX-2 inhibitor, promoted a Type 1 cytokine response, inducing IFNγ, IL-12 and CXCL10 and augmented the vaccination response to tumor challenge (Sharma et al. 2005).

Tumor COX-2 can also modulate MDSC activity through ARG1 in lung carcinoma. MDSC producing high levels of arginase block T cell function by depleting arginine. Until recently, the mechanism that induces ARG1 in MDSC in cancer was unknown. Rodriguez PC et al, utilizing the mouse Lewis lung carcinoma (3LL, that spontaneously arose in the C57BL/6 mice), showed that ARG1 expression was independent of T cell-produced cytokines but rather tumor derived PGE2 maintained ARG1 expression in MDSC. 3LL tumor cells constitutively express COX-1 and COX-2 and produce high levels of PGE2. Genetic or pharmacological inhibition of COX-2 but not COX-1 blocked ARG1 induction *in vitro* and *in vivo*. Signaling through the PGE2 receptor E-prostanoid 4 expressed in MDSC induced ARG1. Furthermore, blocking ARG1 expression using COX-2 inhibitors elicited a lymphocyte-mediated antitumor response. These results demonstrate a new pathway of prostaglandin-induced immune dysfunction and provide a novel mechanism that can help explain the antitumor benefits of COX-2 inhibitors (Rodriguez et al. 2005) that targets the major immune suppressive pathways mediated by MDSC.

The complex nature of interactions between MDSC and Treg cells are yet to be fully defined however it is evident that MDSC promote T reg development *in vivo*. Tumor-reactive T cells have been shown to accumulate in lung cancer tissues but fail to respond because of suppressive tumor cell-derived factors (Yoshino et al. 1992; Batra et al. 2003) and because high proportions of NSCLC tumor infiltrating lymphocytes are CD4+CD25+ T reg cells (Woo et al. 2001). CD4+CD25+ T regulatory (Sakaguchi et al. 2001) cells play an important role in maintenance of immunological self-tolerance. T regulatory cell activities increase in lung cancer, and appear to play a role in suppressing antitumor immune responses. Treg cells actively down regulate the activation and expansion of self-reactive lymphocytes (Sakaguchi 2000). Given that many tumor–associated antigens recognized by autologous T cells are antigenically normal self-constituents, Treg cells engaged in the maintenance of self tolerance may impede the generation and activity of antitumor reactive T cells (Boon et al. 1994; Sakaguchi 2000). Thus, reducing the number of Treg cells or abrogating their activity within the tumor environment may induce effective tumor immunity in otherwise non-responding hosts by activating tumor-specific as well as nonspecific effector cells (Shimizu et al. 1989; Onizuka et al. 1999; Sutmuller et al. 2001). In recent studies we have demonstrated that tumor COX-2 expression contributes to decreased host antitumor immune responses by impacting the frequency and activity of CD4+CD25+FOXP3+ T reg cells (Baratelli et al. 2005; Sharma et al. 2005). Definition of the pathways controlling Treg cell activities will enhance our understanding of limitation of the host antitumor immune responses. We demonstrated that lung tumor-derived COX-2/PGE2 induced expression of the Treg cell-specific transcription factor, Foxp3, and increased Treg cell activity. Assessment of E-prostanoid (EP) receptor requirements revealed that PGE2-mediated induction of Treg cell *Foxp3* gene expression was significantly reduced in the absence of the EP4 receptor and ablated in the absence of the EP2 receptor expression. *In vivo,* COX-2 inhibition reduced Treg cell frequency and activity, attenuated Foxp3 expression in tumor-infiltrating lymphocytes, and decreased tumor burden. Transfer of Treg cells or administration of PGE2 to mice receiving COX-2 inhibitors reversed these effects. Our studies were the first documentation that COX-2 inhibition down regulated tumor induced T regulatory cell activity leading to the restoration of antitumor responses.

2.5 Lung cancer snail knockdown reduces MDSC and increases CD107a activated effector T cells in the tumor microenvironment

We are defining genetic programs in lung cancer that modulate tumor growth and metastases. Cancer cells acquire the ability to progress, invade and metastasize by undergoing the process of epithelial-mesenchymal transition (EMT), by activating transcription factors (for example, Snail, Twist, Zeb, Slug) that repress E-Cadherin, a transmembrane glycoprotein essential for epithelial cell-cell adhesion (Bussemakers et al. 1993; Cano et al. 2000). These transcriptional repressors are normally active during embryogenesis where they program EMT to enable various morphogenetic steps. EMT is involved in tumor progression (Thiery 2002; Jeanes et al. 2008). Snail expression in primary NSCLC has been associated with a shorter overall survival (Yanagawa et al. 2009). Tumor Snail expression has recently been demonstrated to be important in EMT induced metastases in melanoma (Kudo-Saito et al. 2009). We are evaluating the mechanistic role of tumor snail expression that modulates tumor growth and metastases in immune competent mice. Our data (AACR Abstract: Frontiers in Basic Cancer Research, September 14-18 2011., San Francisco) demonstrates that tumor snail expression alters tumor growth and metastasis by impacting MDSC in the tumor microenvironment. 3LL, 3LL Snail knockdown and 3LL control vector cells were implanted in C57BL/6 mice. Compared to controls, 3LL Snail knockdown mice had (i) decreased MDSC, (ii) reduced MDSC as well as the non MDSC populations intracellular expression of ARG1 in the tumors, (iii) increased expression of the CD107a cytolytic marker in tumor infiltrating CD8 T cells and (iv) increased tumor infiltrates of CD4 and CD8 T lymphocytes that elaborated enhanced IFNγ but reduced levels of IL-10 and (v) augmented the frequencies of innate NK effectors and DC. Accompanying the inflammatory signature, Snail knockdown cells demonstrated reduced subcutaneous tumor growth and lung metastases. Current experiments are mechanistically delineating the genetic program(s) induced by tumor Snail knockdown that alter the balance and activity of immune effectors and suppressors in the tumor and the impact of adoptive transfer of MDSC on tumor growth kinetics of Snail knockdown cells. An adequate understanding of the genetic signatures in the tumor and tumor-host interactions that induce immune evasion and promote tumor growth, invasion and metastases will be crucial for the development of effective therapies for lung cancer.

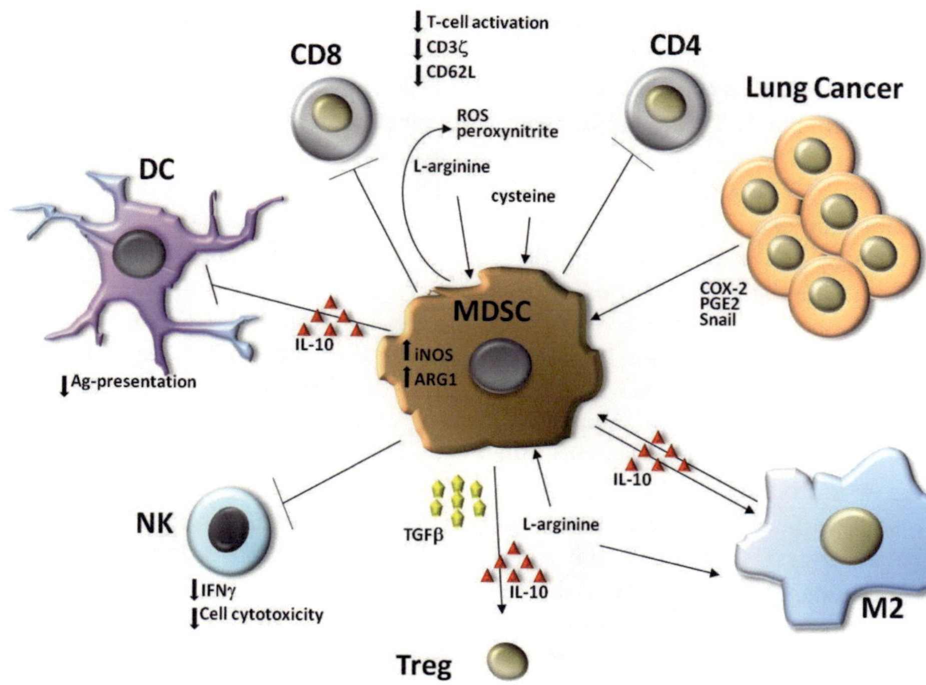

Fig. 2. MDSC accumulation in Lung cancer suppresses antitumor activity MDSC are recruited to and expanded in the tumor through the induction/production of COX-2, PGE2, and Snail in lung cancer. T cell activation is suppressed by MDSC mediated: (i) deprivation of L-arginine and cysteine from the environment, (ii) production of ROS and peroxynitrite, (iii) down regulation of CD62L and the T cell receptor-associated ζ chain and (iv) the induction of Tregs through MDSC IL-10 and TGFβ production. MDSC suppresses NK cell cytotoxicity, NK IFNγ production and induces tumor associated macrophages with a type 2 phenotype. MDSC expansion and IL-10 production inhibits DC antigen presentation.

2.6 Impact of depleting Gr1 or Ly6G myelomonocytic cells on lung cancer growth kinetics

Increases in MDSC evoke strong natural suppressive activity in cancer patients (Young et al. 1997; Kusmartsev et al. 1998) or tumor-bearing mice (Kusmartsev and Ogreba 1989; Subiza et al. 1989; Young et al. 1997). It has been demonstrated that Gr1+CD11b+ immune suppressive cells are capable of inhibiting the T cell proliferative response induced by alloantigens (Schmidt-Wolf et al. 1992), CD3 ligation (Young et al. 1996), or various mitogens (Sugiura et al. 1988; Angulo et al. 1995), and can also inhibit IL-2 utilization (Brooks and Hoskin 1994) as well as NK cell activity (Kusmartsev et al. 1998). These studies indicate that progressive tumor growth is associated with the down-regulation of T cell responses and that the Gr1+CD11b+ myeloid cells are involved in negative immunoregulatory mechanisms in the tumor bearing host. In murine tumor models there is an increase in the MDSC populations in the tumors, spleens, bone marrow and blood as the tumor progresses. In the 3LL lung cancer model as the tumors progress the frequency and activity of immune suppressive cells are enhanced in the tumor microenvironment. We have found that tumors have as much as 45% infiltrates that are predominantly of the Gr1+ CD11b+ immature myeloid phenotype. As has been recently reported for glioblastoma (Fujita et al. 2011) and colon (Mundy-Bosse et al. 2011) murine cancer models, we evaluated the contribution of the Gr1 and Ly6G expressing myelomonocytic cells on 3LL tumor growth kinetics in C57BL/6 mice, by depleting cells expressing these markers with anti-Gr1 (RB6-8C5) or anti-Ly6G (1A8) administered every other day via *i.p* route starting on day 5 post tumor inoculation. Compared to isotype matched control antibody, the anti-Gr1 antibody or anti-Ly6G led to a significant decrease in the $Gr1^{hi}CD11b$ expressing myeloid subset and a subsequent increase in the CD107a expressing CD3T lymphocytes and NK cells in the tumors respectively. Accompanying the decrease in the $Gr1^{hi}CD11b$ expressing myeloid subset was a 8 fold decrease in tumor weight. While the anti-Gr1 antibody reduced both $Gr1^{hi}$ and $Gr1^{lo}$, the anti-Ly6G antibody reduced the $Gr1^{hi}$ subset only. Both these antibodies depleted the Ly6G expressing cells. Although these depletion antibodies impact other Gr1 or Ly6G expressing monocytes, our data suggests that the broad targeting of MDSC along with other myeloid cell types is beneficial in eliciting anticancer effects. This data is consistent with studies by several groups (Fujita et al. 2011; Mundy-Bosse et al. 2011). It would be interesting to evaluate the impact of MDSC depletion on DC and tumor associated macrophages (TAM) functional activity. This may resolve further compensatory pathways of immune suppression. Currently we are evaluating strategies that target the myeloid suppressor subsets in combination with various immune potentiating strategies to increase the antitumor benefit.

2.7 Critical role of antigen presentation in lung cancer: T-cell tolerance versus T-cell priming

Effective antitumor responses require antigen processing cells (APCs), lymphocyte and NK effectors, as well as the elaboration of effector molecules that promote antitumor activity. Although lung cancer cells express tumor antigens, the limited expression of MHC antigens, defective transporter associated with antigen processing (TAP) and lack of costimulatory molecules, make them ineffective APCs (Restifo et al. 1993). Many tumors, including lung cancer, have the capacity to promote immune tolerance and escape host immune surveillance (Chouaib et al. 1997; Smyth and Trapani 2001). Tumors utilize numerous pathways to inhibit immune responses, including reduction in APC activity. The accumulation of MDSC in the tumor microenvironment negatively impacts DC and their APC activity.

The central importance of functional APCs in the immune response against cancer has been well defined (Huang et al. 1994). The study revealed that even highly immunogenic tumors require host APCs for antigen presentation. Thus, host APCs, rather than tumor cells, present tumor antigen. This is consistent with a study indicating that $CD8^{+}$ T-cell responses can be induced *in vivo* by professional APCs that present exogenous antigens in a MHC I-restricted manner (Albert et al. 1998). This has been referred to as cross-priming or representation and may be critical for effective antitumor responses (Bevan 1995). DCs have been demonstrated to be the host APC responsible for cross-priming by presenting epitopes obtained from apoptotic cells (Castellino and Germain 2006).

However, in tumor-bearing hosts, there is a state of T-cell unresponsiveness (Staveley-O'Carroll et al. 1998; Cuenca et al. 2003; Willimsky and Blankenstein 2005). The dominant mechanism underlying the development of antigen-specific T-cell unresponsiveness is thought to be through tumor-antigen processing and presentation by APCs (Sotomayor et al. 2001). The intrinsic APC capacity of tumor cells has little influence over T-cell priming versus tolerance, an important decision that is regulated by bone marrow-derived APCs. DCs, macrophages and B cells are all bone marrow-derived cells that express both MHC and the costimulatory molecules CD80 and CD86 and present tumor antigens to antigen-specific T cells.

Several studies have shown that DCs play a critical role leading to T-cell tolerance versus T-cell priming (Fuchs and Matzinger 1996; Belz et al. 2002; Munn et al. 2002; Steinman et al. 2003), which is dictated by the environmental context in which the DCs encounter the antigen. Antigen capture by DCs in an inflammatory context triggers their maturation to a phenotype capable of generating strong immune responses, whereas antigen capture in a noninflammatory environment leads instead to the development of T-cell tolerance. The tumor microenvironment not only fails to provide the inflammatory signals needed for efficient DC activation, but also inhibits DC differentiation and maturation through IL-10 (Gerlini et al. 2004) and VEGF (Gabrilovich et al. 1996). DCs, which are pivotal for T-cell priming, remain immature and become dysfunctional in hosts bearing growing tumors, acquiring tolerogenic properties that induce T-cell tolerance to tumor antigens. Immature DCs (iDCs) have little or no expression of costimulatory molecules such as CD80, CD86 and CD40 on their surface and produce little or no IL-12, which is required to support T-cell proliferation. iDCs are unable to induce antitumor immune response but can induce T-cell tolerance. If APCs fail to provide an appropriate costimulatory signal for T cells, tolerance or anergy can develop. The importance of restoring APCs with immune-stimulating activity in the tumor microenvironment is crucial. In a recent study ectopic lymph node or tertiary lymphoid structures were retrospectively identified within human non-small-cell lung cancer specimens and demonstrated that there is a correlation of cellular content with clinical outcome (Dieu-Nosjean et al. 2008). The density of DC-Lamp, indicating mature DCs within these structures, is a predictor of long-term survival within their selected lung cancer patient population. The authors observed that a low density of tumor-infiltrating CD4+ and T-bet+ T lymphocytes present in tumors poorly infiltrated by DC-Lamp+ mature DCs appears to provide additional supporting evidence for the prognostic importance of an adaptive immune reaction to a solid tumor.

We have previously demonstrated that elements from the tumor microenvironment can suppress DC function. We found that bone marrow derived DCs stimulated with GM-CSF and IL-4 in the presence of tumor supernatants (TSNs) failed to generate antitumor responses and caused immunosuppressive effects that correlated with enhanced tumor growth. Functional analyses indicated that TSNs cause a decrement in DC capacity to process and present antigens, induce alloreactivity and secrete IL-12. The TSNs caused a reduction in cell surface expression of CD11c, DEC205, MHC I antigen, MHC II antigen, CD80 and CD86, as well as a reduction in TAP 1 and 2 proteins (Sharma et al. 2003).

2.8 IL-7/IL-7Rα-Fc promotes the M1 macrophage phenotype in lung cancer

Although tumor growth and invasion leads to inflammatory responses, the immune system generally develops tolerance to cancer. One way to induce potent immune responses against tumors is to activate key innate and immune effector mechanisms. Toward this end, we are evaluating the utility of chimeric γc homeostatic cytokine, IL-7/IL-7Rα-Fc, to restore host APC and T cell activities dysregulated in cancer patients (Almand et al. 2000; Zou 2005). It is evident from previous studies that intratumoral infiltration by relatively high numbers of activated T lymphocytes (Johnson et al. 2000; Hiraoka et al. 2006) and APC (Dieu-Nosjean et al. 2008) leads to better prognosis in lung cancer patients.

We evaluated the utility of chimeric γc homeostatic cytokine, IL-7/IL-7Rα-Fc, to restore host APC and T cell activities in lung cancer (Andersson et al. 2011). Utilizing murine lung cancer models we determined the antitumor efficacy of IL-7/IL-7Rα-Fc. IL-7/IL-7Rα-Fc administration inhibited tumor growth and increased survival in lung cancer. Accompanying the tumor growth inhibition were increases in APC and T cell activities. In comparison to controls, IL-7/IL-7Rα-Fc treatment of tumor bearing mice led to increased: i) tumor macrophage infiltrates characteristic of M1 phenotype with increased IL-12, iNOS but reduced IL-10 and arginase, ii) frequencies of T and NK cells, iii) T cell activation markers CXCR3, CD69 and CD127,^{low} and iv) effector memory T cells. IL-7/IL-7Rα-Fc treatment abrogated the tumor induced reduction in splenic functional APC activity to T responder cells. Our findings demonstrate that IL-7/IL-7Rα-Fc promotes the afferent M1 macrophage phenotype and the efferent (CXCR3/CXCR3 ligand biological axis) limbs of the immune response for sustained antitumor activity in lung cancer. IL-7/IL-7Rα-Fc provides the cues that address the deficits in the lung tumor microenvironment to achieve the requirements for the inhibition of tumor growth kinetics by: (i) generating sufficient numbers of T cells systemically (ii) increasing the activated T cell infiltrates in the tumor and (iii) activating the innate and immune cells in the tumor to manifest antitumor benefit. Although IL-7/IL-7Rα-Fc is potent at reducing tumor growth kinetics, it does not lead to complete tumor eradication. This may in part be due to the presence of MDSC in the tumor microenvironment that dampens the antitumor activity of IL-7/IL7Rα-Fc and remains to be resolved.

2.9 Drug targets impacting myeloid derived suppressor cells

Several pharmacological approaches that target MDSC are currently being explored in a variety of tumor models. The drugs can be divided into classes based on their ability to control: (i) MDSC differentiation into mature DC and macrophages capable of APC activity (ATRA and Vitamin D3); (ii) MDSC maturation from precursors [(STAT 3 inhibitors, Tyrosine Kinase inhibitors (TKI) (Sunitinib and Sorefnib), Bevacizumab, Anti-BV8 mAb, Amino-Biphosphonates and MMP9 inhibitors]; (iii) MDSC accumulation (Gemcitabine, 5-Fluorouracil (5-FU), CXCR2 and CXCR4 antagonists) and (iv) MDSC function [(ROS scavengers and ARG and NOX inhibitors (Nitroaspirin, PDE-5, COX-2 inhibitors and Cytokines)] (Ugel et al. 2009).

Gabrilovich et al demonstrated that differentiating MDSC to DC and macrophages by using all-trans retinoic acid (ATRA) reduced MDSC numbers and augmented the responses to cancer vaccines. ATRA induced differentiation of MDSC primarily via neutralization of high ROS production in these cells. The mechanism involves specific up-regulation of glutathione synthase and accumulation of glutathione in the MDSC and could be used in developing and monitoring therapeutic application of ATRA (Nefedova et al. 2007).

Recent advances in targeted therapy for cancer have provided small-molecule kinase inhibitors that recognize specific targets on the surface or inside cancer cells. These inhibitors have shown efficacy against several hematopoietic malignancies and solid tumors. Most drugs generally have inhibitory effects on several kinases, including tyrosine kinases (TK) that are critical for the survival, proliferation, migration and invasion of tumor cells. With regards to the effects of TKI on tumor immunity, some studies have demonstrated the immune stimulatory effects of the TKI (eg imatinib) (Wang et al. 2005) whereas others report the immune suppressive effects of the same inhibitor (Seggewiss et al. 2005).

Administration of sunitinib, a receptor TKI, has been shown to reduce the frequency of MDSC and reversing T cell immune suppression in the peripheral blood of patients with metastatic renal cell carcinoma (RCC) and in several murine tumor models. However sunitinib has variable impact at reducing MDSC and restoring T cell activity in the tumor microenvironment that seems to be tumor dependent. The authors suggest that the persistence of MDSC in the tumor following sunitinib treatment in RCC may in part be due to increased GM-CSF expression by the tumors that prolong the survival of MDSC and protect from sunitinib through pSTAT5 pathway. The authors contend that GM-CSF mediated MDSC survival in patient tumors is supported by the observation that GM-CSF produced by RCC cultures protect MDSC from sunitinib induced cell death. However, tumors transduced with GM-CSF in several tumor models have been shown to lead to strong immune dependent rejection. It would be interesting to see in these models the activity of MDSC in the tumor microenvironment of the GM-CSF secreting tumors. Additionally, an alternate explanation for the persistence of MDSC may be associated with increased expression of proangiogenic proteins, such as MMP9, MMP8 and IL-8 produced by tumor stromal cells or infiltrating MDSC (Ko et al. 2010; Finke et al. 2011). More studies are required to evaluate the role of TKI (sunitinib, sorafenib, imatinib and dasatinib) on MDSC activity in the tumor microenvironment and tumor immunity in several tumor models and in clinical samples.

GW2580, a selective molecule kinase inhibitor of colony stimulating factor 1 receptor (CSF1R), blocks the recruitment of CSF1R expressing TAMs as well as MDSC in different tumor models without having an impact on tumor burden (Priceman et al. 2010). PLX3397, another TKI of CSF1R, has also been used to efficiently deplete CD11b+Ly6G-LY6ClowF4/80+ TAMs (70%) without altering the presence of granulocytic MDSC. The treatment of mammary tumor bearing mice with PLX3397 led to a decrease in tumor burden (DeNardo et al. 2011).

Studies by Ping Ying Pan et al have demonstrated that the expression of c-kit ligand [(stem cell factor, (SCF)] by tumor cells may be important for MDSC accumulation in tumor-bearing mice, and that blocking the c-kit ligand/c-kit receptor interaction can reverse MDSC mediated immune suppression. Mice bearing tumor cells with SCF siRNA knockdown exhibited significantly reduced MDSC expansion and restored proliferative responses of tumor-infiltrating T cells. The blockade of SCF receptor (ckit)–SCF interaction by anti-ckit prevented tumor-specific T-cell anergy, Treg development, and tumor angiogenesis. The authors found that the prevention of MDSC accumulation in conjunction with immune activation therapy showed synergistic therapeutic effect when treating mice bearing large tumors. Their data suggests that modulation of MDSC development may be essential to enhance immune therapy against advanced tumors (Pan et al. 2008).

N-acetyl cysteine (NAC) has been proposed as an anti-tumorigenic agent because of its ability to reduce the oxidative stress that promotes genetic instability. NAC treatment of mice with progressively growing tumors have demonstrated therapeutic efficacy (Gao et al. 2007). NAC may have the additional benefit of facilitating T cell activation by increasing extracellular pools of cysteine in the presence of high levels of MDSC in cancer patients. Although NAC targets the cysteine pathway of MDSC mediated T cell suppression, MDSC production of arginase and nitric oxide, can still maintain the suppressive effects of MDSC. However, administration of NAC, an already FDA-approved drug, in combination with other agents that block other MDSC suppressive pathways (ARG1 and NO), maybe more effective at inhibiting MDSC and facilitate the treatment of cancers.

COX-2 is required for PGE2 synthesis; drugs that specifically block COX-2 and reduce PGE2 delay tumor growth by reducing MDSC accumulation. Therefore, inhibition of PGE2 biosynthesis in tumor-bearing mice blocks MDSC generation and subsequently retards tumor progression (Rodriguez et al. 2005; Sinha et al. 2007).

Studies have demonstrated that the chemotherapeutic agent, gemcitabine, enhances T cell responsiveness by reducing the number of MDSC levels in the spleens of murine lung cancer models. In this study, gemcitabine, was administered at a dose similar to the equivalent dose used in patients, was able to specifically reduce the number of MDSC found in the spleens of animals bearing large tumors without significant reductions in CD4+ T cells, CD8+ T cells, NK cells, macrophages, or B cells. The loss of MDSC was accompanied by an increase in the antitumor activity of CD8+ T cells and activated NK cells. Since all measurements on MDSC frequency and activity in this study was performed from the spleens of tumor bearing animals it is not clear from this work as to the extent of depletion of MDSC from the lung tumor microenvironment following gemcitabine treatment and restoration of immune responses in the tumor microenvironment. The authors did observe however, that combining gemcitabine with cytokine immunogene therapy using IFN-β markedly enhanced antitumor efficacy leading to a greater reduction in tumor burden than when either therapy was administered singly (Suzuki et al. 2005).

3. Conclusion and future perspectives

Lung cancer is the most common cause of cancer mortality worldwide for both men and women, causing approximately 1.2 million deaths per year (Jemal et al. 2009). With the existing therapeutic efforts, the long-term survival for lung cancer patients remains low with only 15% surviving for 5 years following diagnosis. Therefore, new therapeutic strategies are needed. One such approach is the development of immune therapy for lung cancer. Immune approaches for lung cancer remain attractive because although surgery, chemotherapy and radiotherapy alone or in combination produce response rates in all histological types of lung cancer, relapse is frequent. Immunologic targeting of lung cancer has the potential for nontoxic and specific therapy. Strategies that harness the immune system to react against tumors can be integrated with existing forms of therapy for optimal responses toward this devastating disease. Immune therapy for lung cancer has potential; however, there have not been improvements in survival with previous regimens. Tumor-induced immune suppression may have contributed to the limited efficacy of the approaches.

Lung cancer growth and invasion into surrounding tissue promotes an inflammatory response that is important for tumor development and progression. Dysregulated inflammation in cancer leads to hypo responsiveness of the tumor. MDSC play a major role of suppressing T cell activation in the lung tumor microenvironment and sustain overall tumor growth, proliferation and metastases. Regulating MDSC recruitment, differentiation/expansion and inhibiting MDSC suppressive function will serve as a multifaceted approach to control lung cancer. Although the broad targeting of MDSC along with other myeloid cell types with anti-Gr1 or anti Ly6G mAbs alone is beneficial in eliciting anticancer effects, the benefit of chemotherapeutic agents that regulate MDSC are evident only when combined with immune therapy and not when administered alone. Cancer immune therapy offers an attractive therapeutic addition, delivering treatment of high specificity, low toxicity and prolonged activity. Despite the identification of a repertoire of tumor antigens, hurdles persist for immune-based therapies. Tumor-induced immune suppression may be contributing to the limited efficacy of the current approaches. Effective immunotherapeutic strategies for lung cancer will result from a basic understanding of the mechanisms that sustain tumor growth kinetics. Strategies that reprogram the tumor niche could alter the inflammatory infiltrate in the lung tumor microenvironment making it permissive for immune destruction of tumors. It is likely that combination therapies that focus on methods to address the immune deficits in the lung cancer microenvironment will be required to develop effective therapies for this disease. Targeting MDSC induced immune suppression is at the forefront of these therapeutic approaches. The future of immune therapy for lung cancer holds promise with novel combined approaches that simultaneously downregulate MDSC suppressor pathways, restore APC immune-stimulating activity, and expand tumor-reactive T cells with γc homeostatic cytokines such as IL-7, IL-15 and IL-21 to generate effective therapy. The optimal way to integrate novel immune targeted combinations will be the major focus of future studies and will require a coordinated and cooperative multidisciplinary effort by the international scientific community. Objective lung cancer regressions and extensions in survival should be correlated with multiple predictive and prognostic molecular and cellular biomarkers of response. This information will prove useful in improving therapy.

4. References

Achiwa, H., Y. Yatabe, et al. (1999). "Prognostic significance of elevated cyclooxygenase 2 expression in primary, resected lung adenocarcinomas." *Clin Cancer Res* 5(5): 1001-5.

Albert, M. L., B. Sauter, et al. (1998). "Dendritic cells acquire antigen from apoptotic cells and induce class I- restricted CTLs." *Nature* 392(6671): 86-9.

Alleva, D. G., C. J. Burger, et al. (1994). "Tumor-induced regulation of suppressor macrophage nitric oxide and TNF-alpha production: role of tumor-derived IL-10, TGF-beta and prostaglandin E2." *The Journal of Immunology* 153: 1674.

Almand, B., J. R. Resser, et al. (2000). "Clinical significance of defective dendritic cell differentiation in cancer." *Clin Cancer Res* 6(5): 1755-66.

Andersson, A., M. K. Srivastava, et al. (2011). "Role of CXCR3 ligands in IL-7/IL-7R{alpha}-Fc-mediated antitumor activity in lung cancer." *Clin Cancer Res* 17(11): 3660-72.

Andreu, P., M. Johansson, et al. (2011). "FcRgamma activation regulates inflammation-associated squamous carcinogenesis." *Cancer* 17(2): 121-34. Epub 2010 Feb 4.

Angulo, I., R. Rodriguez, et al. (1995). "Involvement of nitric oxide in bone marrow-derived natural suppressor activity. Its dependence on IFN-gamma." *J Immunol.* 155(1): 15-26.

Baratelli, F., Y. Lin, et al. (2005). "Prostaglandin E2 induces FOXP3 gene expression and T regulatory cell function in human CD4+ T cells." *J Immunol.* 175(3): 1483-90.

Batra, R. K., Y. Lin, et al. (2003). "Non-small cell lung cancer-derived soluble mediators enhance apoptosis in activated T lymphocytes through an I kappa B kinase-dependent mechanism." *Cancer Res* 63(3): 642-6.

Belz, G. T., G. M. Behrens, et al. (2002). "The CD8alpha(+) dendritic cell is responsible for inducing peripheral self-tolerance to tissue-associated antigens." *J Exp Med.* 196(8): 1099-104.

Bevan, M. J. (1995). "Antigen presentation to cytotoxic T lymphocytes in vivo." *J. Exp. Med.* 182: 639-641.

Boon, T., J.-C. Cerottini, et al. (1994). "Tumor antigens recognized by T lymphocytes." *Annu. Rev. Immunol.* 12: 337-365.

Brooks, J. C. and D. W. Hoskin (1994). "The inhibitory effect of cyclophosphamide-induced MAC-1+ natural suppressor cells on IL-2 and IL-4 utilization in MLR." *Transplantation.* 58(10): 1096-103.

Bussemakers, M. J., A. van Bokhoven, et al. (1993). "Molecular cloning and characterization of the human E-cadherin cDNA." *Mol Biol Rep.* 17(2): 123-8.

Cano, A., M. A. Perez-Moreno, et al. (2000). "The transcription factor snail controls epithelial-mesenchymal transitions by repressing E-cadherin expression." *Nat Cell Biol.* 2(2): 76-83.

Castellino, F. and R. N. Germain (2006). "Cooperation between CD4+ and CD8+ T cells: when, where, and how." *Annu Rev Immunol.* 24: 519-40.

Chouaib, S., C. Assellin-Paturel, et al. (1997). "The host-tumor immune conflict: from immunosuppression to resistance and destruction." *Immunology Today* 18: 493-497.

Condeelis, J. and J. W. Pollard (2006). "Macrophages: obligate partners for tumor cell migration, invasion, and metastasis." *Cell.* 124(2): 263-6.

Cuenca, A., F. Cheng, et al. (2003). "Extra-lymphatic solid tumor growth is not immunologically ignored and results in early induction of antigen-specific T-cell anergy: dominant role of cross-tolerance to tumor antigens." *Cancer Res.* 63(24): 9007-15.

DeNardo, D. G., D. J. Brennan, et al. (2011). "Leukocyte Complexity Predicts Breast Cancer Survival and Functionally Regulates Response to Chemotherapy." *Cancer Discovery* 1(1): 0F52-0F65.

Dieu-Nosjean, M. C., M. Antoine, et al. (2008). "Long-term survival for patients with non-small-cell lung cancer with intratumoral lymphoid structures." *J Clin Oncol.* 26(27): 4410-7.

Dohadwala, M., R. K. Batra, et al. (2002). "Autocrine/paracrine prostaglandin E2 production by non-small cell lung cancer cells regulates matrix metalloproteinase-2 and CD44 in cyclooxygenase-2-dependent invasion." *J Biol Chem* 277(52): 50828-33.

Dohadwala, M., J. Luo, et al. (2001). "Non small cell lung cancer cylooxygenase-2-dependent invasion is mediated by CD44." *J Biol Chem* 276(24): 20809-12.

Finke, J., J. Ko, et al. (2011). "MDSC as a mechanism of tumor escape from sunitinib mediated anti-angiogenic therapy." *Int Immunopharmacol* 11(7): 856-61. Epub 2011 Feb 11.

Fuchs, E. J. and P. Matzinger (1996). "Is cancer dangerous to the immune system?" *Semin Immunol* 8(5): 271-80.

Fujita, M., G. Kohanbash, et al. (2011). "COX-2 blockade suppresses gliomagenesis by inhibiting myeloid-derived suppressor cells." *Cancer Research* 71(7): 2664-74. Epub 2011 Feb 15.

Gabrilovich, D. I., H. L. Chen, et al. (1996). "Production of vascular endothelial growth factor by human tumors inhibits the functional maturation of dendritic cells." *Nat Med* 2(10): 1096-103.

Gabrilovich, D. I. and S. Nagaraj (2009). "Myeloid-derived suppressor cells as regulators of the immune system." *Nat Rev Immunol.* 9(3): 162-74.

Gao, P., H. Zhang, et al. (2007). "HIF-dependent antitumorigenic effect of antioxidants in vivo." *Cancer Cell.* 12(3): 230-8.

Gerlini, G., A. Tun-Kyi, et al. (2004). "Metastatic melanoma secreted IL-10 down-regulates CD1 molecules on dendritic cells in metastatic tumor lesions." *Am J Pathol.* 165(6): 1853-63.

Halak, B. K., H. C. Maguire, Jr., et al. (1999). "Tumor-induced interleukin-10 inhibits type 1 immune responses directed at a tumor antigen as well as a non-tumor antigen present at the tumor site." *Cancer Res* 59(4): 911-7.

Hanson, E. M., V. K. Clements, et al. (2009). "Myeloid-derived suppressor cells down-regulate L-selectin expression on CD4+ and CD8+ T cells." *J Immunol* 183(2): 937-44.

Hida, T., K. Kozaki, et al. (2000). "Cyclooxygenase-2 inhibitor induces apoptosis and enhances cytotoxicity of various anticancer agents in non-small cell lung cancer cell lines." *Clin Cancer Res* 6(5): 2006-11.

Hida, T., Y. Yatabe, et al. (1998). "Increased expression of cyclooxygenase 2 occurs frequently in human lung cancers, specifically in adenocarcinomas." *Cancer Res* 58(17): 3761-4.

Hiraoka, K., M. Miyamoto, et al. (2006). "Concurrent infiltration by CD8+ T cells and CD4+ T cells is a favourable prognostic factor in non-small-cell lung carcinoma." *Br J Cancer.* 94(2): 275-80.

Hosomi, Y., T. Yokose, et al. (2000). "Increased cyclooxygenase 2 (COX-2) expression occurs frequently in precursor lesions of human adenocarcinoma of the lung." *Lung Cancer* 30(2): 73-81.

Huang, A. Y. C., P. Golumbek, et al. (1994). "Role of bone marrow-derived cells in presenting MHC class I-restricted tumor antigens." *Science* 264: 961-965.

Huang, M., S. Sharma, et al. (1996). "Non-small cell lung cancer-derived soluble mediators and prostaglandin E_2 enhance peripheral blood lymphocyte IL-10 transcription and protein production." *J. Immunol.* 157: 5512-5520.

Huang, M., M. Stolina, et al. (1998). "Non-small cell lung cancer cyclooxygenase-2-dependent regulation of cytokine balance in lymphocytes and macrophages: up-regulation of interleukin 10 and down-regulation of interleukin 12 production." *Cancer Res* 58(6): 1208 - 1216.

Jeanes, A., C. J. Gottardi, et al. (2008). "Cadherins and cancer: how does cadherin dysfunction promote tumor progression?" *Oncogene.* 27(55): 6920-9.

Jemal, A., R. Siegel, et al. (2009). "Cancer statistics, 2009." *CA Cancer J Clin.* 59(4): 225-49. Epub 2009 May 27.

Johnson, S. K., K. M. Kerr, et al. (2000). "Immune cell infiltrates and prognosis in primary carcinoma of the lung." *Lung Cancer.* 27(1): 27-35.

Ko, J. S., P. Rayman, et al. (2010). "Direct and differential suppression of myeloid-derived suppressor cell subsets by sunitinib is compartmentally constrained." *Cancer Res* 70(9): 3526-36. Epub 2010 Apr 20.

Kudo-Saito, C., H. Shirako, et al. (2009). "Cancer metastasis is accelerated through immunosuppression during Snail-induced EMT of cancer cells." *Cancer Cell.* 15(3): 195-206.

Kusmartsev, S. A., I. N. Kusmartseva, et al. (1998). "Immunosuppressive cells in bone marrow of patients with stomach cancer." *Adv Exp Med Biol.* 451: 189-94.

Kusmartsev, S. A. and V. I. Ogreba (1989). "[Suppressor activity of bone marrow and spleen cells in C57Bl/6 mice during carcinogenesis induced by 7,12-dimethylbenz(a)anthracene]." *Eksp Onkol.* 11(5): 23-6.

Lewis, C. E. and J. W. Pollard (2006). "Distinct role of macrophages in different tumor microenvironments." *Cancer Res.* 66(2): 605-12.

Li, H., Y. Han, et al. (2009). "Cancer-expanded myeloid-derived suppressor cells induce anergy of NK cells through membrane-bound TGF-beta 1." *J Immunol.* 182(1): 240-9.

Li, H., J. P. Yu, et al. (2007). "CD4 +CD25 + regulatory T cells decreased the antitumor activity of cytokine-induced killer (CIK) cells of lung cancer patients." *J Clin Immunol* 27(3): 317-26.

Lin, M. T., R. C. Lee, et al. (2001). "Cyclooxygenase-2 inducing Mcl-1-dependent survival mechanism in human lung adenocarcinoma CL1.0 cells. Involvement of phosphatidylinositol 3-kinase/Akt pathway." *J Biol Chem* 276(52): 48997-9002.

Liu, C., S. Yu, et al. (2007). "Expansion of spleen myeloid suppressor cells represses NK cell cytotoxicity in tumor-bearing host." *Blood* 109(10): 4336-42.

Lu, T., R. Ramakrishnan, et al. (1172). "Tumor-infiltrating myeloid cells induce tumor cell resistance to cytotoxic T cells in mice." *J Clin INvest* 121(10): 4015-29.

Ma, J., L. Liu, et al. (2010). "The M1 form of tumor-associated macrophages in non-small cell lung cancer is positively associated with survival time." *Bmc* 10: 112.

Maeda, A., K. Hiyama, et al. (1996). "Increased expression of platelet-derived growth factor A and insulin-like growth factor-1 in BAL cells during the development of bleomycin-induced pulmonary fibrosis in mice." *Chest* 109: 780-786.

Mantovani, A., A. Sica, et al. (2005). "Macrophage polarization comes of age." *Immunity.* 23(4): 344-6.

Mantovani, A., A. Sica, et al. (2007). "New vistas on macrophage differentiation and activation." *Eur J Immunol.* 37(1): 14-6.

Mantovani, A., S. Sozzani, et al. (2002). "Macrophage polarization: tumor-associated macrophages as a paradigm for polarized M2 mononuclear phagocytes." *Trends Immunol.* 23(11): 549-55.

Masferrer, J. L., K. M. Leahy, et al. (2000). "Antiangiogenic and antitumor activities of cyclooxygenase-2 inhibitors." *Cancer Res* 60(5): 1306-11.

Mazzoni, A., V. Bronte, et al. (2002). "Myeloid suppressor lines inhibit T cell responses by an NO-dependent mechanism." *J Immunol.* 168(2): 689-95.

Moretta, A., C. Bottino, et al. (2001). "Activating receptors and coreceptors involved in human natural killer cell-mediated cytolysis." *Annu Rev Immunol* 19: 197-223.

Mundy-Bosse, B. L., G. B. Lesinski, et al. (2011). "Myeloid-Derived Suppressor Cell Inhibition of the IFN Response in Tumor-Bearing Mice." *Cancer Research* 71(15): 5101-5110. Epub 2011 Jun 16.

Munn, D. H., M. D. Sharma, et al. (2002). "Potential regulatory function of human dendritic cells expressing indoleamine 2,3-dioxygenase." *Science.* 297(5588): 1867-70.

Nagaraj, S., M. Collazo, et al. (2009). "Regulatory myeloid suppressor cells in health and disease." *Cancer Res* 69(19): 7503-6.

Nefedova, Y., M. Fishman, et al. (2007). "Mechanism of all-trans retinoic acid effect on tumor-associated myeloid-derived suppressor cells." *Cancer Res.* 67(22): 11021-8.

Onizuka, S., I. Tawara, et al. (1999). "Tumor rejection by in vivo administration of anti-CD25 (interleukin-2 receptor alpha) monoclonal antibody." *Cancer Res* 59(13): 3128-33.

Pan, P. Y., G. X. Wang, et al. (2008). "Reversion of immune tolerance in advanced malignancy: modulation of myeloid-derived suppressor cell development by blockade of stem-cell factor function." *Blood* 111(1): 219-28.

Peranzoni, E., S. Zilio, et al. (2010). "Myeloid-derived suppressor cell heterogeneity and subset definition." *Curr Opin Immunol* 22(2): 238-44.

Priceman, S. J., J. L. Sung, et al. (2010). "Targeting distinct tumor-infiltrating myeloid cells by inhibiting CSF-1 receptor: combating tumor evasion of antiangiogenic therapy." *Blood* 115(7): 1461-71.

Restifo, N. P., F. Esquivel, et al. (1993). "Identification of human cancers deficient in antigen processing." *J. Exp. Med.* 177: 265-272.

Riedl, K., K. Krysan, et al. (2004). "Multifaceted roles of cyclooxygenase-2 in lung cancer." *Drug Resist Updat* 7(3): 169-84.

Rodriguez, P. C., C. P. Hernandez, et al. (2005). "Arginase I in myeloid suppressor cells is induced by COX-2 in lung carcinoma." *J Exp Med.* 202(7): 931-9 Epub 2005 Sep 26.

Sakaguchi, S. (2000). "Regulatory T cells: key controllers of immunologic self-tolerance." *Cell* 101(5): 455-8.

Sakaguchi, S., N. Sakaguchi, et al. (2001). "Immunologic tolerance maintained by CD25+ CD4+ regulatory T cells: their common role in controlling autoimmunity, tumor immunity, and transplantation tolerance." *Immunol Rev* 182: 18-32.

Schmidt-Wolf, I. G., S. Dejbakhsh-Jones, et al. (1992). "T-cell subsets and suppressor cells in human bone marrow." *Blood.* 80(12): 3242-50.

Seggewiss, R., K. Lore, et al. (2005). "Imatinib inhibits T-cell receptor-mediated T-cell proliferation and activation in a dose-dependent manner." *Blood.* 105(6): 2473-9. Epub 2004 Nov 30.

Serafini, P., R. Carbley, et al. (2004). "High-dose granulocyte-macrophage colony-stimulating factor-producing vaccines impair the immune response through the recruitment of myeloid suppressor cells." *Cancer Res.* 64(17): 6337-43.

Sharma, S., M. Stolina, et al. (2003). "Tumor Cyclooxygenase 2-dependent Suppression of Dendritic Cell Function." *Clin Cancer Res* 9(3): 961-8.

Sharma, S., S. C. Yang, et al. (2005). "Tumor cyclooxygenase-2/prostaglandin E2-dependent promotion of FOXP3 expression and CD4+ CD25+ T regulatory cell activities in lung cancer." *Cancer Res.* 65(12): 5211-20.

Sharma, S., L. Zhu, et al. (2005). "COX-2 inhibition promotes IFN gamma-dependent enhancement of anti-tumor responses." *J Immunol.*

Shimizu, J., T. Suda, et al. (1989). "Induction of tumor-specific in vivo protective immunity by immunization with tumor antigen-pulsed cells." *J Immunol* 142: 1053-1059.

Sica, A. and V. Bronte (2007). "Altered macrophage differentiation and immune dysfunction in tumor development." *J Clin Invest* 117(5): 1155-66.

Sica, A., P. Larghi, et al. (2008). "Macrophage polarization in tumour progression." *Semin Cancer Biol.* 18(5): 349-55 Epub 2008 Mar 26.

Sinha, P., V. K. Clements, et al. (2007). "Cross-talk between myeloid-derived suppressor cells and macrophages subverts tumor immunity toward a type 2 response." *J Immunol.* 179(2): 977-83.

Sinha, P., V. K. Clements, et al. (2007). "Prostaglandin E2 promotes tumor progression by inducing myeloid-derived suppressor cells." *Cancer Res* 67(9): 4507-13.

Smyth, M. J., M. W. Teng, et al. (2006). "CD4+CD25+ T regulatory cells suppress NK cell-mediated immunotherapy of cancer." *J Immunol.* 176(3): 1582-7.

Smyth, M. J. and J. A. Trapani (2001). "Lymphocyte-mediated immunosurveillance of epithelial cancers?" *Trends Immunol* 22(8): 409-11.

Sotomayor, E. M., I. Borrello, et al. (2001). "Cross-presentation of tumor antigens by bone marrow-derived antigen-presenting cells is the dominant mechanism in the induction of T-cell tolerance during B-cell lymphoma progression." *Blood.* 98(4): 1070-7.

Srivastava, M. K., P. Sinha, et al. (2010). "Myeloid-derived suppressor cells inhibit T-cell activation by depleting cystine and cysteine." *Cancer Res* 70(1): 68-77.

Staveley-O'Carroll, K., E. Sotomayor, et al. (1998). "Induction of antigen-specific T cell anergy: An early event in the course of tumor progression." *Proc Natl Acad Sci U S A* 95(3): 1178-83.

Steinman, R. M., D. Hawiger, et al. (2003). "Tolerogenic dendritic cells." *Annu Rev Immunol.* 21: 685-711 Epub 2001 Dec 19.

Stolina, M., S. Sharma, et al. (2000). "Specific inhibition of cyclooxygenase 2 restores antitumor reactivity by altering the balance of IL-10 and IL-12 synthesis." *J Immunol* 164(1): 361-70.

Subiza, J. L., J. E. Vinuela, et al. (1989). "Development of splenic natural suppressor (NS) cells in Ehrlich tumor-bearing mice." *Int J Cancer.* 44(2): 307-14.

Sugiura, K., M. Inaba, et al. (1988). "Wheat germ agglutinin-positive cells in a stem cell-enriched fraction of mouse bone marrow have potent natural suppressor activity." *Proc Natl Acad Sci U S A.* 85(13): 4824-6.

Sutmuller, R. P., L. M. van Duivenvoorde, et al. (2001). "Synergism of cytotoxic T lymphocyte-associated antigen 4 blockade and depletion of CD25(+) regulatory T cells in antitumor therapy reveals alternative pathways for suppression of autoreactive cytotoxic T lymphocyte responses." *J Exp Med* 194(6): 823-32.

Suzuki, E., V. Kapoor, et al. (2005). "Gemcitabine selectively eliminates splenic Gr-1+/CD11b+ myeloid suppressor cells in tumor-bearing animals and enhances antitumor immune activity." *Clin Cancer Res* 11(18): 6713-21.

Talmadge, J. E. (2007). "Pathways mediating the expansion and immunosuppressive activity of myeloid-derived suppressor cells and their relevance to cancer therapy." *Clin Cancer Res.* 13(18 Pt 1): 5243-8.

Thiery, J. P. (2002). "Epithelial-mesenchymal transitions in tumour progression." *Nat Rev Cancer.* 2(6): 442-54.

Tsujii, M. and R. Dubois (1995). "Alterations in cellular adhesion and apoptosis in epithelial cells overexpressing prostaglandin endoperoxide synthase-2." *Cell* 83: 493-501.

Tsujii, M., S. Kawano, et al. (1998). "Cyclooxygenase regulates angiogenesis induced by colon cancer cells." *Cell* 93(5): 705-16.

Ugel, S., F. Delpozzo, et al. (2009). "Therapeutic targeting of myeloid-derived suppressor cells." *Curr Opin Pharmacol* 9(4): 470-81.

Wang, H., F. Cheng, et al. (2005). "Imatinib mesylate (STI-571) enhances antigen-presenting cell function and overcomes tumor-induced CD4+ T-cell tolerance." *Blood.* 105(3): 1135-43. Epub 2004 Sep 28.

Willimsky, G. and T. Blankenstein (2005). "Sporadic immunogenic tumours avoid destruction by inducing T-cell tolerance." *Nature.* 437(7055): 141-6.

Wolff, H., K. Saukkonen, et al. (1998). "Expression of cyclooxygenase-2 in human lung carcinoma." *Cancer Res* 58(22): 4997-5001.

Woo, E. Y., C. S. Chu, et al. (2001). "Regulatory CD4(+)CD25(+) T cells in tumors from patients with early-stage non-small cell lung cancer and late-stage ovarian cancer." *Cancer Res* 61(12): 4766-72.

Yanagawa, J., T. C. Walser, et al. (2009). "Snail promotes CXCR2 ligand-dependent tumor progression in non-small cell lung carcinoma." *Clin Cancer Res.* 15(22): 6820-9. Epub 2009 Nov 3.

Yoshino, I., T. Yano, et al. (1992). "Tumor-reactive T-cells accumulate in lung cancer tissues but fail to respond due to tumor cell-derived factor." *Cancer Research* 52(4): 775-81.

Young, M. R., M. A. Wright, et al. (1996). "Suppression of T cell proliferation by tumor-induced granulocyte-macrophage progenitor cells producing transforming growth factor-beta and nitric oxide." *J Immunol.* 156(5): 1916-22.

Young, M. R., M. A. Wright, et al. (1997). "Myeloid differentiation treatment to diminish the presence of immune-suppressive CD34+ cells within human head and neck squamous cell carcinomas." *J Immunol.* 159(2): 990-6.

Zhang, Y., Q. Liu, et al. (2009). "Fas signal promotes lung cancer growth by recruiting myeloid-derived suppressor cells via cancer cell-derived PGE2." *J Immunol.* 182(6): 3801-8.

Zou, W. (2005). "Immunosuppressive networks in the tumour environment and their therapeutic relevance." *Nat Rev Cancer.* 5(4): 263-74.

8

Immunobiology of Monocytes/Macrophages in Hepatocellular Carcinoma

Dong-Ming Kuang* and Limin Zheng
Key Laboratory of Gene Engineering of the Ministry of Education, State Key Laboratory of Biocontrol, School of Life Sciences, Sun Yat-sen University, Guangzhou, P. R. China

1. Introduction

Hepatocellular carcinoma (HCC) is the fifth most common cancer worldwide and characterized by progressive development, high postsurgical recurrence and extremely poor prognosis [1–3]. The dismal outcome has been attributed to the highly vascular nature of HCC, which increases the propensity to spread and invade into neighboring or distant sites [4, 5]. Therefore, it is considered an urgent task to identify key prognostic factors of HCC and to elucidate the mechanisms of disease progression.

HCC is usually present in inflamed fibrotic and/or cirrhotic liver with extensive leukocyte infiltration [6, 7]. Thus, the immune status at different tumor sites can largely influence the biological behavior of HCC [6, 8, 9]. Several recent studies have shown that high infiltration of intratumoral regulatory T cells is associated with reduced survival and increased invasiveness in HCC [10, 11]. These findings are in accordance with the general view that the tumor microenvironment induces tolerance [12–14]. However, there is substantial evidence that the inflammatory response associated with cancers can also promote HCC progression by stimulating angiogenesis and tissue remodeling [6, 15, 16]. These findings strongly indicate that, besides inducing immune tolerance, HCC may also reroute the pro-inflammatory immune response into a tumor-promoting direction.

Macrophages (Mφs) constitute a major component of the leukocyte infiltrate in tumors. These cells are derived from circulating monocytes, and, in response to environmental signals, they acquire special phenotypic characteristics with diverse functions [17–19]. Recent studies have found that tumor environments co-opt the normal development of Mφs to dynamically activate the recruited monocytes in different niches of HCC. The malignant cells can thereby avoid initiation of potentially dangerous Mφ functions and create favorable conditions for tumor progression [20, 21]. Notably, the density of activated monocytes in the peritumoral stroma is selectively associated with vascular invasion and poor prognosis in HCC patients, whereas the increased infiltration of suppressive Mφs in the cancer nests is only correlated with the reduced survival of patients [22]. Thus, immune functional data of activated monocytes/Mφs in distinct cancer environments are essential for understanding their roles and potential mechanisms in HCC immunopathogenesis.

---

* Corresponding Author

In this chapter, we will summarize the current knowledge about the tumor immune microenvironment of HCC and the role of monocytes/Mφs in HCC progression, paying particular attention to the tissue micro-localization and phenotype of these cells. Additionally, we will describe the poly-directional communications between monocytes/Mφs and other stroma cells, including cytotoxic T cells, regulatory T cells, TH17/TC17 cells as well as neutrophils, and how activated monocytes in HCC repurpose the inflammatory response away from antitumor immunity and toward tissue remodeling and pro-angiogenic pathways. Finally, possible implications for the design of novel monocyte/Mφ-based immunotherapeutic strategies will be discussed.

2. Immune microenvironments of human HCC

After several decades of neglect, tumor microenvironments are once again an area of active research interest in cancer [23–25]. The biology of cancer cannot be understood simply by underlining the significance of the malignant cells but instead must encompass the contributions of the cancer microenvironment to tumorigenesis and disease progression.

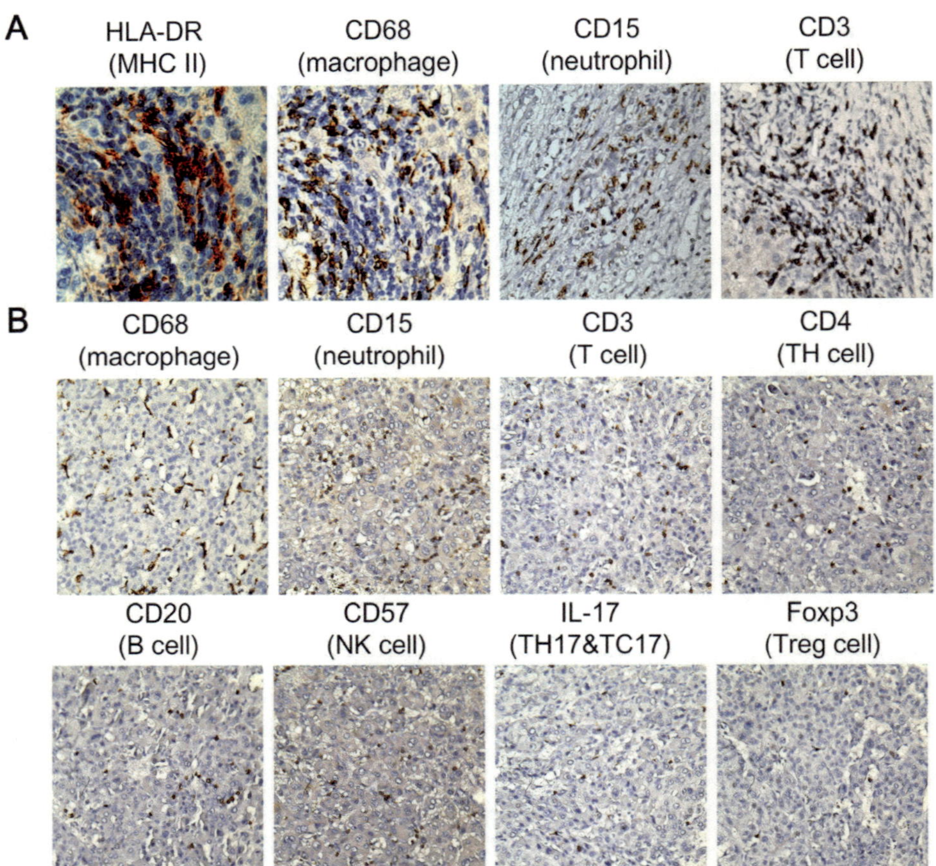

Fig. 1. **Infiltration patterns of immune cells in HCC samples.** Paraffin-embedded HCC sections were stained with indicated antibodies. The micrographs show the stained peritumoral stroma (A) and cancer nest (B).

Human HCC microenvironments, composed of non-cancer cells and their stroma (Figure 1), are now recognized as a major factor influencing the disease progression [6, 21]. Although normal stromal environment is non-permissive for HCC progression, hepatoma cells can modulate adjacent stroma to generate a supportive microenvironment. This includes the ability to alter the ratios of effectors to regulatory T cells and to affect the functions of APCs and the expression of co-signaling molecules, which in turn creates an immunosuppressive network to promote tumor progression and immune evasion [10, 21, 26]. However, there is also emerging evidence that the pro-inflammatory response at the tumor stroma can be rerouted in a tumor-promoting direction [15, 16]. These observations suggest that different tumor microenvironments can create either immune suppression or activation at distinct sites to promote tumor progression.

2.1 Immune responses against HCC

In HCC, several lines of evidence have suggest a positive role of immune system, e.g., by controlling hepatoma growth [7, 27–29]. Indeed, data from clinical investigations have revealed that HCC patients with an increased intratumoral accumulation of cytotoxic $CD8^+$ T lymphocytes had a superior 5-year survival rate and a prolonged recurrence-free survival after liver resection [11, 30]. In contrast, HCC-infiltrating $CD4^+$ T lymphocytes exhibited a $CD25^{high}Foxp3^+$ phenotype that was a predictor of poor overall survival of patients, indicating distinct roles of different tumor-infiltrating lymphocyte subsets in HCC [10, 11]. The important role of $CD8^+$ T cells in HCC control is further supported by studies in hepatoma-bearing mice; and interferon (IFN)-γ, perforin and granzyme B produced by $CD8^+$ T cells had been shown to be several major effector mechanisms for apoptosis of hepatoma cells [21, 31, 32].

Of note, the tumor-specific antigens (TSAs) in HCC patients are currently still under investigation. At present, several tumor-associated antigens (TAAs) of HCC have been identified, which has been recently introduced [7, 33]. In brief, several shared tumor antigens could also be recognized as antigens targeted by cytotoxic $CD8^+$ T cells in HCC, e.g., human telomerase-reverse transcriptase (hTERT) or NY-ESO-1. Expression of these antigens has been reported for other malignancies as well. Other antigens are expressed specifically in HCC and are also recognized by cells of the immune system, e.g., α-fetoprotein (AFP) or Glypican-3. The latter two antigens belong to the family of oncofetal antigens that are expressed only during ontogenesis. Although the exact mechanisms underlying are not yet clear, re-expression of such antigens is often observed in HCC. Thus, further research is also required to determine the frequency, immunodominance and strength of the immune responses induced against different TAAs.

Besides tumor-specific cytotoxic $CD8^+$ T cells, the natural killer (NK) cells have also been implicated in a successful immune response against HCC, e.g., by direct lysis of malignant cells [34]. Indeed, an increased preoperative NK cell activity that related to the expression of perforin and granzyme B was correlated with prolonged recurrence-free survival in HCC patients [35]. Contrarily, the NK cell dysfunction was shown to predict the poor survival of HCC patients after resection [36]. Other studies also showed that the stimulation of antigen-present cells (APCs) or natural killer T cells (NKT cells) can lead to an activation of NK cells and clearance of hepatoma cells in mice [37, 38].

Increased levels of B cells have been observed in several types of human tumor, and studies in mice indicate that, depending on microenvironment, tumor-infiltrating B cells are capable of being pro- or anti-tumorigenic [39, 40]. The role of B cells in human HCC is unclear thus far. B cell-derived autoantibodies against several antigens have been described in mouse models of HCC as well as in HCC patients [41, 42]. Additional studies showed that monoclonal antibodies against Glypican-3 were able to induce antibody-dependent cellular cytotoxicity (ADCC) and thus lysis of human hepatoma cells in vitro and in mice [43]. However, the importance of ADCC and antibodies in general in the natural immune response against HCC has not been investigated so far.

2.2 Immune responses promote HCC progression

Although immune system can exhibit vigorous anti-hepatoma activities in vitro, HCC-specific immune responses fail to control tumor progression in most patients. Clinical and experimental studies have demonstrated that the growth of HCC is closely associated with impaired differentiation and maturation of APCs, particularly Mφs and dendritic cells (DCs) [20, 44, 45]. Also, phenotypic and functional analyses of APCs from HCC patients have revealed that tumor cells or tumor-derived factors do favor differentiation of monocytes into tumor-associated Mφs (TAMs) [20] or tolerogenic semi-mature DCs (TDCs) [46]. Also, such abnormal development of APCs in the HCC microenvironment could intensely impact the infiltration and function of other immune cells in tumor in situ, which will be expounded in the 3rd section of this chapter.

Suppression of immune responses by regulatory T (Treg) cells is one of the major mechanisms for the induction and maintenance of self-tolerance [12, 13]. Recent studies reported increased numbers of Treg cells in the peripheral blood and tumor-infiltrating lymphocytes (TILs) in patients with ovarian or liver cancers, which impaired cell-mediated immunity and promoted disease progression [10, 11, 47, 48]. Experimental depletion of Treg cells in several types of tumor-bearing mice could successfully improve tumor clearance and enhance the efficacy of immunotherapy [49, 50]. In parallel, depletion of $CD4^{+}CD25^{+}$ Treg cells could effectively enhance T-lymphocyte and NK-cell effector function in advanced stage HCC patients [51, 52]. These data together suggest that Treg cells may impair cell-mediated immune responses to HCC. At present, the precise underlying mechanism by which Treg cells accumulate at the tumor site in HCC patients is also unknown.

A direct role in HCC progression has also been shown for other cells of the immune system. For example, high infiltration of intratumoral neutrophils has been shown to predict a reduced recurrence-free survival time of HCC patients after liver resection [53]. Of note, neutrophils at the tumor edge induced angiogenesis progression and thus indirectly enhanced cancer growth [9]. This observation becomes especially intriguing in light of the finding that peritumoral neutrophils can be recruited by the pro-inflammatory cytokine interleukin (IL)-17. IL-17 is produced by T cells, termed TC17 or TH17, in the $CD8^{+}$ or $CD4^{+}$ T cell compartment in tumor environments, respectively [54, 55]. Indeed, IL-17-producing cells accumulate in tumors from patients with HCC and that their levels are positively correlated with microvessel density in tissues and poor survival in HCC patients [56]. It should be noted that, in several types of human cancer, high level of IL-17 in tumors in situ can predict improved survival of patients and associates with increased infiltration of cytotoxic $CD8^{+}$ T cells [57, 58]. Therefore, a better understanding of the network of tumor immune environments might provide a novel strategy for the rational design of anticancer therapies.

3. Polarization of monocytes in HCC microenvironments

APCs are critical for initiating and maintaining tumor-specific T-cell responses [21, 46]. DCs are considered the most effective APCs for primary immune responses [59]; Mφs markedly outnumber other APCs and represent an abundant population of APCs in solid tumors [60]. Monocytes can give rise to either DCs or Mφs in human tumors. In HCC patients, increased HLA-DR^{+} monocytes in liver are associated with metastatic phenotype [6]. Thus, polarization of monocytes in the cancer environments is essential for understanding their roles in HCC immunopathogenesis.

3.1 Differentiation of monocyte-derived Mφs in HCC microenvironments

Mφs are essential components of host defense and act as both APCs and effector cells [19]. Under the influence of local conditions, they acquire specialized phenotypic characteristics with diverse functional programs [16–18]. Mφs constitute a major component of the leukocyte infiltrate of tumors, and the TAMs are derived almost entirely from circulating blood monocytes [17–19]. Mφs in normal or inflamed tissues exhibit spontaneous antitumor activity, whereas TAMs are polarized M2 cells that suppress antitumor immunity and promote tumor progression [61]. Those findings agree with clinical studies showing that a high density of TAM is associated with poor prognosis in most solid tumors [22, 62]. Although the precise underlying mechanisms are not yet clear, it is generally assumed that the tumor microenvironment is critical determinants of the phenotype of local Mφs. Tumor-derived factors, including IL-10 and transforming growth factor (TGF)-β, "educate" the newly recruited monocytes to take on a M2 phenotype and perform a protumoral role [63, 64]. In contrast, over-expression or local delivery of IL-12 can reestablish the antitumor activity of Mφs, and in that case a high density of TAMs is correlated with a marked reduction in tumor growth [65, 66]. Such opposing effects of Mφs on tumor progression indicate that selective modulation of Mφ polarization might serve as a novel strategy for cancer therapy. However, such an approach is hampered by the fact that the mechanisms by which tumor microenvironments educate Mφs to perform specific tasks have not been fully elucidated.

In HCC patients, soluble factors derived from hepatoma cells, including extracellular matrix components hyaluronan fragments [20], effectively induced the formation of TAMs. Interestingly, kinetic analysis revealed 2 opposing functional stages in the TAM life cycle: monocytes are rapidly activated during a narrow time window, 4 to 16 hours after their first exposure to hepatoma cell culture supernatants, and afterward the same cells become exhausted and their production of cytokines is extinguished, with the exception of IL-10 [20, 21]. Because TAMs are derived from blood monocytes, such sequential pre-activation and exhaustion of cells may reflect a novel immune-escape mechanism by which tumors dynamically regulate the functions of migrating monocytes at distinct tumoral sites. More precisely, this means that during their first exposure to the tumor microenvironment, the newly recruited monocytes may be transiently activated while they are approaching the stroma surrounding the tumor, with the aim of minimizing their potential to damage tumor cells. Thereafter, when these Mφs are in close proximity to the tumor cells, they become exhausted and thus fail to mount an effective antitumor immune response. This notion is supported by the observations in human HCC tissues, indicating that most CD68-positive cells are smaller and show high expression of HLA-DR in the peritumoral stromal region, whereas they exhibit a HLA-DR^{low}IL-10^{high} phenotype in the cancer nest (Figure 3 in Ref. 20).

Of note, similar activation patterns of monocytes/Mφs were detected in ovarian and lung cancer [20, 67].

Monocytes/Mφs in the peritumoral stroma of HCC had an activated phenotype with increased expression of HLA-DR, CD80, and CD86 [6]. Data from in vivo observations showed that such tumor-activated monocytes also expressed significant level of B7-H1 (PD-L1) [8, 21]; and autocrine TNF-α and IL-10, but not IFN-γ, released from activated monocytes, stimulated monocyte B7-H1 expression [21, 68]. Furthermore, in vitro study using recombinant TNF-α and IL-10 indicated that IL-10 was essential for B7-H1 induction and that pro-inflammatory TNF-α acted synergistically with anti-inflammatory IL-10 to enhance B7-H1 expression on monocytes. In addition, a positive correlation between IL-17-producing cells and B7-H1-expressing Mφs was also observed in the peritumoral stroma of HCC tissues (Figure 1 in Ref. 8). Although culture supernatants derived from hepatoma cells also induced B7-H1 expression on monocytes, IL-17 additionally increased hepatoma-mediated monocyte B7-H1 expression. Similar regulatory effect of IL-17 on APCs was also observed in hepatitis [69]. These findings reveal a fine-tuned collaborative action between different types of immune cells in the peritumoral stroma of HCC, which reroutes the monocyte inflammatory response into immunosuppression.

TAMs in the cancer nests of HCC exhibited an exhausted suppressive phenotype; they are strongly impaired with regard to various functions related to inflammation [20, 21]. However, in contact with autologous T cells, these suppressive Mφs recuperate their capabilities to produce low level of IL-12 in tumors, and thereby activate T cells to produce IFN-γ, which in turn leads to IDO expression in Mφs and ultimately impairs the antitumor T cell immunity (Zhao Q, et al. J Immunol. doi: 10.4049/jimmunol.1100164). These findings give important new insights into the collaborative action of tumor stroma cells that is exercised to counteract the normal development of Mφs in distinct HCC environments.

3.2 Differentiation of monocyte-derived DCs in HCC microenvironments

DCs are the most potent "professional" APCs, and they are responsible for integrating a variety of incoming signals and orchestrating the immune response [59]. Bidirectional interactions between DCs and T cells initiate either an immunogenic or a tolerogenic pathway, both of which play crucial roles in autoimmune diseases and tumor immunity [70, 71]. It is generally assumed that these two contrasting functions of DCs are associated with the maturation stages of the cells: fully mature DCs (mDCs) are efficient activators of naive T cells, whereas immature DCs (iDCs) have been implicated for anergy induction. Furthermore, an intermediate stage of maturation was recently described in which the cells are referred to as semi-mature DCs [72]. These DCs expressed high levels of MHC class II and co-stimulatory molecules, even though they exhibited an IL-12^{low}IL-10^{high} phenotype [73]. It was also observed that the semi-mature DCs can induce tolerance by generating regulatory T cells and/or T cell anergy [74].

In HCC patients, soluble factors derived from hepatoma cells drove human monocytes to become tolerogenic DCs (TDCs) that exhibited a semi-mature phenotype with a 2- to 5-fold increase in expression of CD83, CD86, and HLA-DR, and a distinctive IL-12^{low}IL-10^{high} cytokine production profile [46]. Upon encountering T cells, the TDCs triggered rapid down-regulation of CD3ε and TCR-α/β and subsequent apoptosis in autologous T cells.

Consistent with these results, accumulation of immunosuppressive DCs coincided with CD3ε down-regulation and T cell deletion in the cancer nests of human HCC tumors (Figure 2 and 4 in Ref. 46). The impaired T cell function was mediated by factor(s) released by live TDCs after direct interaction with lymphocytes. Also, the TDC-induced effect on T cells was markedly reduced by blocking of NADPH oxidase but not by inhibition of arginase, inducible NO synthase (iNOS), indoleamine 2, 3-dioxygenase (IDO), or IFN-γ. These observations indicate that tumor microenvironments educate DCs to adopt a semi-mature phenotype, which in turn aids tumor immune escape by causing defects in the CD3/TCR complex and deletion of T cells. In addition, besides triggering T cell apoptosis, hepatoma-exposed DCs also play an important role in expanding intratumoral Treg cells [45].

4. Cross talks between monocytes/Mφs and other stroma cells in HCC tissues

Tumor progression is now recognized as the product of evolving crosstalk between different cell types within the tumor and its stroma [23, 24]. HCC environments can alter the normal development of Mφs that is intended to trigger transient early activation of monocytes in the peritumoral region, which in turn induces formation of suppressive TAMs in the cancer nests [20, 21]. In this section, we will describe several recent findings about the cross talks between monocytes/Mφs and other stroma cells, paying particular attention to the tissue micro-localization and phenotype of these cells in HCC.

4.1 Activated monocytes in the peritumoral stroma of HCC foster immune privilege and disease progression through B7-H1

B7-H1 is a cell-surface glycoprotein belonging to the B7 family of co-signaling molecules with a profound regulatory effect on T cell responses [75]. Studies in mouse models have revealed that expression of B7-H1 helped dormant tumor cells to evade cytotoxic T cell responses [14]. In human HCC, B7-H1$^+$ monocytes/Mφs and CD8$^+$ T cells were both accumulated in the peritumoral stroma of HCC tissues, which suggests that these monocytes/Mφs promote tumor progression by impairing T cell immunity (Figure 1, 3-5 in Ref. 21). Supporting this hypothesis, a significantly larger portion of the tumor-infiltrating cytotoxic T cells was found to express the B7-H1 receptor PD-1 [8, 21, 68]. Moreover, HCC-infiltrating T cells co-cultured with HCC-derived monocytes exhibited an impaired production of IFN-γ, and blockade of B7-H1 by pre-incubation of tumor monocytes with the mAb MIH1 could markedly enhance the ability of tumor T cells to produce that cytokine. Consistent with these data, only PD-1$^+$ cytotoxic T cells isolated from HCC tissues exhibited attenuated production of IFN-γ, IL-2, and TNF-a as well as low cytotoxic potential [21]. These findings, together with regulatory mechanism of B7-H1 in monocytes/Mφs (Section 2A), suggest that there is a fine-turned collaborative action between immune activation and immunosuppression in tumor microenvironments. Soluble factors derived from hepatoma cells [21], as well as IL-17 released by TH17 and TC17 [54, 55], can trigger transient activation of newly recruited monocytes in the peritumoral stroma area of HCC, and thereby induce the monocytes to produce significant amount of cytokines, including TNF-α, IL-23, IL-1β, and IL-10, which in turn leads to the expression of B7-H1 protein on their surface and ultimately impairs the antitumor T cell immunity.

4.2 Activated monocytes in the peritumoral stroma of HCC promote expansion of memory IL-17-producing T cells

Although cancer patients exhibit a generalized immunosuppressive status, substantial evidence indicates that the inflammatory reaction at a tumor site can promote tumor growth and progression. HCC is usually derived from inflamed cirrhotic liver with extensive leukocyte infiltration. Recent study has shown that TH17 cells were highly enriched in HCC and their levels were positively correlated with micro-vessel density in tissues and poor survival in HCC patients [56]. In contrast to the classical TH17 cells that hardly express IFN-γ, almost half of the IL-17-producing $CD4^+$ T cells we isolated from HCC tissues were able to simultaneously produce IFN-γ, suggesting that the tumor microenvironment can profoundly determine the phenotype of such cells [54–56]. In addition, the IL-17-producing cells often predominantly accumulate in the peritumoral stroma rather than in the cancer nests of HCC [54, 55]. A significant correlation between the levels of $CD68^+$ cells and $IL\text{-}17^+$ lymphocytes was found in the peritumoral stroma of HCC (Figure 1 in Ref. 54). However, there was no such correlation in intratumoral tissue, suggesting that Mφs in different parts of HCC play disparate roles in IL-17-producing T cell expansion.

Most of the $CD68^+$ cells in the peritumoral stroma had a smaller volume and showed marked expression of HLA-DR, which implies that they were newly recruited and activated monocytes. In contrast, most Mφs in the cancer nests were negative for HLA-DR (Figure 2). Accordingly, hepatoma-activated monocytes were significantly superior to the suppressive tumor Mφs in inducing expansion of both TH17 ($CD4^+$ IL-17-producing T cells) and TC17 ($CD8^+$ IL-17-producing T cells) cells from circulating memory T cells in vitro with phenotypic features similar to those isolated from HCC, and these monocytes secreted a set of key pro-inflammatory cytokines, including IL-1β, IL-6, and IL-23, that triggered proliferation of functional TH17 cells. In addition, inhibition of monocytes/Mφs inflammation in liver markedly reduced the level of tumor-infiltrating $IL\text{-}17^+$ cells and tumor growth in vivo [54]. Therefore, the pro-inflammatory IL-17-producing cells are

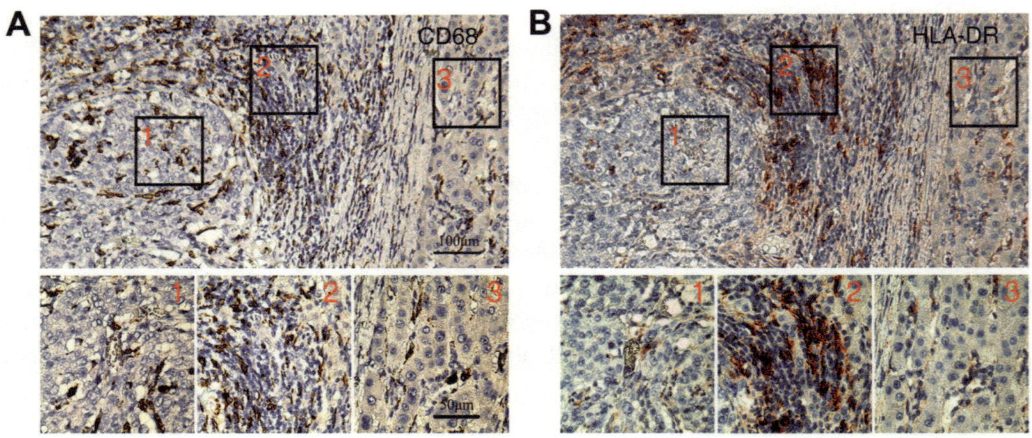

Fig. 2. **Distinct activation patterns of monocytes/Mφs in HCC samples.** Adjacent sections of paraffin-embedded HCC samples were stained with an anti-CD68 (A) or anti-HLA-DR (B). The micrographs at higher magnification show the stained cancer nest (1), peritumoral stroma (2), and adjacent normal tissue (3).

generated and regulated by a fine-tuned collaborative action between different types of immune cells in distinct HCC microenvironments, and allow the inflammatory response of activated monocytes to be rerouted in a tumor-promoting direction. Selectively modulating the "context" of inflammatory response in tumors might provide a novel strategy for anticancer therapy.

4.3 Peritumoral neutrophils link inflammatory response to disease progression by fostering angiogenesis in HCC

Most monocytes/Mφs in the peritumoral stroma of HCC exhibit an activated phenotype that favors the generation of IL-17-producing cells in the same area, and their levels were correlated with disease progression in HCC patients [54]. Interestingly, another important myeloid cell population, namely tumor-associated neutrophils (TANs), was also enriched predominantly in the peritumoral stroma of HCC tissues, and their levels were well correlated with IL-17-producing cell density in the same area (Figure 2 in Ref. 9). Data from both clinical sample analysis and experimental studies showed that functional IL-17^{+} cells in the peritumoral stroma stimulated epithelial cells to produce CXC chemokines that induced neutrophil trafficking to tumors [9]. Thereafter, exposure of neutrophils to HCC environment resulted in sustained survival of cells [76]. The accumulated neutrophils in the peritumoral stroma were the major source of MMP-9, which in turn triggered the angiogenic switch at the adjacent invading edge [9]. These data, therefore, provide direct evidence that neutrophils play an important role in human tumor progression by serving as a link between the pro-inflammatory response and angiogenesis in the tumor milieu. This notion is supported by the findings that the density of neutrophils in the peritumoral stroma was correlated with advanced disease stages and could serve as an independent predictor of poor survival in HCC patients (Figure 1 in Ref. 9). Consistent with these results, tumor angiogenesis is often more active at the invading edge, which is close to the peritumoral stroma, than intratumoral areas.

4.4 Activated CD69^{+} T cells foster immune privilege by regulating Mφ IDO expression in the cancer nest of HCC

IDO is a rate-limiting enzyme for tryptophan catabolism. In humans and mice, IDO inhibits antigen-specific T cell proliferation in vitro and suppresses T cell responses to fetal alloantigens during murine pregnancy [71, 77, 78]. Expression of IDO is often induced or maintained by many inflammatory cytokines, of which IFN-γ is the most potent [71]. In addition to being expressed in APCs, most human cancers also express high levels of IDO protein which correlates with poor prognosis in some cases [78]. In contrast, low or rare IDO expression is observed in most mouse and human tumor-cell lines, possibly due to the lack of a complete cancer microenvironment in cell lines in vitro [78, 79]. At present, little is known about the regulating mechanisms of IDO in TAMs at stroma of human tumors in situ.

Experimental studies indicate that the IDO proteins are selectively high expressed by Mφ in several types of human tumors, including HCC (Zhao Q, et al. J Immunol. doi: 10.4049/jimmunol.1100164). However, exposure to hepatoma cell culture supernatants did not elicit the IDO expression in monocytes/Mφs, which suggests that additional factors within the tumor milieu are required for inducing IDO expression in tumor Mφs. CD69 is an immunoregulatory molecule expressed by early activated leukocytes at sites of chronic inflammation and $CD69^+$ T cells have been found to promote human tumor progression [80, 81]. Upon encountering autologous $CD69^+$ T cells, tumor Mφs acquired capabilities to produce greatly higher amount of IDO protein. The T cells isolated from the HCC tissues expressed significant CD69 molecules than those on paired circulating and non-tumor-infiltrating T cells; and these tumor-derived $CD69^+$ T cells could induce considerable IDO in monocytes. Interestingly, the tumor-associated monocytes/Mφ isolated from HCC tissues or generated by in vitro culture effectively activated circulating T cells to express CD69. IL-12 derived from tumor Mφ was required for early T cell activation and subsequent IDO expression (Zhao Q, et al. J Immunol. doi: 10.4049/jimmunol.1100164). Consistent with this, another recent study has shown that intratumoral delivery of exogenous IL-12 could elicit an IFN-γ-dependent IDO counter-regulation in mouse model [82]. Moreover, the conditioned medium form IDO^+ Mφ effectively suppressed T cell responses in vitro; an effect which could be reversed by adding extrinsic IDO substrate tryptophan or by pre-treating Mφs with an IDO-specific inhibitor 1-MT. Such an active induction of immune-tolerance should be considered for the rational design of effective immune-based anti-cancer therapies.

4.5 Increased intratumoral Treg cells are related to intratumoral Mφs and poor prognosis in HCC patients

Treg cell-mediated immunosuppression is a crucial strategy of tumor immune evasion and a main obstacle for successful cancer immunotherapy [12]. Several recent studies have demonstrated that $FoxP3^+$ Treg cells with immunosuppressive properties were concentrated within HCC tumors and that the intratumoral prevalence of $FoxP3^+$ Treg cells was associated with disease progression and poor prognosis [10, 11]. However, the source of Treg cells in HCC is still unclear. By analyzing the association between the densities of Treg cells and Mφs in HCC tissue, Zhou et al observed that the elevated intratumoral $FoxP3^+$ Treg population was correlated with high-intratumoral Mφ density in HCC patients [26]. Depletion of liver Mφs thus decreased the frequency of liver $FoxP3^+$ Treg cells in hepatoma-bearing mice. Additionally, Mφs exposed to TSNs from hepatoma-derived cell lines augmented the $FoxP3^+$ Treg population, partially via IL-10. However, in the absence of Mφs, culture supernatants derived from hepatoma cells could not increase the percentage of $FoxP3^+$ Treg cells upon anti-CD3/CD28 stimulation. These data indicated that HCC-associated immunosuppressive Mφs can increase the intratumoral $FoxP3^+$ Treg population.

Cross talks between monocytes/Mφs and other stroma cells are summarized in Figure 3. Notably, the regulatory mechanisms of monocytes/Mφs are less well understood in human HCC. Besides interacting with TH17, TC17, Treg, and $CD69^+$ T cells, tumor-associated monocytes/Mφs also secrete molecules (eg, TGF-β, osteopontin), which directly induced epithelial-mesenchymal transition or transformation (EMT) of cancer cells [83]. Moreover, one of our latest finding indicated that monocytes/Mφs isolated from human HCC tissues induced NK cell dysfunction via a 2B4/CD48 interaction (Wu et al. Unpublished data). In addition, although not directly related to HCC, tumor-infiltrating Treg cells can trigger production of IL-10 by Mφs, which in turn stimulates such cells to express B7-H4 in an autocrine manner and renders them immunosuppressive via the B7-H4 molecules [84]. Therefore, manipulating the involved molecules may open new avenues for developing novel immune-based therapies to enhance antitumor immunity in human cancer.

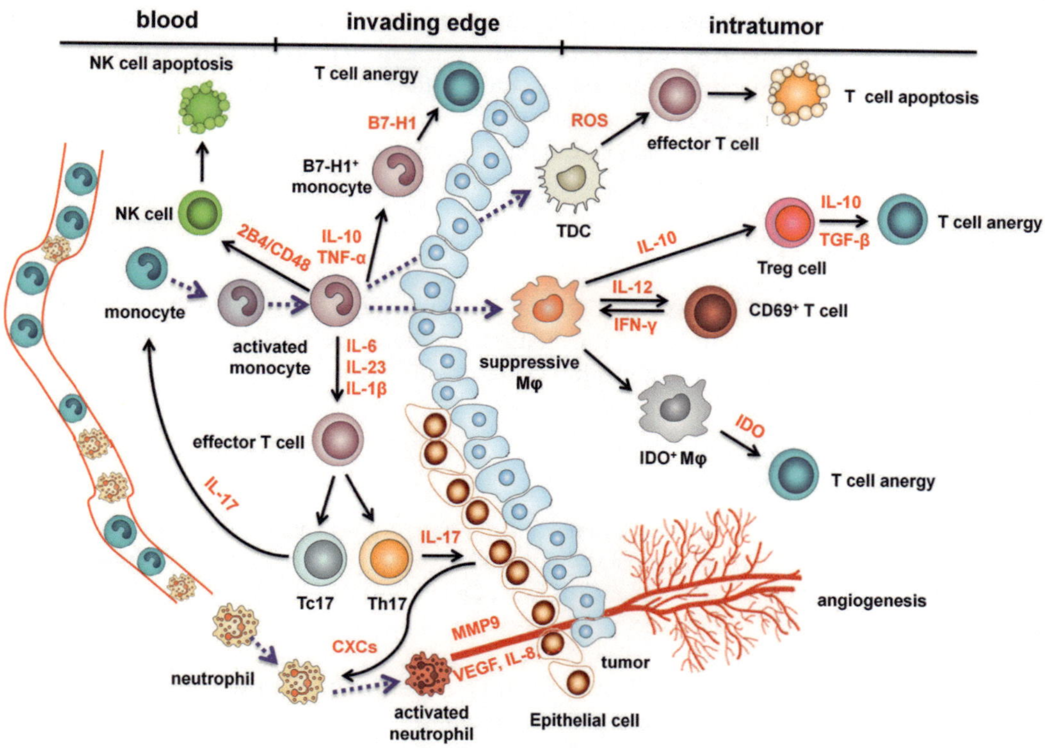

Fig. 3. Map of Cross talks between monocytes/Mφs and other immune cells in distinct niches of HCC.

5. Summary

Much research has been focused on tumor-mediated immunosuppression over the past decade. However, in spite of the generalized immunosuppressive status in cancer patients, many malignancies arise at sites of chronic inflammation, and inflammatory mediators are often produced in tumors [85, 86]. Human HCC tissues can be anatomically classified into areas of intratumoral and peritumoral stroma, each with distinct compositions and functional properties [20, 21, 54, 55]. Intratumoral environments of HCC usually contain abundant immunosuppressive molecules and cells to inhibit the T cell responses and create conditions that are conducive to tumor growth [20, 26]. In contrast, the peritumoral stromal areas of HCC contain a significant amount of leukocyte infiltrate, which are thereby situated close to the advancing edge of a tumor [21, 54]. Monocytes/Mφs represent an abundant population of APCs in HCC. Soluble factors derived from hepatoma cells can alter the normal developmental process of Mφs that is intended to dynamically regulate monocyte activation at distinct sites [20]. Hepatoma-activated monocytes in the peritumoral stroma induce sequential expansion of memory TH17 and TC17 cells and infiltration of neutrophils to promote inflammation and angiogenesis at invading tumor edge [54, 55]. Of note, these activated monocytes also express high level of B7-H1 to inhibit tumor-specific T cell immunity [21], and in that way repurpose the inflammatory response away from anti-tumor immunity (the sword) and towards tissue remodeling and pro-angiogenic pathways (a plowshare). Furthermore, interactions between suppressive Mφs and T cells in the cancer nest of HCC lead to Mφ IDO expression and Treg cell expansion [26]. Thus, it is not inflammation per se but inflammatory "context" that determines the ability of pro-inflammatory factors to facilitate or prevent tumor growth. Studying the mechanisms that can selectively modulate the functional activities of monocytes/Mφs might provide a novel strategy for anticancer therapy.

6. Acknowledgment

This work was supported by the Fundamental Research Funds for the Central Universities (11lgzd12) and project grants from the National Natural Science Foundation of China (81000915 and 81171882) and the Education Department of Guangdong Province (LYM10008 and sybzzxm201108).

7. References

[1] Llovet JM, Burroughs A, Bruix J. Hepatocellular carcinoma. Lancet. 2003;362:1907-17.

[2] Schwartz M, Roayaie S, Konstadoulakis M. Strategies for the management of hepatocellular carcinoma.Nat Clin Pract Oncol. 2007;4:424-32.

[3] Bruix J, Llovet JM. Prognostic prediction and treatment strategy in hepatocellular carcinoma. Hepatology. 2002;35:519-24.

[4] Poon RT, Ng IO, Lau C, et al. Tumor microvessel density as a predictor of recurrence after resection of hepatocellular carcinoma: a prospective study. J Clin Oncol. 2002;20:1775-85.

[5] Semela D, Dufour JF. Angiogenesis and hepatocellular carcinoma. J Hepatol. 2004;41:864-80.

[6] Budhu A, Forgues M, Ye QH, et al. Prediction of venous metastases, recurrence, and prognosis in hepatocellular carcinoma based on a unique immune response signature of the liver microenvironment. Cancer Cell. 2006;10:99-111.

[7] Flecken T, Spangenberg HC, Thimme R. Immunobiology of hepatocellular carcinoma. Langenbecks Arch Surg. DOI: 10.1007/s00423-011-0783-x.

[8] Zhao Q, Xiao X, Wu Y, et al. Interleukin-17-educated monocytes suppress cytotoxic T-cell function through B7-H1 in hepatocellular carcinoma patients. Eur J Immunol. 2011;41:2314-22.

[9] Kuang DM, Zhao Q, Wu Y, et al. Peritumoral neutrophils link inflammatory response to disease progression by fostering angiogenesis in hepatocellular carcinoma. J Hepatol. 2011;54:948-55.

[10] Fu J, Xu D, Liu Z, et al. Increased regulatory T cells correlate with CD8 T-cell impairment and poor survival in hepatocellular carcinoma patients. Gastroenterology. 2007;132:2328-39.

[11] Gao Q, Qiu SJ, Fan J, et al. Intratumoral balance of regulatory and cytotoxic T cells is associated with prognosis of hepatocellular carcinoma after resection. J Clin Oncol. 2007;25:2586-93.

[12] Zou W. Regulatory T cells, tumour immunity and immunotherapy. Nat Rev Immunol. 2006;6:295-307.

[13] Rabinovich GA, Gabrilovich D, Sotomayor EM. Immunosuppressive strategies that are mediated by tumor cells. Annu Rev Immunol. 2007;25:267-96.

[14] Zou W. Immunosuppressive networks in the tumour environment and their therapeutic relevance. Nat Rev Cancer. 2005;5:263-74.
[15] Mantovani A, Allavena P, Sica A, et al. Cancer-related inflammation. Nature. 2008;454:436-44.
[16] Mosser DM, Edwards JP. Exploring the full spectrum of macrophage activation. Nat Rev Immunol. 2008;8:958-69.
[17] Lewis CE, Pollard JW. Distinct role of macrophages in different tumor microenvironments. Cancer Res. 2006;66:605-12.
[18] Pollard JW. Tumour-educated macrophages promote tumour progression and metastasis. Nat Rev Cancer. 2004;4:71-8.
[19] Gordon S, Taylor PR. Monocyte and macrophage heterogeneity. Nat Rev Immunol. 2005;5:953-64.
[20] Kuang DM, Wu Y, Chen N, et al. Tumor-derived hyaluronan induces formation of immunosuppressive macrophages through transient early activation of monocytes. Blood. 2007;110:587-95.
[21] Kuang DM, Zhao Q, Peng C, et al. Activated monocytes in peritumoral stroma of hepatocellular carcinoma foster immune privilege and disease progression through PD-L1. J Exp Med. 2009;206:1327-37.
[22] Ding T, Xu J, Wang F, et al. High tumor-infiltrating macrophage density predicts poor prognosis in patients with primary hepatocellular carcinoma after resection. Hum Pathol. 2009;40:381-9.
[23] Mueller MM, Fusenig NE. Friends or foes - bipolar effects of the tumor stroma in cancer. Nat Rev Cancer. 2004;4:839-49.
[24] Tlsty TD, Coussens LM. Tumor stroma and regulation of cancer development. Annu Rev Pathol. 2006;1:119-150.
[25] Ahmed F, Steele JC, Herbert JM, et al. Tumor stroma as a target in cancer. Curr Cancer Drug Targets. 2008;8:447-453.
[26] Zhou J, Ding T, Pan W, et al. Increased intratumoral regulatory T cells are related to intratumoral macrophages and poor prognosis in hepatocellular carcinoma patients. Int J Cancer. 2009;125:1640-8.
[27] Doskali M, Tanaka Y, Ohira M, et al. Possibility of adoptive immunotherapy with peripheral blood-derived $CD3^{-}CD56^{+}$ and $CD3^{+}CD56^{+}$ cells for inducing antihepatocellular carcinoma and antihepatitis C virus activity. J Immunother. 2011;34:129-38.
[28] Abushahba W, Balan M, Castaneda I, et al. Antitumor activity of type I and type III interferons in BNL hepatoma model. Cancer Immunol Immunother. 2010;59:1059-71.
[29] Mizukoshi E, Nakamoto Y, Arai K, et al. Comparative analysis of various tumor-associated antigen-specific t-cell responses in patients with hepatocellular carcinoma. Hepatology. 2011;53:1206-16.
[30] Unitt E, Marshall A, Gelson W, et al. Tumour lymphocytic infiltrate and recurrence of hepatocellular carcinoma following liver transplantation. J Hepatol. 2006;45:246-53.
[31] Hiroishi K, Eguchi J, Baba T, et al. Strong CD8(+) T-cell responses against tumor-associated antigens prolong the recurrence-free interval after tumor treatment in patients with hepatocellular carcinoma. J Gastroenterol. 2010;45:451-8.
[32] Komita H, Homma S, Saotome H, et al. Interferon-gamma produced by interleukin-12-activated tumor infiltrating CD8+T cells directly induces apoptosis of mouse hepatocellular carcinoma. J Hepatol. 2006;45:662-72.

[33] Breous E, Thimme R. Potential of immunotherapy for hepatocellular carcinoma. J Hepatol. 2011;54:830-4.
[34] Caligiuri MA. Human natural killer cells. Blood. 2008;112:461-9.
[35] Taketomi A, Shimada M, Shirabe K, et al. Natural killer cell activity in patients with hepatocellular carcinoma: a new prognostic indicator after hepatectomy. Cancer. 1998;83:58-63.
[36] Chuang WL, Liu HW, Chang WY. Natural killer cell activity in patients with hepatocellular carcinoma relative to early development and tumor invasion. Cancer. 1990;65:926-30.
[37] Miyagi T, Takehara T, Tatsumi T, et al. CD1d-mediated stimulation of natural killer T cells selectively activates hepatic natural killer cells to eliminate experimentally disseminated hepatoma cells in murine liver. Int J Cancer. 2003;106:81-9.
[38] Nedvetzki S, Sowinski S, Eagle RA, et al. Reciprocal regulation of human natural killer cells and macrophages associated with distinct immune synapses. Blood. 2007;109:3776-85.
[39] Andreu P, Johansson M, Affara NI, et al. FcRgamma activation regulates inflammation-associated squamous carcinogenesis. Cancer Cell. 2010;17:121-34.
[40] de Visser KE, Korets LV, Coussens LM. De novo carcinogenesis promoted by chronic inflammation is B lymphocyte dependent. Cancer Cell. 2005;7:411-23.
[41] Chen X, Fu S, Chen F, et al. Identification of tumor-associated antigens in human hepatocellular carcinoma by autoantibodies. Oncol Rep. 2008;20:979-85.
[42] Heo CK, Woo MK, Yu DY, et al. Identification of autoantibody against fatty acid synthase in hepatocellular carcinoma mouse model and its application to diagnosis of HCC. Int J Oncol. 2010;36:1453-9.
[43] Nakano K, Orita T, Nezu J, et al. Anti-glypican 3 antibodies cause ADCC against human hepatocellular carcinoma cells. Biochem Biophys Res Commun. 2009;378:279-84.
[44] Beckebaum S, Zhang X, Chen X, et al. Increased levels of interleukin-10 in serum from patients with hepatocellular carcinoma correlate with profound numerical deficiencies and immature phenotype of circulating dendritic cell subsets. Clin Cancer Res. 2004;10:7260-9.
[45] Li L, Li SP, Min J, et al. Hepatoma cells inhibit the differentiation and maturation of dendritic cells and increase the production of regulatory T cells. Immunol Lett. 2007;114:38-45.
[46] Kuang DM, Zhao Q, Xu J, et al. Tumor-educated tolerogenic dendritic cells induce CD3epsilon down-regulation and apoptosis of T cells through oxygen-dependent pathways. J Immunol. 2008;181:3089-98.
[47] Wei S, Kryczek I, Edwards RP, et al. Interleukin-2 administration alters the CD4+FOXP3+ T-cell pool and tumor trafficking in patients with ovarian carcinoma. Cancer Res. 2007;67:7487-94.
[48] Curiel TJ, Coukos G, Zou L, et al. Specific recruitment of regulatory T cells in ovarian carcinoma fosters immune privilege and predicts reduced survival. Nat Med. 2004;10:942-9.
[49] Shimizu J, Yamazaki S, Sakaguchi S. Induction of tumor immunity by removing CD25+CD4+ T cells: a common basis between tumor immunity and autoimmunity. J Immunol. 1999;163:5211-18.

[50] Steitz J, Bruck J, Lenz J, et al. Depletion of CD25(+) CD4(+) T cells and treatment with tyrosinase-related protein 2-transduced dendritic cells enhance the interferon alpha-induced. CD8(+) T-cell-dependent immune defense of B16 melanoma. Cancer Res. 2001;61:8643-6.
[51] Ghiringhelli F, Menard C, Puig PE, et al. Metronomic cyclophosphamide regimen selectively depletes CD4+CD25+ regulatory T cells and restores T and NK effector functions in end stage cancer patients. Cancer Immunol Immunother. 2007;56:641-8.
[52] Mahnke K, Schonfeld K, Fondel S, et al. Depletion of CD4+CD25+ human regulatory T cells in vivo: kinetics of Treg depletion and alterations in immune functions in vivo and in vitro. Int J Cancer. 2007;120:2723-33.
[53] Li YW, Qiu SJ, Fan J, et al. Intratumoral neutrophils: a poor prognostic factor for hepatocellular carcinoma following resection. J Hepatol. 2011;54:497-505.
[54] Kuang DM, Peng C, Zhao Q, et al. Activated monocytes in peritumoral stroma of hepatocellular carcinoma promote expansion of memory T helper 17 cells. Hepatology. 2010;51:154-64.
[55] Kuang DM, Peng C, Zhao Q, et al. Tumor-activated monocytes promote expansion of IL-17-producing CD8+ T cells in hepatocellular carcinoma patients. J Immunol. 2010;185:1544-9.
[56] Zhang JP, Yan J, Xu J, et al. Increased intratumoral IL-17-producing cells correlate with poor survival in hepatocellular carcinoma patients. J Hepatol. 2009;50:980-9.
[57] Zou W, Restifo NP. T(H)17 cells in tumour immunity and immunotherapy. Nat Rev Immunol. 2010;10:248-56.
[58] Kryczek I, Banerjee M, Cheng P, et al. Phenotype, distribution, generation, and functional and clinical relevance of Th17 cells in the human tumor environments. Blood. 2009;114:1141-9.
[59] Banchereau J, Briere F, Caux C, et al. Immunobiology of dendritic cells. Annu Rev Immunol. 2000;18:767-811.
[60] Kryczek I, Zou L, Rodriguez P, et al. B7-H4 expression identifies a novel suppressive macrophage population in human ovarian carcinoma. J Exp Med. 2006;203:871-81.
[61] Mantovani A, Sozzani S, Locati M, et al. Macrophage polarization: tumor-associated macrophages as a paradigm for polarized M2 mononuclear phagocytes. Trends Immunol. 2002;23:549-55.
[62] Chen JJ, Lin YC, Yao PL, et al. Tumor-associated macrophages: the double-edged sword in cancer progression. J Clin Oncol. 2005;23:953-64.
[63] Katakura T, Miyazaki M, Kobayashi M, et al. CCL17 and IL-10 as effectors that enable alternatively activated macrophages to inhibit the generation of classically activated macrophages. J Immunol. 2004;172:1407-13.
[64] Maeda H, Kuwahara H, Ichimura Y, et al. TGF-beta enhances macrophage ability to produce IL-10 in normal and tumor-bearing mice. J Immunol. 1995;155:4926-32.
[65] Satoh T, Saika T, Ebara S, et al. Macrophages transduced with an adenoviral vector expressing interleukin 12 suppress tumor growth and metastasis in a preclinical metastatic prostate cancer model. Cancer Res. 2003;63:7853-60.
[66] Watkins SK, Egilmez NK, Suttles J, et al. IL-12 rapidly alters the functional profile of tumorassociated and tumor-infiltrating macrophages in vitro and in vivo. J Immunol. 2007;178:1357-62.
[67] Hagemann T, Wilson J, Burke F, et al. Ovarian cancer cells polarize macrophages toward a tumor-associated phenotype. J Immunol. 2006;176:5023-32.

[68] Wu K, Kryczek I, Chen L, et al. Kupffer cell suppression of CD8+ T cells in human hepatocellular carcinoma is mediated by B7-H1/programmed death-1 interactions. Cancer Res. 2009;69:8067-75.
[69] Zhang JY, Zhang Z, Lin F, et al. Interleukin-17-producing CD4(+) T cells increase with severity of liver damage in patients with chronic hepatitis B. Hepatology. 2010;51:81-91.
[70] Vlad G, Cortesini R, Suciu-Foca N. License to heal: bidirectional interaction of antigen-specific regulatory T cells and tolerogenic APC. J Immunol. 2005;174:5907-14.
[71] Mellor AL, Munn DH. IDO expression by dendritic cells: tolerance and tryptophan catabolism. Nat Rev Immunol. 2004;4:762-74.
[72] Reis e Sousa C. Dendritic cells in a mature age. Nat Rev Immunol. 2006;6:476-83.
[73] Rutella S, Danese S, Leone G. Tolerogenic dendritic cells: cytokine modulation comes of age. Blood. 2006;108:1435-40.
[74] Verginis P, Li HS, Carayanniotis G. Tolerogenic semimature dendritic cells suppress experimental autoimmune thyroiditis by activation of thyroglobulin-specific CD4+CD25+ T cells. J Immunol. 2005;174:7433-39.
[75] Zou W, Chen L. Inhibitory B7-family molecules in the tumour microenvironment. Nat Rev Immunol. 2008;8:467-77.
[76] Wu Y, Zhao Q, Peng C, et al. Neutrophils promote motility of cancer cells via a hyaluronan-mediated TLR4/PI3K activation loop. J Pathol. 2011;225:438-47.
[77] Terness P, Chuang JJ, Opelz G. The immunoregulatory role of IDO-producing human dendritic cells revisited. Trends Immunol. 2006;27:68-73.
[78] Uyttenhove C, Pilotte L, Théate I, et al. Evidence for a tumoral immune resistance mechanism based on tryptophan degradation by indoleamine 2, 3-dioxygenase. Nat Med. 2003;9:1269-1274.
[79] Godin-Ethier J, Pelletier S, Hanafi LA, et al. Human activated T lymphocytes modulate IDO expression in tumors through Th1/Th2 balance. J Immunol. 2009;183:7752-60.
[80] Wald O, Izhar U, Amir G, et al. CD4+CXCR4highCD69+T cells accumulate in lung adenocarcinoma. J Immunol. 2006;177:6983-90.
[81] Han Y, Guo Q, Zhang M, et al. CD69+ CD4+ CD25- T cells, a new subset of regulatory T cells, suppress T cell proliferation through membrane-bound TGF-beta 1. J Immunol. 2009;182:111-20.
[82] Gu T, Rowswell-Turner RB, Kilinc MO, et al. Central role of IFNgamma-indoleamine 2, 3-dioxygenase axis in regulation of interleukin-12-mediated antitumor immunity. Cancer Res. 2010;70:129-38.
[83] Cheng J, Huo DH, Kuang DM, et al. Human macrophages promote the motility and invasiveness of osteopontin-knockdown tumor cells. Cancer Res. 2007;67:5141-7.
[84] Kryczek I, Wei S, Zou L, et al. Cutting edge: induction of B7-H4 on APCs through IL-10: novel suppressive mode for regulatory T cells. J Immunol. 2006;177:40-44.
[85] Karin M, Lawrence T, Nizet V. Innate immunity gone awry: linking microbial infections to chronic inflammation and cancer. Cell. 2006;124:823-35.
[86] Vakkila J, Lotze MT. Inflammation and necrosis promote tumour growth. Nat Rev Immunol. 2004;4:641-8.

9

Macrophages and Microglia in Brain Malignancies

Cristina Riccadonna and Paul R. Walker
Geneva University Hospitals and University of Geneva, Switzerland

1. Introduction

Tumour and myeloid cell interactions that occur in the brain are exposed to unique microenvironmental conditions. While tumour outgrowth ultimately has a major impact, the intrinsic properties of the brain initially impose the framework on which subsequent cellular interactions must build. The particularities of the brain are partly anatomical, with strictly controlled traffic of cells and molecules from the blood by virtue of the blood brain barrier (BBB). But they are also due to a unique cellular composition not found outside the nervous system; this includes the neurons and glial cells which have potent immunoregulatory properties. Taken together, these factors have been used to attempt to explain the "immune privilege" of the brain, which is often used to describe low level adaptive immune responses. But in addition immune privilege also impacts on, and is influenced by, the brain myeloid cells which are the subject of this chapter.

Our understanding of immune privilege must be defined and put into context, since it was originally used in the restricted field of the extended survival of allografts in the brain compared with that achieved in other sites (Barker & Billingham, 1977; Medawar, 1948). Over the years, the concept and terminology has often been used to apply to any situation of low or absent immune reactivity in the brain. Indeed, this seemed consistent with the overriding need to control inflammatory reactions in the brain because of their potentially deleterious consequences to critical neuronal functions with low regenerative capacity. Moreover, immune privilege also seemed consistent with an apparent isolation of the brain behind the BBB, and the absence of draining lymphatics and immune competent cells from much of the brain. However, this over simplistic interpretation of the brain as an immune privileged site has now been reassessed to define it as an immune specialized site, where immune cells are poised to respond to injury and infection, but in a highly regulated way (Carson et al., 2006; Galea et al., 2007). A further complexity of this updated concept of immune privilege is that this status is not uniform throughout the brain, and in addition, the myeloid cell populations are distinct in different brain regions. As argued by Perry and colleagues (Galea et al., 2007), the brain parenchyma is the brain compartment that exhibits most features associated with immune privilege. Other brain regions with distinct immune properties are the ventricles containing the choroid plexus and the cerebrospinal fluid (CSF), the meninges, and the perivascular space. Brain tumours can of course potentially invade any or all of these brain sites, but how this influences interactions with myeloid cells has not generally been defined. However, it should be noted that most experimentally induced or grafted tumours are in the brain parenchyma, and so the initial contact will be with parenchymal myeloid cells. For the same reason, although most of the neuroimmunology described in this chapter could apply more generally to the central nervous system, we refer more specifically to the brain, to maintain a direct link to the vast majority of available information on malignancies.

2. The myeloid cells of the brain

Myeloid cells are abundantly present in the healthy brain, representing between 5% and 20% of cells, depending on the specific location. Their histological appearance, their origin, and potentially their functions are distinct from those found in other tissues. The phenotypic classification of brain myeloid cells by defined markers is challenging, which has led to imprecise or changing nomenclature over the years. This terminology arose from histological studies around a century ago, which distinguished the small, ramified microglial cell of the parenchyma from the larger "macroglial" cells such as the astrocytes, oligodendrocytes and ependymal cells, as recently reviewed (Ransohoff & Cardona, 2010). Parenchymal microglial cells are considered to be the resident macrophages of the brain. Those myeloid cells populating other brain compartments are generally referred to as macrophages, prefixed with their localization (choroid plexus, meningeal, perivascular) (Hickey et al., 1992; Matyszak et al., 1992). Confusingly, the term microglia has also sometimes been used for these cell types (or even dendritic-like cells, or perivascular cells), although as we shall discuss, recent studies indicate that the origin of these macrophages is distinct from parenchymal microglia, and so in this chapter we retain the term microglia only for parenchymal cells.

Type	Location	Phenotype	Functions
Parenchymal microglia	Within the parenchyma, not directly associated with vessels	Ramified to amoeboid, $CD11b^{+}$, $CD45^{low}$, MHC II^{low}	Ramified: parenchymal surveillance, synaptic housekeeping. Amoeboid: see text.
Perivascular macrophages	Associated with the blood vessels in the parenchyma	Amoeboid or dendritic, $CD11b^{+}$, $CD45^{high}$, MHC II^{+}	Phagocytosis, antigen presentation, blood brain barrier component.
Meningeal macrophages	Associated with the pial vasculature and the subarachnoid space	Amoeboid or dendritic, $CD11b^{+}$, $CD45^{high}$, MHC II^{+}	Phagocytosis, antigen presentation, blood brain barrier component.
Choroid plexus macrophages	Choroid plexus	Amoeboid or dendritic, $CD11b^{+}$, $CD45^{high}$, MHC II^{+}	Phagocytosis, antigen presentation.

Table 1. Principal myeloid populations in the healthy brain.

Myeloid cells of each type in the listed location are identified in all species analysed (generally humans, rat, and mouse). The phenotypic markers may be species-specific. The function is often presumed rather than experimentally demonstrated in all species.

2.1 Parenchymal microglial cells – Origins and phenotypic definition

The origins of microglial cells have been debated for many decades. The difficulties in reaching definitive conclusions are partially linked to the lack of unique markers to differentiate the microglia from other myeloid cells, and the inherent plasticity of myeloid cells to differentiate or modulate expression of many key markers (Geissmann et al., 2010; Santambrogio et al., 2001). From the 1990's accumulating evidence finally assigned microglia to the myeloid lineage (Prinz & Mildner, 2011; Ransohoff & Cardona, 2010), thus distancing them from the neuroectoderm derived macroglia. The subsequent question that has been more elusive to answer is whether microglia derive from the bone marrow. Here a distinction must be made between the principle origin of parenchymal microglial cells in embryonic development, and their potential replenishment in the adult. Compelling evidence based on in vivo lineage tracing studies in mice indicated that microglia form an ontogenically distinct population in the mononuclear phagocyte system. The microglia that populate the adult brain parenchyma derive from myeloid progenitors in the yolk sac. This first primitive hematopoiesis temporally precedes and it is distinct from the definitive hematopoietic wave which gives rise to circulating hematopoietic precursors, including monocytes (Ginhoux et al., 2010).

The mechanism by which the parenchymal microglial population is replenished during adult life or in pathological situations has been challenging to elucidate. First, as will be discussed, it is difficult to unambiguously differentiate parenchymal microglia from other macrophages. Second, the use of radiation bone marrow chimeras to conveniently replace bone marrow stem cells with labelled donor cells inevitably introduces artefacts such as vessel damage, and abnormal proportions and fluxes of donor stem cells in the circulation. With these limitations in mind, initial data suggested replenishment from bone marrow precursors (Flugel et al., 2001). However, elegant experiments based on parabiosis rather than radiation indicated that self-renewal within the brain is sufficient to maintain the adult parenchymal microglial population (Ajami et al., 2007). Nevertheless, in certain pathologies, repopulation from bone-marrow derived precursors remains a possibility (Soulet & Rivest, 2008).

The original definition of parenchymal microglia was based on morphology and localization in brain parenchyma. Specific markers are clearly essential to objectively compare findings between research groups, and to manipulate microglial cells in vitro. However, most markers are shared with other tissue macrophage populations, thus CD11b/CD18 (integrin αMβ2) is expressed, as well as F4/80 in mouse microglia. Constitutive expression of MHC class II, and costimulatory molecules is generally low on parenchymal microglia. The low expression of many myeloid markers may be reinforced by neuron-microglial-cell inhibitory signalling through cell surface and soluble ligands (Ransohoff & Cardona, 2010). The principal tool to distinguish parenchymal microglia from other brain macrophages has been the level of CD45 expression (leukocyte common antigen, Ly-5): microglia are characterized by low CD45 expression, whereas other macrophages are $CD45^{high}$ (Ford et al., 1995). However, this distinction can only be achieved by flow cytometry, not by immunohistochemistry. Parenchymal microglia of human origin are more problematic to identify, and no markers have been consistently described to discriminate among the two cell populations (Wu et al., 2010). Moreover, non-pathogical human brain tissue is infrequently studied, and so it is unclear what proportion of parenchymal microglia compared with other activated macrophage populations is to be expected. Nevertheless, at least one study has suggested that human parenchymal microglia can be identified as $CD11b^{+}$, $CD45^{low}$, and unlike other brain macrophages, negative for CD14 (Parney et al., 2009).

2.2 Non-microglial brain macrophages – Origins and phenotypic definition

The myeloid populations in non-parenchymal regions of the brain are phenotypically closer to their extracranial counterparts than parenchymal microglia (Hickey et al., 1992). Moreover, whilst cranial irradiation does not deplete parenchymal microglial cells, other myeloid cells are radiosensitive and are readily replenished from bone marrow precursors within about 4 to 8 weeks (Chinnery et al., 2010; Hickey & Kimura, 1988).

A wide diversity of phenotypes, in humans and rodents, is reported for choroid plexus myeloid cells: from classical tissue macrophages, to dendritic or "dendriform" like cells (Chinnery et al., 2010; Matyszak et al., 1992; McMenamin, 1999; Serot et al., 2000). In human tissue, there was an absence of co-stimulatory molecule expression (CD40, CD80, CD86) on these cells (Serot et al., 2000), but this was not studied in rodent origin choroid plexus derived cells. Similarly, in the meninges, pleomorphic myeloid cells with either macrophage or dendritic cell like features can be identified (Chinnery et al., 2010; McMenamin, 1999; McMenamin et al., 2003).

The non-parenchymal site that has been the most thoroughly studied is the perivascular space, with myeloid cells strategically located to engage in dialogue with both blood-born immigrants and parenchymal residents. Moreover, these perivascular myeloid cells are proposed to contribute to BBB function (Bechmann et al., 2007). Phenotypically, perivascular myeloid cells can be macrophage-like or dendriform, although often this is based only on morphology, as dendritic cell specific markers have not been used in all studies (Flaris et al., 1993; Platten & Steinman, 2005).

2.3 Functions of microglia and brain macrophages in the healthy and diseased brain

The spectrum of functional activities reported for myeloid cells in the brain is as wide as for conventional tissue macrophages, and will depend upon the stimulus or pathology that is inducing activation. Although the focus of this chapter is to understand myeloid cells and brain tumours, other pathologies (especially autoimmune and neurodegenerative diseases) have furnished a lot of basic information about myeloid cell function. These findings are therefore discussed first before considering the impact of malignancy on these complex cellular interactions.

Attributing functions specifically to "microglial cells" or "brain macrophages" necessitates clarification of certain basic assumptions about the identity of these cells. A microglial cell assumes its overall morphology, its specific phenotype and its functions largely because of its localization in the brain parenchyma. If we wish to isolate brain myeloid cells using CD45 staining intensity to differentiate microglia from other macrophages, we must accept the inherent limitations of this marker which is not necessarily expressed at a constant level in different in vivo pathologies, or in vitro. Moreover, cells cultured in vitro will be exposed to a microenvironment totally distinct from the brain parenchyma, and when cultured in serum containing medium, will be exposed to known microglial activators such as fibrinogen (Adams et al., 2007). These issues were thoroughly and quantitatively addressed using gene expression analysis of microglia activated by LPS/IFN-γ in vitro versus in vivo, with similar experiments performed for peritoneal and brain infiltrating macrophages (Schmid et al., 2009). This important study showed that brain-resident microglia are heterogeneous, with very different gene expression patterns after stimulation in vitro and in vivo. Furthermore, the brain micro-environment was a more important factor in determining gene expression than the origin of the myeloid cells tested. The "microglia" and "brain macrophage" functions that we will now describe must therefore be interpreted with these complexities of terminology in mind, together with the limitations of in vitro tests that may not recapitulate the significantly overlapping properties of these cells in the in vivo brain microenvironment.

2.3.1 Transition of parenchymal microglia from "resting" to "activated"

In the healthy brain, parenchymal microglial cells are termed "resting" cells, morphologically identified as ramified cells with small soma and fine cellular processes. However, so called resting microglia have been proposed to be actively involved in maintaining synaptic integrity, indicating a different functional status than would be expected from a macrophage, as recently discussed (Graeber, 2010). With the advent of two-photon microscopy able to visualize microglia in situ in the living mouse, the term "resting" is even more directly seen to be a misnomer, as these cells are dynamically surveying their microenvironment (Davalos et al., 2005; 2008; Nimmerjahn et al., 2005). Time-lapse imaging experiments demonstrated that microglial processes are motile and continuously (over periods of a few minutes) extend and retract to survey neighbouring astrocytes, neuronal cell bodies, and blood vessels. Upon tissue damage or signals that might mimic infection (application of LPS), microglia were capable of targeted movement of their processes towards the injured site, leading to a barrier of intertwined processes between damaged and healthy tissue (Davalos et al., 2005). Although not directly demonstrated, it is likely that the same processes can occur in malignant pathologies. A key signal that promoted this microglial activation was ATP, binding to the purinergic $P2Y_{12}$ receptor on microglia. The source of ATP mediating these effects is proposed to be from both damaged cells and ATP-induced ATP release from astrocytes.

Microglial cell activation results in changes in morphology and function that are postulated to be directly linked to the consequences of initial chemoattraction by ATP (Orr et al., 2009). Extracellular ATP can be degraded to adenosine by microglia expressed ectonucleotidases, such as CD39 and CD73, which then leads to activation of the adenosine A2A receptor and process retraction by the microglia. Further activation of the microglial cell will occur when those elements maintaining their "resting" (but surveillant) status are removed. Since many of these inhibitory signals come from neurons, if tissue damage has perturbed neuronal function, this will remove or limit negative signalling, such as that mediated by CD200 (Chitnis et al., 2007; Hoek et al., 2000) or CX_3CL1 (fractaline) (Cardona et al., 2006). The activated microglial cell becomes amoeboid in shape, motile, and phagocytic, i.e., very similar to other macrophages.

2.3.2 Functions of activated microglia and brain macrophages

Microglia not only change in morphology upon activation, but also increase in number. Indeed, unlike most tissue macrophages, brain-resident microglia have a high potential for proliferation (Ajami et al., 2007; Graeber et al., 1998). Microglial functions can be potent, and so can either be beneficial or pathogenic according to the tissue targeted and when it is targeted. The products released by fully activated microglial cells include reactive oxygen species, nitric oxide (NO), and tumour necrosis factor (TNF), all of which can damage neurons and glial cells (Block et al., 2007), although whether this is directly linked to neurodegenerative disease is disputed by some (Graeber & Streit, 2010). The other side of the spectrum of microglial cell function is that of neuroprotection, in which there is abundant evidence for beneficial functions (Glezer et al., 2007; Hanisch & Kettenmann, 2007). Probably most functions of an activated microglial cell could be carried out by other brain macrophages, and so unless specifically stated otherwise, the references to microglial cell function do not exclude this possibility.

Migration. Proliferation is not sufficient to explain the high density of microglia around brain lesions; migration is also necessary (Carbonell et al., 2005a; 2005b). One study, using focal laser injury in ex vivo retinal explants, suggested that transition to a migratory phenotype could occur whilst microglia remain in the "resting" ramified morphology (Lee et al., 2008). However, in most pathologies, migratory microglia will be amoeboid and "activated". Microglial migration is under control of several types of receptors: those found on other macrophages, as well as receptors such as purinergic receptors generally found on neural cells. Capacity to migrate towards certain stimuli is generally assessed using in vitro assays, and so their relative importance awaits in vivo validation. Among the key chemokine-chemokine receptor interactions, CCL21 produced by damaged neurons can attract microglia via CXCR3 (Biber et al., 2001); CX3CL1 (fractaline) produced by neurons and astrocytes signals through CX3CR1 on microglia (Cardona et al., 2006; Liang et al., 2009); stromal cell derived factor-1α (SDF-1α) binds to $CXCR4^{+}$ microglia (X. Wang et al., 2008); and monocyte chemotactic protein 1 (MCP-1, CCL2) produced by many brain cells, including microglia themselves, signals through CCR2 (Simpson et al., 1998). The multiple non-chemokine receptors expressed by activated microglial cells facilitate migration towards other categories of stimuli present in the brain, including neurotransmitters, cannabinoids, lysophosphatidic acid (LSA), opioids, bradykinin, and various growth factors. These have recently been comprehensively reviewed (Kettenmann et al., 2011).

Phagocytosis. A major function of activated microglia is phagocytosis: it is essential during brain development, for homeostatic debris clearance in the normal brain, and can tilt the balance towards neuroprotection or neurodegeneration. It can also provide a link to adaptive immune responses if phagocytosed antigenic proteins are processed and presented to T cells. Activated microglial cells can express a wide array of phagocytic receptors, both those responsible for pathogen recognition and clearance, and those facilitating removal of apoptotic cells (Kettenmann et al., 2011; Neumann et al., 2009). Of the former category, Toll like receptors (TLRs) 1-9, Fc receptors, scavenger receptors, and complement receptors can be expressed, ligation of which will generally lead to an inflammatory response, with release of TNF, IL-1 and nitric oxide. Receptors of the latter category include TREM2 (triggering receptor expressed on myeloid cells-2), purine receptors (some of which are not found on other macrophages), and phosphatidylserine receptors. Ligation of this category of receptors can lead to anti-inflammatory signalling and release of TGF-β and IL-10.

Antigen presentation. As microglia are certainly sentinel cells of the brain parenchyma, and they are the most abundant phagocyte, are they also antigen presenting cells (APCs) for T cells? A prerequisite is expression of MHC class II (for CD4 T cells) and MHC class I (for CD8 T cells), and costimulatory molecules. The level of expression of these molecules is totally dependent upon the activating and inhibitory factors perceived by the microglial cell (Aloisi et al., 2000). The antigen presenting capacity as tested in vitro (sometimes ex vivo) on

CD4 T cells can vary from full to partial activation, to apoptosis induction (Ford et al., 1996; Frei et al., 1994; Matyszak et al., 1999; Platten & Steinman, 2005). The status of microglia as APC in vivo, in different pathologies, is therefore a key question. Accumulating evidence from rodent experimental autoimmune encephalomyelitis (EAE) models has now identified that the principal cell able to present antigen to restimulate infiltrating CD4 T cells resides in the perivascular space (Hickey & Kimura, 1988; McMahon et al., 2005), or the meninges (Bartholomaus et al., 2009). Unlike parenchymal microglia, these perivascular myeloid cells are radiosensitive, and may even have dendritic morphology and CD11c expression. The role of the parenchymal microglial cells in these EAE models was proposed to be to augment pathology by the release of T cell stimulating cytokines and toxic mediators such as IL-12, IL-23, osteopontin, and reactive oxygen species (Heppner et al., 2005; Platten & Steinman, 2005).

Antigen presentation of exogenously acquired antigens on MHC class I molecules (cross-presentation) is essential for CD8 T cell immune responses, but is an inefficient process in most cells. In vivo, certain subsets of dendritic cells (that are CD11c^{+}CD8^{+} in the mouse) are considered to be the principle cross-presenting APC (Lin et al., 2008), but these have not been reported in the brain. However, one study showed that in the adult mouse, microglia can take up soluble ovalbumin and present processed antigen to CD8 T cells (Beauvillain et al., 2008), albeit with modest efficiency. These results are similar to earlier studies in the rat, although in this study the authors suggested that antigen presentation was very feeble and should be considered as compromised (Flugel et al., 1999). A further cross-presenting brain APC candidate is a ramified, radioresistant cell found in the parenchyma of mice that is CD11b^{+}CD11c^{+}MHCII^{-}, termed a "brain DC" by the authors, but with a very similar phenotype to microglial cells. When activated in vivo with IFN-γ, then tested in vitro for stimulation of ovalbumin specific CD8 (and CD4) T cells, this APC could present and cross-present soluble ovalbumin (Gottfried-Blackmore et al., 2009). The in vivo significance of these cells and their relation to other myeloid cells in the brain awaits clarification.

The most stringent task for an APC is to prime naïve T cells. Since naïve T cells normally recirculate between blood and secondary lymphoid tissue, this can only occur efficiently in the T cell zones of lymph node (or spleen). Therefore, an APC having captured antigen in the brain must be able to migrate to the lymph node, which is facilitated by expression of the chemokine receptor CCR7, promoting lymph node entry through the high endothelial venules in response to a CCL21 chemokine gradient. Murine microglia have been reported to express CCR7 (Dijkstra et al., 2006), but functional homing experiments were not performed. Indirect evidence points towards dendritic cells (DCs) as being the principle APC candidate to migrate from the brain to lymph nodes (Hatterer et al., 2006; Hatterer et al., 2008; Karman et al., 2004), although definitive tracking of cell migration required intracranial injection of dendritic cells that may not precisely recapitulate endogenous cell behaviour.

2.4 Brain tumours in humans and animal models

Cellular heterogeneity has long been accepted to be a hallmark of most brain tumours, and even the earliest histological studies suggested that myeloid cells might be present in the tumour stroma and peritumoural regions. Multiple histological types of primary and metastatic brain tumour are described and are expected to vary in their myeloid cell involvement. The commonest primary brain tumours are astrocytomas (Schwartzbaum et al., 2006) and of these, the high grade malignant gliomas (WHO grade III and IV) are particularly lethal. Malignant glioma is profoundly resistant to conventional treatment modalities, and complete surgical resection is impossible because of their inaccessible location and highly infiltrative growth characteristics. Thus, even with the best resection possible and combined regimens of radiotherapy with new generation chemotherapy, the median survival of patients with glioblastoma multiforme (GBM: WHO grade IV glioma) is 14.6 months (Stupp et al., 2009). For animal studies, the use of xenografted human glioma in immunodeficient mice cannot be expected to induce normal myeloid cell responses as the whole immune network is perturbed in the host mice. Instead, animal brain tumour models have focused on either orthotopically implanted models, historically often in rats (Barth & Kaur, 2009), but increasing in mouse models such as GL261 glioma, syngeneic to C57BL/6 mice (Szatmari et al., 2006) There is also considerable interest in the use of genetically engineered mouse models that may better recapitulate the pathology and heterogeneity of human glioma (Huse & Holland, 2009). However, these models were often designed and exploited for genetic studies; they have only recently been investigated for immunological parameters.

2.4.1 Identification of microglia and macrophages in brain tumours

Although thorough characterization of brain tumour associated myeloid cells had to await the advent of monoclonal antibodies, an early pioneering study determined that glioblastomas, meningiomas, medulloblastomas, and metastatic tumours were all infiltrated by Fc receptor-positive cells, i.e., predominately myeloid cells (Wood & Morantz, 1979). These macrophages or microglia were particularly abundant in glioblastoma, representing a mean content of 41% (range 5-78%) of the tumour tissue digested to give a single-cell suspension. Subsequent studies were able to profit from monoclonal antibodies to better define myeloid cells, not only in suspension, but also in tissue sections. In histological sections, quantification is somewhat more challenging and difficult to compare between studies, but reports from several groups using panels of different antibodies described significant myeloid cell infiltration in low grade glioma (Rossi et al., 1988; Shinonaga et al., 1988), high grade glioma (Rossi et al., 1987; 1989; Shinonaga et al., 1988), as well as metastatic brain tumours (Shinonaga et al., 1988). Moreover, although flow cytometric analysis on single-cell suspensions of digested human tumour confirmed these findings, they did not allow an unequivocal distinction of microglia and other brain macrophages (Parney et al., 2009; Watters et al., 2005). Some of the histological studies on microglia and macrophage infiltration attempted to make correlations of type or intensity of myeloid cell infiltration and tumour type or grade (Nishie et al., 1999; Roggendorf et al., 1996; Rossi et al., 1988; 1987): there was a tendency for greater infiltration of high grade tumours such as glioblastoma. Higher myeloid cell infiltration was proposed to correlate with peritumoural oedema (Shinonaga et al., 1988), but not with survival in one early study (Rossi et al., 1989). Our contemporary understanding of the complexity of the myeloid cell compartment in the brain that we have discussed in section 2 predicts that correlation of survival and simple myeloid cell phenotyping and quantification is improbable. A more recent study on a larger series of patients with glioblastoma examined polymorphisms in the gene encoding the CX3CR1 chemokine receptor, expressed on microglial cells and used in their migration

(Rodero et al., 2008). Based on genetic analysis of 230 patients, and immunohistochemistry of over 100 patients, expression of one common allelic variant was significantly associated with prolonged survival after surgery (23.5 vs 14.1 months; $P < .0001$), as well as reduced microglia/macrophage infiltration.

In common with many other domains of cancer research, relevant animal models have played a major role in advancing our understanding of brain myeloid cells. For brain tumours in particular, the inaccessibility of the tumour site in patients often restricts studies to a single tumour sample, rodent models have therefore been widely exploited. Studies of myeloid cells infiltrating rat gliomas allowed intensity of CD45 expression on $CD11b^+$ cells to be used to distinguish parenchymal microglia from other brain macrophages. The microglia and macrophage content varied somewhat according to the model (C6, 9L, RG-2), with $CD45^{low}$ microglial cells present in peritumoural areas and in the hemisphere contralateral to the tumour, and $CD45^{high}$ macrophages infiltrating the tumour bed (Badie & Schartner, 2001). In another study, orthotopically implanted Rat 9L glioma was also studied by immunohistochemistry, and compared with an intracranial carcinoma; both were comparably infiltrated by microglia or macrophages (Morioka et al., 1992). Mouse glioma models have similarly been assessed for myeloid cell infiltration. In GL261 glioma, the infiltrate was predominately $CD11b^+F4/80^+CD45^{high}$, considered as macrophages rather than microglia by the authors (Nakagawa et al., 2007). We have also analysed orthotopic GL261 glioma, a representative immune infiltrate is shown in Fig. 1. In the SMA-560 model, $CD11b^+$ cells were identified by immunohistochemistry (Uhl et al., 2004). A further study used an orthotopically implanted PDGF-driven glioma model to study myeloid cells (along with other immune cells) longitudinally (Kennedy et al., 2009). The frequency of $CD11b^+CD45^+$ cells was measured, without distinguishing the level of CD45 expression. These macrophages/microglia increased from 1.1% during the early phase, to 5.6% during the late stage. A further category of tumour model in which myeloid cells have been documented is genetically engineered "spontaneous" gliomas. The GFAP-V^{12}HA-*ras* model is of particular interest, because astrocytomas form spontaneously in these mice, without the trauma (and potential microglial cell activation) associated with intracranial implantation (Ding et al., 2001; Shannon et al., 2005). We have explored immune parameters in these mice, analyzing the immune infiltrate from earliest stages of pathology, but without appearance of symptoms in mice (4, 8, and 12 weeks), to mice bearing advanced tumours producing symptoms (Tran Thang et al., 2010). Although there was a significant lymphocyte infiltrate in asymptomatic mice (at 12 weeks), myeloid cell augmentation correlated with appearance of terminal symptoms. Microglia ($CD11b^+CD45^{low}$) approximately doubled in number at this stage, whereas the previously minor population of $CD11b^+CD45^{high}$ macrophages increased by more than 50 fold, becoming the major myeloid subset in the brain. The intriguing correlation of terminal progression of the brain tumour and the presence of these macrophages clearly raises issues about their origin and likely function; this is the subject of ongoing investigations. Myeloid cells were also investigated in another genetically engineered glioma model, in which de novo gliomas were generated by intracerebroventricuar transfection of *NRas* and a short hairpin RNA against *P53* using the Sleeping Beauty transposon system (Fujita et al., 2011; 2010). The brain tumours of these mice were infiltrated by $CD11b^+$ cells, although the authors focused particularly on the myeloid derived suppressor cell (MDSC) component, as described in section 3.2 below.

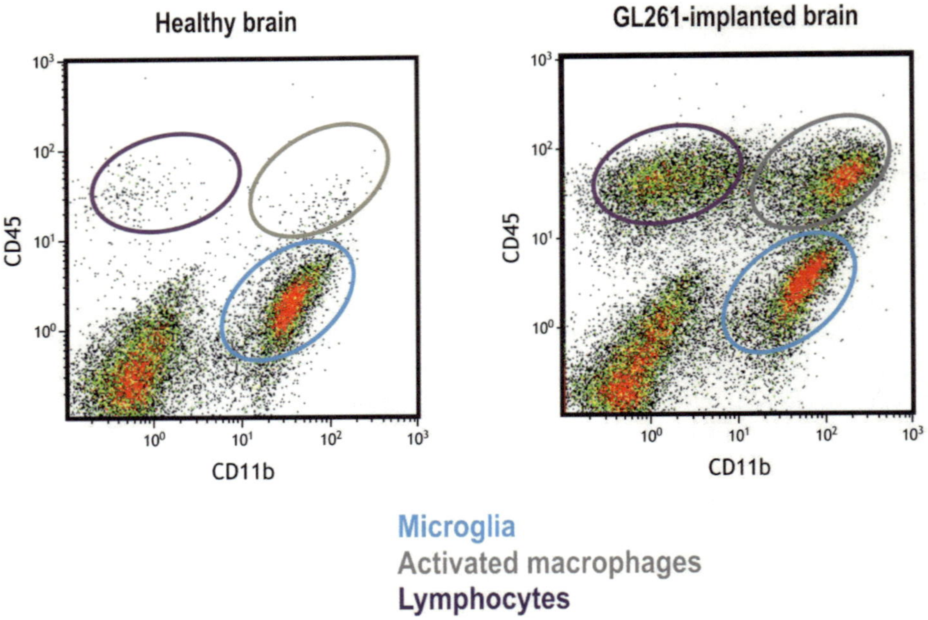

Fig. 1. Leucocyte populations in brain of healthy and tumour-bearing mice.

Leucocytes isolated from brains of healthy (left) and glioma bearing mice (right) were stained for CD45 and CD11b markers, and analysed by flow cytometry. The only highly represented leucocytes in healthy brain are $CD11b^+CD45^{low}$ microglia. In mice bearing advanced brain tumours, there is also an infiltrate of $CD11b^+CD45^{high}$ macrophages and $CD11b^-CD45^{high}$ lymphocytes.

2.4.2 Additional myeloid cell populations in brain tumours

Studies of various malignancies in patients and in tumour-bearing mice demonstrated that the heterogeneous cells known as MDSCs can accumulate in secondary lymphoid tissue and at the tumour site (Gabrilovich & Nagaraj, 2009). The MDSC population includes immature macrophages, granulocytes and DCs, and these cells have the potential to suppress T cell immune responses. Proposed mechanisms differ in lymphoid tissue and the tumour site, but include reactive oxygen species, arginase 1 activity and nitric oxide production. Phenotypically, they are usually defined as $CD11b^+GR1^+$ in mice (although subsets exist); in humans, phenotyping is more complex but MDSCs may include $CD14^-CD11b^+CD33^+$ cells.

In patients with malignant glioma, MDSCs were detected in peripheral blood (Raychaudhuri et al., 2011; Rodrigues et al., 2010), and the phenotype could also be induced by exposure of normal monocytes to glioma cell lines (Rodrigues et al., 2010). However, the presence of MDSCs infiltrating human brain tumours has not yet been described.

In rodents, presence of MDSCs within the brain tumour bed has been documented in several models. An early study using the T9 glioma model in Fischer 344 rats demonstrated that suppressive cells expressing both the rat granulocyte marker His48 and CD11b/c accumulated in the spleen and in the intracranial tumour bed (Prins et al., 2002). Moreover, this accumulation was enhanced by subcutaneous vaccination with irradiated glioma cells. These cells were further investigated in a recent study, in the same model, in which bone marrow replacement confirmed that the brain infiltrating MDSCs were of bone marrow origin (Jia et al., 2010). Functionally, nitric oxide was determined to be the main suppressive molecule.

In mice, MDSCs were described in both the GL261 orthotopically implanted glioma (Umemura et al., 2008), as well in genetically engineered models (Fujita et al., 2011; 2010; Tran Thang et al., 2010). The definition of MDSCs infiltrating GL261 glioma was discussed in some detail (Umemura et al., 2008). The authors concluded that there is substantial overlap with other tumour associated macrophages, and that moreover, these cells have considerable plasticity in their function and phenotype according to the microenvironment in which they function. These issues are probably central to most myeloid cells associated with tumours. A rather simpler observation of the presence of $CD11b^{+}GR1^{+}CD45^{high}$ cells was made in the GFAP-V^{12}HA-*ras* model of spontaneous astrocytoma (Tran Thang et al., 2010), but without further phenotyping or functional tests. However, elevated proportions of these cells were present in only a minority of ill mice. This may be a reflection of the inherent heterogeneity of tumours in this model (the genetic background is outbred, and tumours appear after stochastic accumulation of genetic mutations that vary between mice), or it may signify that MDSCs are of only minor functional significance in this model. In contrast, in the genetically induced glioma models studied by the Okada group (Fujita et al., 2011; 2010), $CD11b^{+}Ly6G^{high}$ MDSCs were a major component of the brain tumour infiltrate, which was also explored functionally. Depletion of $Ly6G^{+}$ cells prolonged survival of mice developing gliomas, as did COX-2 blockade with nonsteroidal anti-inflammatory drugs. The latter approach may have acted at two levels: by inhibiting the MDSC differentiation factor prostaglandin E_2, and by limiting MDSC recruitment to the brain tumour site by reducing levels of the MDSC chemoattractant CCL2.

A final type of myeloid cell that may be specifically recruited to brain tumours is an immunosuppressive $CD11b^{+}$ DC. In the context of glioma, this cell type has been most thoroughly investigated in the GL261 mouse glioma model (Biollaz et al., 2009). The brain infiltrating dendritic cells were shown to be of bone marrow origin using bone marrow chimeric mice, and they had little or no expression of costimulatory molecules (CD40, B7.1, B7.2) and GR1. Functional tests in vitro showed that brain infiltrating DCs could induce regulatory T cells from naïve CD4 T cells, but were inefficient at inducing alloreactive or antigen specific CD4 T cell proliferation. Of particular interest was that the immunosuppressive functions of these GL261 infiltrating DCs were predominately found when the tumour was growing intracranially, but not with the same tumour implanted subcutaneously. Moreover, the overall tumour infiltrate and microenvironment was entirely different in the brain: intracranial GL261 had higher levels of DCs, regulatory T cells and TGF-β, and mice had shorter survival. Overall, this important study indicates how brain tumour-immune system interactions are a consequence of both the tumour and the specialized site of the brain.

2.4.3 Microglia and macrophage function in the contest of malignant glioma

The overall consequences of the appearance of malignant glioma in the brain have been extensively studied in patients as well as in animal models; there is progressive invasive (but non-metastatic) growth, no evidence for spontaneous immune-mediated regression, but substantial evidence for local immunosuppression (Walker et al., 2003). The local microenvironment is of course complex, and a product of multiple cell type and site-specific factors. The role of certain cells infiltrating the tumour is unambiguous, such as Foxp3$^+$CD4$^+$ regulatory T cells that infiltrate both human and mouse glioma (Walker et al., 2009). Myeloid cells are less simple to define, but the unique myeloid cells constitutively present in the brain are likely to be central players in shaping the developing tumour stroma, potentially being the precursors of other brain macrophages, and able to influence the function of other immigrant myeloid cells (as described in section 2.4.2 above). Ultimately, in advanced tumours, myeloid cells of all origins will become the major non-tumoural component of the brain tumour bed (Fig. 2). Indeed, multiple chemokines secreted by glioma cells are known to attract microglia and other myeloid cells. These include CCL21 (Biber et al., 2001; Zhai et al., 2011), MCP-3 (Okada et al., 2009), stromal cell derived factor-1α (SDF-1α) (Rempel et al., 2000; X. Wang et al., 2008), and MCP-1 (Fujita et al., 2011; Platten et al., 2003). Moreover, the latter two factors may be particularly efficacious at attracting myeloid cells to hypoxic areas of the tumour. Whether myeloid cells associated with brain tumours are a cause or a consequence of tumour progression is still controversial. Indeed both pro- and anti-tumoural functions can be demonstrated on isolated cells, but in vivo there are complex mixed populations, functioning in a microenvironment totally different from that created in vitro. The conceptual framework for understanding these functions has developed both from neuroscience and macrophage biology. Myeloid cells in brain tumours may appear to display some aspects of microglial cell function, i.e., anti-inflammatory and

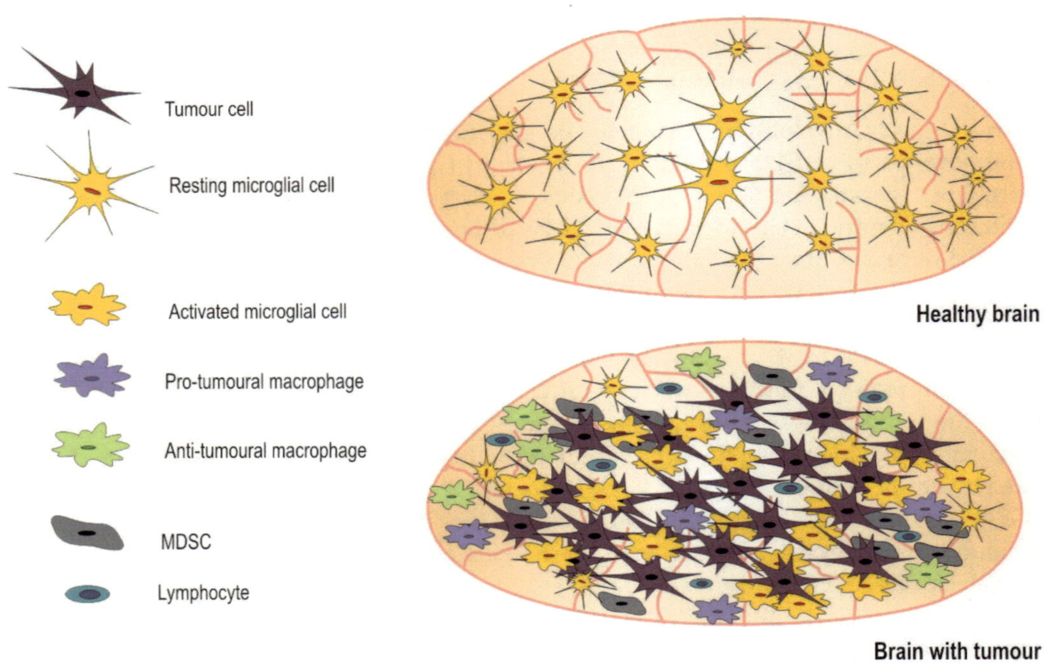

Fig. 2. Heterogenous myeloid and lymphoid cells infiltrate tumour bearing brain.

In healthy brain (top), the principle immune cells of the parenchyma are the microglia, which are resting, but active in brain surveillance. Appearance of malignancy (bottom) promotes activation of resident microglia and infiltration of diverse myeloid and lymphoid cells with potential for pro- and anti-tumoural functions (see text).

housekeeping roles, appropriate for maintaining healthy brain function (Kettenmann et al., 2011), but not for combating a lethal tumour. On the other hand, it is tempting to model brain myeloid cells on current concepts of macrophage plasticity, in which classically activated macrophages (M1) may promote anti-tumoural responses, whereas alternatively activated macrophages (M2) are predicted to be pro-tumoural (Biswas & Mantovani, 2010). This polarization concept is certainly helpful, as long as it can be associated with the specific dialect of neuroimmunology.

Anti-tumoural functions of microglia and brain macrophages. Microglial cells and brain macrophages have the potential to exert anti-tumour effects, and this has been demonstrated in vitro (Hwang et al., 2009; Rosales, 1996). Normal rodent microglial cells can release nitric oxide and Cathepsin B, which together can promote glioma cell apoptosis, whilst sparing normal cultured astrocytes (Hwang et al., 2009). However, constitutive function of microglial cells in vivo is unlikely to achieve the same effect. Nevertheless, global depletion of CD11b$^+$ cells in mice intracranially implanted with GL261 glioma resulted in increased tumour growth (Galarneau et al., 2007). The mechanisms were not fully elucidated, but were suggested to be T-cell independent. Moreover, the immune infiltrate was characterized as a type 1 response, with CD11b$^+$ cells being the main source of TNF, with also high levels of MCP-1 and IL-1β. Levels of type 2 cytokines IL-4 and IL-10 were low. One complexity in the interpretation of this study is that myeloid cell depletion (achieved by systemic administration of ganciclovir in CD11b-HSVTK mice) was incomplete, only up to 45%. Therefore, the result may be a consequence of the preferential elimination of pro-tumoural myeloid cells. This may also account for an apparently contradictory result in a more recent study using a virtually identical model, in which CD11b+ cell depletion reduced GL261 glioma growth (Zhai et al., 2011). The principle difference was that in this latter study, ganciclovir was administered intracranially, which would be assumed to give more efficient depletion of brain myeloid cells.

Regarding brain APC, we have observed presentation of brain tumour antigens in different murine models. However, the cell type responsible for this function was not defined. In the MT539 murine glioma, brain APC were responsible for cross-presenting glioma derived antigens to CD8 T cells, and retaining them in the brain parenchyma (Calzascia et al., 2003). In a different model, tumour-specific CD8 T cell activation in the cervical lymph node was measured after intracranial tumour implantation, and in this case we determined that the responsible cells that had migrated from the brain were radiosensitive, and thus were not parenchymal microglia (Calzascia et al., 2005). In another independent study using a different mouse tumour model, presentation of tumour antigen to T cell populations including CD4 T cells was observed (Plautz et al., 2000). Overall, these observations indicate that the brain is either equipped or can recruit cells with potential to directly (cytotoxicity) or indirectly (antigen presentation) act against tumours, but in the most malignant tumours, these functions may be subverted or overwhelmed by pro-tumoural elements.

Pro-tumoural effects of brain myeloid cells. Pro-tumoural effects of microglia and brain macrophages can be indirect or direct. In the former case, brain myeloid cells can participate in creating an immunosuppressive microenvironment, thus blocking immunity that could act against the tumour. In the latter case, they can directly act on the tumour or its microenvironment to promote tumour growth and invasion. As mentioned in the above subsection, overall support for the pro-tumoural role of brain myeloid cells can be concluded from one of the two CD11b$^+$ cell depletion studies (Zhai et al., 2011), but such an approach is arguably too extreme to either apply therapeutically, or to interpret in depth given myeloid cell heterogeneity. Based on the observations in malignant glioma that tumours progress in the presence of abundant myeloid cell infiltration (Nishie et al., 1999; Roggendorf et al., 1996; Rossi et al., 1988; Rossi et al., 1987), we will examine the evidence that this infiltrate supports tumour growth.

Many pro-tumoural effects of myeloid cells can be associated with M2 polarization. Although one group studying the GL261 model has suggested that the glioma associated myeloid cells are not readily characterized by such terminology (Umemura et al., 2008), the concept can also applied less rigidly to determine the overall balance of the infiltrate. Indeed, another study on GL261 glioma claimed that the polarization balance of the tumour associated $CD11b^+$ microglia or macrophages (mostly amoeboid) was distinctly towards a pro-tumoural M2 phenotype, with strong expression of IL-10 and arginase 1, both associated with dampening inflammation and T cell immunity. In human glioma, a histological study noted a malignancy-correlated infiltration of microglia or macrophages expressing the M2 associated markers CD163 and CD204 (Komohara et al., 2008). This infiltration was also associated with glioma production of M-CSF, and the proliferation index of the tumour. Based on additional in vitro experiments in which glioma supernatant induced CD163 and CD204 expression on macrophages, it was proposed, although not directly demonstrated, that glioma derived M-CSF is a key factor in M2 macrophage polarization.

Several studies from the Heimberger group have chronicled the in vitro functions of myeloid cells isolated from patients with malignant glioma (Hussain et al., 2006a; 2006b). These glioma associated microglia/macrophages expressed multiple toll like receptors, MHC class II, but low levels of co-stimulatory molecules. They did not support T cell proliferative responses, and they did not constitutively express significant levels of inflammatory or anti-inflammatory cytokines when tested ex vivo. Phagocytic function was detectable in these experiments, however, other studies on rat microglia indicated that continued presence of glioma cells may inhibit this process (Voisin et al., 2010).

Early demonstrations of microglia or macrophage modulation by glioma cells generally relied on co-culture with cell lines. More recent concepts in oncology have proposed that cancers, including glioma, arise from a small population of cells with stem-like properties, which can self-renew to produce tumourigenic daughter cells and more differentiated but non-tumourigenic cells (Singh et al., 2004). Glioma stem-like cells can be enriched in neurosphere cultures; these have now been assessed for their impact on human microglia and macrophage function (Wu et al., 2010). Supernatants from glioma stem-like cells were more potent at promoting monocyte recruitment than bulk glioma cells, potentially through CSF-1 and CCL2, and they inhibited macrophage phagocytosis. However, these supernatants also induced pro-tumoural characteristics, some of which may have been driven by phosphorylated *STAT3* expression in monocytes. Treated macrophages and microglia secreted immunosuppressive cytokines (IL-10, TGF-β1, IL-23) and potentiated inhibition of T cell responses. Moreover, these functions were enhanced when glioma stem-like cells were cultured under hypoxic conditions (Wei et al., 2011). Overall, these studies suggest that glioma stem-like cells acquire their central role in tumour malignancy not only through their intrinisic stem-like properties and ability to thrive in hypoxic areas of the tumour, but also by recruiting myeloid cells, recently confirmed in vivo (Yi et al., 2011), and reinforcing their pro-tumoural effects.

The lethality of malignant glioma is not due to metastasis as for most solid tumours, but due to its capacity to invade healthy brain tissue. This invasiveness is facilitated by metalloproteinases that degrade extracellular matrix. Membrane type 1 metalloprotease (MT1-MMP) is highly expressed in human glioma as well as in rodent models, and expression is concentrated within myeloid cells at the tumour borders. These cells were shown to be of amoeboid morphology and were derived from endogenous microglia (Markovic et al., 2009; Sliwa et al., 2007). In elegant in vivo and ex vivo experiments, membrane type 1 metalloprotease (MT1-MMP) was shown to be induced in microglial cells by soluble glioma-derived factors that were dependent on microglial expression of the toll-like receptor adapter protein MyD88 and the p38 MAPK pathway. Glioma growth was promoted by microglial MT1-MMP activation of glioma-derived pro-MMP-2, whereas reduction in glioma volume was achieved either in MyD88-/- mice, or after microglial cell ablation (Markovic et al., 2009). A further route by which microglia can promote invasion is through TGF-β release, which can subsequently induce metalloproteinase release from glioma cells (Wesolowska et al., 2008). Although many cells (including glioma cells) can produce TGF-β in vivo, in vitro invasion tests with microglial and C6 rat glioma co-cultures showed that microglial cells were an important source. This latter observation, although not the specific subject of this study, also confirms the likely contribution of microglial derived TGF-β to the immunosuppressive tumour microenvironment.

A further major pro-tumoural role of brain microglial cells and macrophages is achieved through their promotion of angiogenesis, a process essential for tumour progression. In an in vivo orthotopic mouse glioma model, hypoxia exposed glioma cells recruited $CD11b^+$ myeloid cells in a hypoxia-inducible factor (HIF) 1 and SDF-1α dependent manner (Du et al., 2008). Matrix metalloproteinase (MMP)-9 expression by these macrophages promoted angiogenesis by converting VEGF from a sequestered to a bioavailable state. Another central cytokine linked to angiogenesis in glioma is TNF, which can induce both VEGF (Ryuto et al., 1996) and MMP9 (Esteve et al., 2002). Although TNF is considered a product of M1 polarized cells, its expression was nevertheless described in perivascular and intratumoural macrophages in human glioma (Roessler et al., 1995) as well as in $CD11b^+CD45^{high}$ macrophages infiltrating GL261 mouse glioma (Nakagawa et al., 2007). Angiogenesis may also be driven indirectly, through microglia/macrophage stimulated release of angiogenic factors from the glioma cells. In this regard, several studies in human glioblastoma correlated microglia/macrophage macrophage infiltration of glioma with the angiogenic factor IL-8 (Hong et al., 2009; Nishie et al., 1999; X. B. Wang et al., 2011), and in some cases vessel density (Nishie et al., 1999; X. B. Wang et al., 2011).

2.4.4 Therapeutic modulation of microglia and macrophage in brain malignancy

The balance of pro- and anti-tumour functions of brain microglia and macrophages is clearly not favourable in progressive brain tumours, and so their modulation could be an attractive therapeutic strategy. In view of their essential roles of microglial cell function in the healthy brain, ablation of all brain myeloid cells would appear unwise. Multiple possibilities for modulation of cancer promoting macrophages are being explored in non-cerebral malignancies. In this section we will concentrate on approaches already developed in brain tumours: blocking the infiltration of certain myeloid cells, targeting of key transcription factors, re-polarization with strong stimuli and TGF-β inhibition (Fig.3).

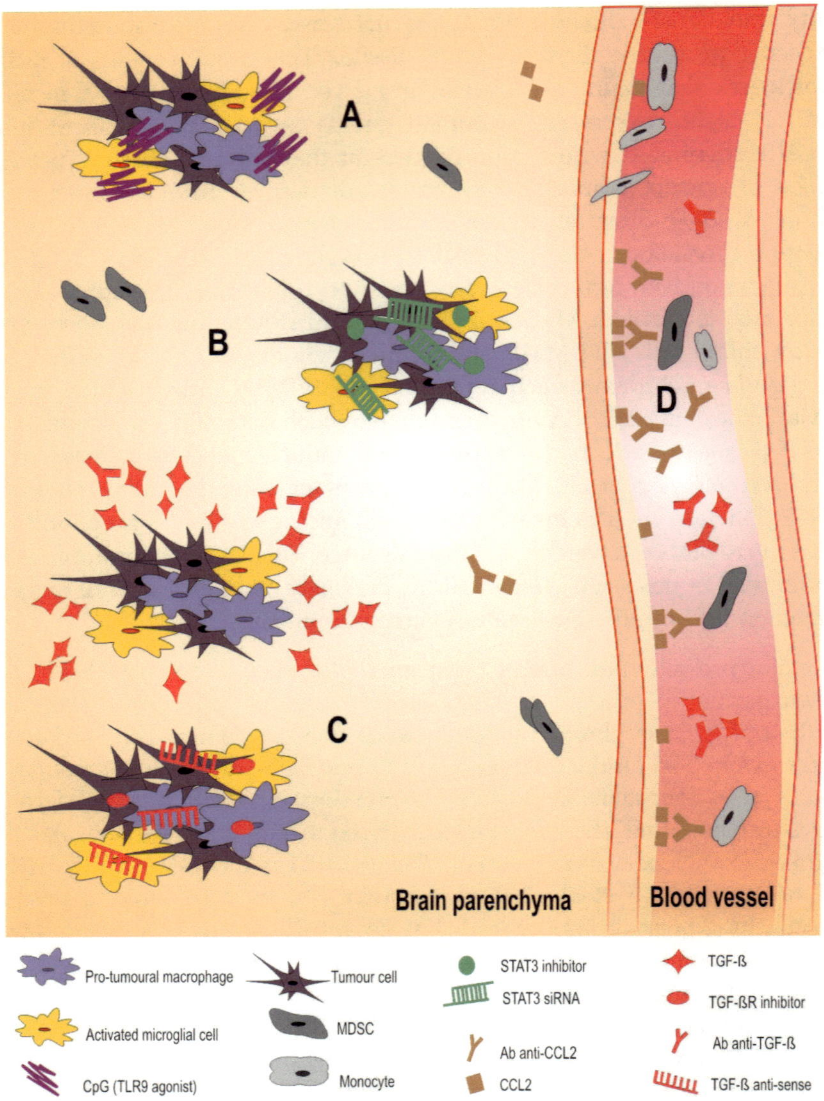

Fig. 3. Therapeutic approaches to modulate myeloid cells in brain tumours.

Examples of therapies having a major impact on myeloid cells are indicated. Promotion of M1 anti-tumoural polarization of brain myeloid cells can be achieved by use of the TLR9 agonist CpG (A) and by inhibition of STAT3 in multiple cell types (B). Inhibition of TGFβ or its signaling diminishes immunosuppression and tumour progression by acting on multiple target cells (C). Infiltration of pro-tumoural monocytes/macrophages and MDSCs can be reduced by antibody blockade of the MCP-1/CCL2 (D).

Blocking infiltration of pro-tumoural myeloid cells. Antibody inhibition of a myeloid cell chemoattractant is a straightforward and attractive approach to block immigration of deleterious cells. Based on the observations that MCP-1/CCL2 is expressed by human glioma and is associated with glioma aggressiveness and macrophage infiltration in animal models (Platten et al., 2003), antibody blockade was tested as a mono- and combination therapy (Zhu et al., 2010). Macrophage and MDSC infiltration was decreased (but not abolished) in GL261 mouse glioma and a human xenografted model, although resident $CD11b^{+}CD45^{low}$ microglia were less affected, perhaps because of limited antibody penetration into the tumour bed. Survival was only modestly increased, but this significantly improved in combination with the alkylating chemotherapy agent temozolomide. Such approaches may have a role in modulating infiltrating macrophages, but if a high proportion of pro-tumoural macrophages are derived from brain resident macrophages, efficacy will be limited.

STAT3 inhibition. Although not a myeloid cell specific approach, targeting signal transducer and activator of transcription 3 (STAT3) is predicted to influence many immunosuppressive and pro-tumoural factors in the brain tumour microenvironment. Inhibition of STAT3 can be achieved with small molecular inhibitors, and is a particularly attractive therapeutic target in cancers such as glioma, because activated STAT3 is detected both in the tumour cells and in the infiltrating immune cells. Treating human microglia/macrophages isolated from glioma with a STAT3 inhibitor induced costimulatory molecule and type 1 cytokine expression (Hussain et al., 2007). Another compound that inhibits STAT3 is the plant-derived corosolic acid (Fujiwara et al., 2010). In vitro studies on human monocyte-derived macrophages showed that this compound prevented M2 macrophage polarization, as measured by inhibition of CD163 expression and IL-10 secretion (M2 markers); it also augmented glioblastoma cell apoptosis (Fujiwara et al., 2010). In mouse models, a STAT3 inhibitor or small interfering RNA blocked "immunosuppressive polarization"(principally IL-10 and IL-6 secretion) of microglia stimulated by glioma cell supernatant (Zhang et al., 2009). Furthermore, in orthotopic GL261 murine glioma in vivo, intratumoural STAT3 siRNA injection augmented TNF mRNA expression, and prolonged survival (Zhang et al., 2009).

TLR Agonists. Pathogen stimulation of myeloid cells through pathogen recognition receptors such as toll like receptors (TLRs) can result in strong M1 polarization that would potentially be useful in anti-tumour immunity, but is not generally achieved during chronic tumour growth. However, it is predicted that use of synthetic TLR agonists can mimic such pathogen induced activation. CpG oligonucleotides as agonists of the intracellularly expressed TLR9 have been investigated in many glioma preclinical models as well as in patients. Intratumoural injection of CpG oligonucleotides in orthotopic rat glioma models reduced tumour volume and elicited therapeutic immunity in a proportion of animals. These successful preclinical experiments have led to a clinical trial, but the clinical results showed only marginal benefit (Carpentier et al., 2010). Indeed, other preclinical studies gave very variable results, ranging from tumour rejection to enhancement of tumour volume (Ginzkey et al., 2010). A recent approach has tried to improve the targeting of CpG oligonucleotides by conjugating CpG oligonucleotides to carbon nanotubes that are preferentially taken up by brain myeloid cells after intratumoural injection (Zhao et al., 2010). In vitro experiments showed that monocytes were efficiently stimulated by the conjugated CpG to express high levels of type 1 cytokines (including IL-12 and TNF). In vivo, GL261 mouse glioma was eradicated by conjugated CpG injection in half of the mice. Overall, there seems to be considerable promise in the approach of stimulating brain myeloid cells with TLR agonists to reorient their functional polarization, although optimization to improve efficacy of the next generation of clinical trials will be essential.

TGF-β inhibition. The central role of TGF-β in promoting tumour progression makes it a highly relevant therapeutic target in brain malignancy. The multiple targets and sources of this cytokine makes interpretation of its therapeutic modulation complex, since of TGF-β acts directly on tumour cells, as well as on pro- and anti-tumoural myeloid and other immune cells. TGF-β inhibition through systemic application of neutralizing antibody (1D11) enhanced efficacy of therapeutic vaccination in mouse GL261 glioma, and promoted a type 1 immune response, although it was not effective as a single modality treatment (Ueda et al., 2009). In a further study, the same 1D11 antibody was tested on both subcutaneous and intracranial GL261; in the former site, there was total tumour regression, whereas the orthotopic glioma merely showed reduced invasion (Hulper et al., 2011) These results suggest that it will be challenging to achieve full efficacy with systemic use of blocking antibodies for tumours localised in the brain. Local TGF-β inhibition has been tested with intratumoural delivery of synthetic antisense oligonucleotides: in a rat intracranial glioma model this showed therapeutic benefit when combined with tumour vaccination (Liu et al., 2007). However, when tested clinically as a monotherapy in recurrent high grade glioma, the clinical effects were disappointing (Bogdahn et al., 2011). A potentially simpler approach is with small molecules targeting TGF-β receptor signalling pathways: these are predicted to have better penetration of the brain tumour bed. Early preclinical studies with a systemically delivered TGF-β receptor I kinase inhibitor (SD-208) indicated survival benefit on mice bearing syngeneic SMA-560 brain tumours; this also correlated with enhanced infiltration of $CD11b^+$ cells (in addition to $CD8^+$ T cells and NK cells) (Uhl et al., 2004). Similar approaches are currently being tested in clinical trials. Overall, targeting TGF-β or its effects may be a valuable way of restoring antitumoural polarization of myeloid and other elements in brain tumours, particularly in the context of multimodal therapies.

3. Conclusion

The myeloid cells populating the brain in health and in malignant disease show a heterogeneity mirroring that found in other tissues, but the microglial cells have particularities that are found in no other tissue macrophages. Their unique features are most striking in the normal brain, when "resting" but highly surveillant ramified microglia are the principle myeloid cell of the brain parenchyma. Is this only of interest for neuroscience, or does it also impact on brain cancer, in which the myeloid infiltrate of advanced cerebral malignancies may superficially resemble that of extracranial tumours? Analysis of lower grade tumours in patients, or early stages of gliomagenesis in animal models reveals that endogenous parenchymal microglia are clearly detectable, and thus shape the microenvironment that influences tumour progression and the function of immune cells immigrating from the periphery. For primary brain tumours, endogenous microglia will also be the first to detect the malignant lesion, and it is possible that their default response of dampening inflammation leaves opportunity for tumour progression.

Do these factors influence how we should treat brain tumours? We suggest that the particularities of the brain and its resident protective cells should be respected in treatment design. Pro-tumoural myeloid cells that we may wish to target will generally be of two sources: immigrating cells from the blood, and proliferating and differentiating microglia. Most systemically used drugs that aim to block myeloid cell infiltration will only efficiently target the former cells. The alternative approach of repolarizing pro-tumoural cells to release high levels of inflammatory cytokines may be promising, but it may not be advisable to convert all brain myeloid cells to highly pro-inflammatory cells, since uncontrolled brain inflammation can be as dangerous as the cancer we are aiming to treat.

Current results from treatment approaches for malignant glioma that impact on myeloid cells should offer hope, but should also impose caution. For example, the therapeutic potential of strong macrophage stimuli such as CpG is highly encouraging in certain preclinical trials. But what we now need to understand is why it is not always successful - either in different preclinical models, as well as for many patients in clinical trials. If we can better define those cells and polarizations that are deleterious, we can envisage better targeting of therapeutic agents to improve efficacy and safety of the next generation of cancer therapies.

4. References

Adams, R. A.; Bauer, J.; Flick, M. J.; Sikorski, S. L.; Nuriel, T.; Lassmann, H.; Degen, J. L. & Akassoglou, K. (2007). The fibrin-derived gamma377-395 peptide inhibits microglia activation and suppresses relapsing paralysis in central nervous system autoimmune disease. *J Exp Med,* Vol.204, No.3, pp. 571-582

Ajami, B.; Bennett, J. L.; Krieger, C.; Tetzlaff, W. & Rossi, F. M. (2007). Local self-renewal can sustain CNS microglia maintenance and function throughout adult life. *Nat Neurosci,* Vol.10, No.12, pp. 1538-1543

Aloisi, F.; Ria, F. & Adorini, L. (2000). Regulation of T-cell responses by CNS antigen-presenting cells: different roles for microglia and astrocytes. *Immunol Today,* Vol.21, No.3, pp. 141-147

Badie, B. & Schartner, J. (2001). Role of microglia in glioma biology. *Microsc Res Tech,* Vol.54, No.2, pp. 106-113

Barker, C. F. & Billingham, R. E. (1977). Immunologically privileged sites. *Adv Immunol,* Vol.25, pp. 1-54

Barth, R. F. & Kaur, B. (2009). Rat brain tumor models in experimental neuro-oncology: the C6, 9L, T9, RG2, F98, BT4C, RT-2 and CNS-1 gliomas. *J Neurooncol,* Vol.94, No.3, pp. 299-312

Bartholomaus, I.; Kawakami, N.; Odoardi, F.; Schlager, C.; Miljkovic, D.; Ellwart, J. W.; Klinkert, W. E.; Flugel-Koch, C.; Issekutz, T. B.; Wekerle, H. & Flugel, A. (2009). Effector T cell interactions with meningeal vascular structures in nascent autoimmune CNS lesions. *Nature,* Vol.462, No.7269, pp. 94-98

Beauvillain, C.; Donnou, S.; Jarry, U.; Scotet, M.; Gascan, H.; Delneste, Y.; Guermonprez, P.; Jeannin, P. & Couez, D. (2008). Neonatal and adult microglia cross-present exogenous antigens. *Glia,* Vol.56, No.1, pp. 69-77

Bechmann, I.; Galea, I. & Perry, V. H. (2007). What is the blood-brain barrier (not)? *Trends Immunol,* Vol.28, No.1, pp. 5-11

Biber, K.; Sauter, A.; Brouwer, N.; Copray, S. C. & Boddeke, H. W. (2001). Ischemia-induced neuronal expression of the microglia attracting chemokine Secondary Lymphoid-tissue Chemokine (SLC). *Glia,* Vol.34, No.2, pp. 121-133

Biollaz, G.; Bernasconi, L.; Cretton, C.; Puntener, U.; Frei, K.; Fontana, A. & Suter, T. (2009). Site-specific anti-tumor immunity: differences in DC function, TGF-beta production and numbers of intratumoral Foxp3+ Treg. *Eur J Immunol,* Vol.39, No.5, pp. 1323-1333

Biswas, S. K. & Mantovani, A. (2010). Macrophage plasticity and interaction with lymphocyte subsets: cancer as a paradigm. *Nat Immunol,* Vol.11, No.10, pp. 889-896

Block, M. L.; Zecca, L. & Hong, J. S. (2007). Microglia-mediated neurotoxicity: uncovering the molecular mechanisms. *Nat Rev Neurosci,* Vol.8, No.1, pp. 57-69

Bogdahn, U.; Hau, P.; Stockhammer, G.; Venkataramana, N. K.; Mahapatra, A. K.; Suri, A.; Balasubramaniam, A.; Nair, S.; Oliushine, V.; Parfenov, V.; Poverennova, I.; Zaaroor, M.; Jachimczak, P.; Ludwig, S.; Schmaus, S.; Heinrichs, H. & Schlingensiepen, K. H. (2011). Targeted therapy for high-grade glioma with the TGF-beta2 inhibitor trabedersen: results of a randomized and controlled phase IIb study. *J neurooncol.,* Vol.81, No.2, pp.149-162

Calzascia, T.; Di Berardino-Besson, W.; Wilmotte, R.; Masson, F.; de Tribolet, N.; Dietrich, P. Y. & Walker, P. R. (2003). Cutting edge: cross-presentation as a mechanism for efficient recruitment of tumor-specific CTL to the brain. *J Immunol,* Vol.171, No.5, pp. 2187-2191

Calzascia, T.; Masson, F.; Di Berardino-Besson, W.; Contassot, E.; Wilmotte, R.; Aurrand-Lions, M.; Ruegg, C.; Dietrich, P. Y. & Walker, P. R. (2005). Homing phenotypes of tumor-specific CD8 T cells are predetermined at the tumor site by crosspresenting APCs. *Immunity,* Vol.22, No.2, pp. 175-184

Carbonell, W. S.; Murase, S.; Horwitz, A. F. & Mandell, J. W. (2005a). Migration of perilesional microglia after focal brain injury and modulation by CC chemokine receptor 5: an in situ time-lapse confocal imaging study. *J Neurosci,* Vol.25, No.30, pp. 7040-7047

Carbonell, W. S.; Murase, S. I.; Horwitz, A. F. & Mandell, J. W. (2005b). Infiltrative microgliosis: activation and long-distance migration of subependymal microglia following periventricular insults. *J Neuroinflammation,* Vol.2, No.1, pp. 5

Cardona, A. E.; Pioro, E. P.; Sasse, M. E.; Kostenko, V.; Cardona, S. M.; Dijkstra, I. M.; Huang, D.; Kidd, G.; Dombrowski, S.; Dutta, R.; Lee, J. C.; Cook, D. N.; Jung, S.; Lira, S. A.; Littman, D. R. & Ransohoff, R. M. (2006). Control of microglial neurotoxicity by the fractalkine receptor. *Nat Neurosci,* Vol.9, No.7, pp. 917-924

Carpentier, A.; Metellus, P.; Ursu, R.; Zohar, S.; Lafitte, F.; Barrie, M.; Meng, Y.; Richard, M.; Parizot, C.; Laigle-Donadey, F.; Gorochov, G.; Psimaras, D.; Sanson, M.; Tibi, A.; Chinot, O. & Carpentier, A. F. (2010). Intracerebral administration of CpG oligonucleotide for patients with recurrent glioblastoma: a phase II study. *Neuro Oncol,* Vol.12, No.4, pp. 401-408

Carson, M. J.; Doose, J. M.; Melchior, B.; Schmid, C. D. & Ploix, C. C. (2006). CNS immune privilege: hiding in plain sight. *Immunol Rev,* Vol.213, pp. 48-65

Chinnery, H. R.; Ruitenberg, M. J. & McMenamin, P. G. (2010). Novel characterization of monocyte-derived cell populations in the meninges and choroid plexus and their rates of replenishment in bone marrow chimeric mice. *J Neuropathol Exp Neurol,* Vol.69, No.9, pp. 896-909

Chitnis, T.; Imitola, J.; Wang, Y.; Elyaman, W.; Chawla, P.; Sharuk, M.; Raddassi, K.; Bronson, R. T. & Khoury, S. J. (2007). Elevated neuronal expression of CD200 protects Wlds mice from inflammation-mediated neurodegeneration. *Am J Pathol,* Vol.170, No.5, pp. 1695-1712

Davalos, D.; Grutzendler, J.; Yang, G.; Kim, J. V.; Zuo, Y.; Jung, S.; Littman, D. R.; Dustin, M. L. & Gan, W. B. (2005). ATP mediates rapid microglial response to local brain injury in vivo. *Nat Neurosci,* Vol.8, No.6, pp. 752-758

Davalos, D.; Lee, J. K.; Smith, W. B.; Brinkman, B.; Ellisman, M. H.; Zheng, B. & Akassoglou, K. (2008). Stable in vivo imaging of densely populated glia, axons and blood vessels in the mouse spinal cord using two-photon microscopy. *J Neurosci Methods,* Vol.169, No.1, pp. 1-7

Dijkstra, I. M.; de Haas, A. H.; Brouwer, N.; Boddeke, H. W. & Biber, K. (2006). Challenge with innate and protein antigens induces CCR7 expression by microglia in vitro and in vivo. *Glia,* Vol.54, No.8, pp. 861-872

Ding, H.; Roncari, L.; Shannon, P.; Wu, X.; Lau, N.; Karaskova, J.; Gutmann, D. H.; Squire, J. A.; Nagy, A. & Guha, A. (2001). Astrocyte-specific expression of activated p21-ras results in malignant astrocytoma formation in a transgenic mouse model of human gliomas. *Cancer Res,* Vol.61, No.9, pp. 3826-3836

Du, R.; Lu, K. V.; Petritsch, C.; Liu, P.; Ganss, R.; Passegue, E.; Song, H.; Vandenberg, S.; Johnson, R. S.; Werb, Z. & Bergers, G. (2008). HIF1alpha induces the recruitment of bone marrow-derived vascular modulatory cells to regulate tumor angiogenesis and invasion. *Cancer Cell,* Vol.13, No.3, pp. 206-220

Esteve, P. O.; Chicoine, E.; Robledo, O.; Aoudjit, F.; Descoteaux, A.; Potworowski, E. F. & St-Pierre, Y. (2002). Protein kinase C-zeta regulates transcription of the matrix metalloproteinase-9 gene induced by IL-1 and TNF-alpha in glioma cells via NF-kappa B. *J Biol Chem,* Vol.277, No.38, pp. 35150-35155

Flaris, N. A.; Densmore, T. L.; Molleston, M. C. & Hickey, W. F. (1993). Characterization of microglia and macrophages in the central nervous system of rats: definition of the differential expression of molecules using standard and novel monoclonal antibodies in normal CNS and in four models of parenchymal reaction. *Glia,* Vol.7, No.1, pp. 34-40

Flugel, A.; Bradl, M.; Kreutzberg, G. W. & Graeber, M. B. (2001). Transformation of donor-derived bone marrow precursors into host microglia during autoimmune CNS inflammation and during the retrograde response to axotomy. *J Neurosci Res,* Vol.66, No.1, pp. 74-82

Flugel, A.; Labeur, M. S.; Grasbon-Frodl, E. M.; Kreutzberg, G. W. & Graeber, M. B. (1999). Microglia only weakly present glioma antigen to cytotoxic T cells. *Int J Dev Neurosci,* Vol.17, No.5-6, pp. 547-556

Ford, A. L.; Foulcher, E.; Lemckert, F. A. & Sedgwick, J. D. (1996). Microglia induce CD4 T lymphocyte final effector function and death. *J Exp Med,* Vol.184, No.5, pp. 1737-1745

Frei, K.; Lins, H.; Schwerdel, C. & Fontana, A. (1994). Antigen presentation in the central nervous system. The inhibitory effect of IL-10 on MHC class II expression and production of cytokines depends on the inducing signals and the type of cell analyzed. *J Immunol,* Vol.152, No.6, pp. 2720-2728

Fujita, M.; Kohanbash, G.; Fellows-Mayle, W.; Hamilton, R. L.; Komohara, Y.; Decker, S. A.; Ohlfest, J. R. & Okada, H. (2011). COX-2 blockade suppresses gliomagenesis by inhibiting myeloid-derived suppressor cells. *Cancer Res,* Vol.71, No.7, pp. 2664-2674

Fujita, M.; Scheurer, M. E.; Decker, S. A.; McDonald, H. A.; Kohanbash, G.; Kastenhuber, E. R.; Kato, H.; Bondy, M. L.; Ohlfest, J. R. & Okada, H. (2010). Role of type 1 IFNs in antiglioma immunosurveillance--using mouse studies to guide examination of novel prognostic markers in humans. *Clin Cancer Res,* Vol.16, No.13, pp. 3409-3419

Fujiwara, Y.; Komohara, Y.; Ikeda, T. & Takeya, M. (2010). Corosolic acid inhibits glioblastoma cell proliferation by suppressing the activation of signal transducer and activator of transcription-3 and nuclear factor-kappa B in tumor cells and tumor-associated macrophages. *Cancer science,* Vol.102, No.1, pp. 206-211

Gabrilovich, D. I. & Nagaraj, S. (2009). Myeloid-derived suppressor cells as regulators of the immune system. *Nat Rev Immunol,* Vol.9, No.3, pp. 162-174

Galarneau, H.; Villeneuve, J.; Gowing, G.; Julien, J. P. & Vallieres, L. (2007). Increased glioma growth in mice depleted of macrophages. *Cancer Res,* Vol.67, No.18, pp. 8874-8881

Galea, I.; Bechmann, I. & Perry, V. H. (2007). What is immune privilege (not)? *Trends Immunol,* Vol.28, No.1, pp. 12-18

Geissmann, F.; Gordon, S.; Hume, D. A.; Mowat, A. M. & Randolph, G. J. (2010). Unravelling mononuclear phagocyte heterogeneity. *Nat Rev Immunol,* Vol.10, No.6, pp. 453-460

Ginhoux, F.; Greter, M.; Leboeuf, M.; Nandi, S.; See, P.; Gokhan, S.; Mehler, M. F.; Conway, S. J.; Ng, L. G.; Stanley, E. R.; Samokhvalov, I. M. & Merad, M. (2010). Fate mapping analysis reveals that adult microglia derive from primitive macrophages. *Science,* Vol.330, No.6005, pp. 841-845

Ginzkey, C.; Eicker, S. O.; Marget, M.; Krause, J.; Brecht, S.; Westphal, M.; Hugo, H. H.; Mehdorn, H. M.; Steinmann, J. & Hamel, W. (2010). Increase in tumor size following intratumoral injection of immunostimulatory CpG-containing oligonucleotides in a rat glioma model. *Cancer Immunol Immunother,* Vol.59, No.4, pp. 541-551

Glezer, I.; Simard, A. R. & Rivest, S. (2007). Neuroprotective role of the innate immune system by microglia. *Neuroscience,* Vol.147, No.4, pp. 867-883

Gottfried-Blackmore, A.; Kaunzner, U. W.; Idoyaga, J.; Felger, J. C.; McEwen, B. S. & Bulloch, K. (2009). Acute in vivo exposure to interferon-gamma enables resident brain dendritic cells to become effective antigen presenting cells. *Proc Natl Acad Sci U S A,* Vol.106, No.49, pp. 20918-20923

Graeber, M. B. (2010). Changing face of microglia. *Science,* Vol.330, No.6005, pp. 783-788

Graeber, M. B.; Lopez-Redondo, F.; Ikoma, E.; Ishikawa, M.; Imai, Y.; Nakajima, K.; Kreutzberg, G. W. & Kohsaka, S. (1998). The microglia/macrophage response in the neonatal rat facial nucleus following axotomy. *Brain Res,* Vol.813, No.2, pp. 241-253

Graeber, M. B. & Streit, W. J. (2010). Microglia: biology and pathology. *Acta Neuropathol,* Vol.119, No.1, pp. 89-105

Hanisch, U. K. & Kettenmann, H. (2007). Microglia: active sensor and versatile effector cells in the normal and pathologic brain. *Nat Neurosci,* Vol.10, No.11, pp. 1387-1394

Hatterer, E.; Davoust, N.; Didier-Bazes, M.; Vuaillat, C.; Malcus, C.; Belin, M. F. & Nataf, S. (2006). How to drain without lymphatics? Dendritic cells migrate from the cerebrospinal fluid to the B-cell follicles of cervical lymph nodes. *Blood,* Vol.107, No.2, pp. 806-812

Hatterer, E.; Touret, M.; Belin, M. F.; Honnorat, J. & Nataf, S. (2008). Cerebrospinal fluid dendritic cells infiltrate the brain parenchyma and target the cervical lymph nodes under neuroinflammatory conditions. *PLoS One,* Vol.3, No.10, pp. e3321

Heppner, F. L.; Greter, M.; Marino, D.; Falsig, J.; Raivich, G.; Hovelmeyer, N.; Waisman, A.; Rulicke, T.; Prinz, M.; Priller, J.; Becher, B. & Aguzzi, A. (2005). Experimental autoimmune encephalomyelitis repressed by microglial paralysis. *Nat Med,* Vol.11, No.2, pp. 146-152

Hickey, W. F. & Kimura, H. (1988). Perivascular microglial cells of the CNS are bone marrow-derived and present antigen in vivo. *Science,* Vol.239, No.4837, pp. 290-292

Hickey, W. F.; Vass, K. & Lassmann, H. (1992). Bone marrow-derived elements in the central nervous system: an immunohistochemical and ultrastructural survey of rat chimeras. *J Neuropathol Exp Neurol,* Vol.51, No.3, pp. 246-256

Hoek, R. M.; Ruuls, S. R.; Murphy, C. A.; Wright, G. J.; Goddard, R.; Zurawski, S. M.; Blom, B.; Homola, M. E.; Streit, W. J.; Brown, M. H.; Barclay, A. N. & Sedgwick, J. D. (2000). Down-regulation of the macrophage lineage through interaction with OX2 (CD200). *Science,* Vol.290, No.5497, pp. 1768-1771

Hong, T. M.; Teng, L. J.; Shun, C. T.; Peng, M. C. & Tsai, J. C. (2009). Induced interleukin-8 expression in gliomas by tumor-associated macrophages. *J Neurooncol,* Vol.93, No.3, pp. 289-301

Huse, J. T. & Holland, E. C. (2009). Genetically engineered mouse models of brain cancer and the promise of preclinical testing. *Brain Pathol,* Vol.19, No.1, pp. 132-143

Hussain, S. F.; Kong, L. Y.; Jordan, J.; Conrad, C.; Madden, T.; Fokt, I.; Priebe, W. & Heimberger, A. B. (2007). A novel small molecule inhibitor of signal transducers and activators of transcription 3 reverses immune tolerance in malignant glioma patients. *Cancer Res,* Vol.67, No.20, pp. 9630-9636

Hussain, S. F.; Yang, D.; Suki, D.; Aldape, K.; Grimm, E. & Heimberger, A. B. (2006a). The role of human glioma-infiltrating microglia/macrophages in mediating antitumor immune responses. *Neuro Oncol,* Vol.8, No.3, pp. 261-279

Hussain, S. F.; Yang, D.; Suki, D.; Grimm, E. & Heimberger, A. B. (2006b). Innate immune functions of microglia isolated from human glioma patients. *J Transl Med,* Vol.4, pp. 15

Hülper, P.; Schulz-Schaeffer, W.; Dullin, C.; Hoffmann, P.; Harper, J.; Kurtzberg, L.; Lonning, S.; Kugler, W; Lakomek, M. & Erdlenbruch, B. (2011). Tumor localization of an anti-TGF-ß antibody and its effects on gliomas. *International Journal of Oncology,* Vol. 38, pp. 51-59

Hwang, S. Y.; Yoo, B. C.; Jung, J. W.; Oh, E. S.; Hwang, J. S.; Shin, J. A.; Kim, S. Y.; Cha, S. H. & Han, I. O. (2009). Induction of glioma apoptosis by microglia-secreted molecules: The role of nitric oxide and cathepsin B. *Biochim Biophys Acta,* Vol.1793, No.11, pp. 1656-1668

Jia, W.; Jackson-Cook, C. & Graf, M. R. (2010). Tumor-infiltrating, myeloid-derived suppressor cells inhibit T cell activity by nitric oxide production in an intracranial rat glioma + vaccination model. *J Neuroimmunol,* Vol.223, No.1-2, pp. 20-30

Karman, J.; Ling, C.; Sandor, M. & Fabry, Z. (2004). Initiation of immune responses in brain is promoted by local dendritic cells. *J Immunol,* Vol.173, No.4, pp. 2353-2361

Kennedy, B. C.; Maier, L. M.; D'Amico, R.; Mandigo, C. E.; Fontana, E. J.; Waziri, A.; Assanah, M. C.; Canoll, P.; Anderson, R. C.; Anderson, D. E. & Bruce, J. N. (2009). Dynamics of central and peripheral immunomodulation in a murine glioma model. *BMC Immunol,* Vol.10, pp. 11

Kettenmann, H.; Hanisch, U. K.; Noda, M. & Verkhratsky, A. (2011). Physiology of microglia. *Physiol Rev,* Vol.91, No.2, pp. 461-553

Komohara, Y.; Ohnishi, K.; Kuratsu, J. & Takeya, M. (2008). Possible involvement of the M2 anti-inflammatory macrophage phenotype in growth of human gliomas. *J Pathol,* Vol.216, No.1, pp. 15-24

Lee, J. E.; Liang, K. J.; Fariss, R. N. & Wong, W. T. (2008). Ex vivo dynamic imaging of retinal microglia using time-lapse confocal microscopy. *Invest Ophthalmol Vis Sci,* Vol.49, No.9, pp. 4169-4176

Liang, K. J.; Lee, J. E.; Wang, Y. D.; Ma, W.; Fontainhas, A. M.; Fariss, R. N. & Wong, W. T. (2009). Regulation of dynamic behavior of retinal microglia by CX3CR1 signaling. *Invest Ophthalmol Vis Sci,* Vol.50, No.9, pp. 4444-4451

Lin, M. L.; Zhan, Y.; Villadangos, J. A. & Lew, A. M. (2008). The cell biology of cross-presentation and the role of dendritic cell subsets. *Immunol Cell Biol,* Vol.86, No.4, pp. 353-362

Liu, Y.; Wang, Q; Kleinschmidt-DeMasters, B.K.; Franzusoff, A.; Ng, K. & Lillehei, K.O. (2007). TGF-β2 inhibition augments the effect of tumor vaccine and improves the survival of animals with pre-established brain tumors. *Journal of neuro-oncology,* Vol.81, No.2, pp.149-162

Markovic, D. S.; Vinnakota, K.; Chirasani, S.; Synowitz, M.; Raguet, H.; Stock, K.; Sliwa, M.; Lehmann, S.; Kalin, R.; van Rooijen, N.; Holmbeck, K.; Heppner, F. L.; Kiwit, J.; Matyash, V.; Lehnardt, S.; Kaminska, B.; Glass, R. & Kettenmann, H. (2009). Gliomas induce and exploit microglial MT1-MMP expression for tumor expansion. *Proc Natl Acad Sci U S A,* Vol.106, No.30, pp. 12530-12535

Matyszak, M. K.; Denis-Donini, S.; Citterio, S.; Longhi, R.; Granucci, F. & Ricciardi-Castagnoli, P. (1999). Microglia induce myelin basic protein-specific T cell anergy or T cell activation, according to their state of activation. *Eur J Immunol,* Vol.29, No.10, pp. 3063-3076

Matyszak, M. K.; Lawson, L. J.; Perry, V. H. & Gordon, S. (1992). Stromal macrophages of the choroid plexus situated at an interface between the brain and peripheral immune system constitutively express major histocompatibility class II antigens. *J Neuroimmunol,* Vol.40, No.2-3, pp. 173-181

McMahon, E. J.; Bailey, S. L.; Castenada, C. V.; Waldner, H. & Miller, S. D. (2005). Epitope spreading initiates in the CNS in two mouse models of multiple sclerosis. *Nat Med,* Vol.11, No.3, pp. 335-339

McMenamin, P. G. (1999). Distribution and phenotype of dendritic cells and resident tissue macrophages in the dura mater, leptomeninges, and choroid plexus of the rat brain as demonstrated in wholemount preparations. *J Comp Neurol,* Vol.405, No.4, pp. 553-562

McMenamin, P. G.; Wealthall, R. J.; Deverall, M.; Cooper, S. J. & Griffin, B. (2003). Macrophages and dendritic cells in the rat meninges and choroid plexus: three-dimensional localisation by environmental scanning electron microscopy and confocal microscopy. *Cell Tissue Res,* Vol.313, No.3, pp. 259-269

Medawar, P. B. (1948). Immunity to homologous grafted skin; the fate of skin homografts transplanted to the brain, to subcutaneous tissue, and to the anterior chamber of the eye. *Br J Exp Pathol,* Vol.29, No.1, pp. 58-69

Morioka, T.; Baba, T.; Black, K. L. & Streit, W. J. (1992). Inflammatory cell infiltrates vary in experimental primary and metastatic brain tumors. *Neurosurgery,* Vol.30, No.6, pp. 891-896

Nakagawa, J.; Saio, M.; Tamakawa, N.; Suwa, T.; Frey, A. B.; Nonaka, K.; Umemura, N.; Imai, H.; Ouyang, G. F.; Ohe, N.; Yano, H.; Yoshimura, S.; Iwama, T. & Takami, T.

(2007). TNF expressed by tumor-associated macrophages, but not microglia, can eliminate glioma. *Int J Oncol,* Vol.30, No.4, pp. 803-811

Neumann, H.; Kotter, M. R. & Franklin, R. J. (2009). Debris clearance by microglia: an essential link between degeneration and regeneration. *Brain,* Vol.132, No.Pt 2, pp. 288-295

Nimmerjahn, A.; Kirchhoff, F. & Helmchen, F. (2005). Resting microglial cells are highly dynamic surveillants of brain parenchyma in vivo. *Science,* Vol.308, No.5726, pp. 1314-1318

Nishie, A.; Ono, M.; Shono, T.; Fukushi, J.; Otsubo, M.; Onoue, H.; Ito, Y.; Inamura, T.; Ikezaki, K.; Fukui, M.; Iwaki, T. & Kuwano, M. (1999). Macrophage infiltration and heme oxygenase-1 expression correlate with angiogenesis in human gliomas. *Clin Cancer Res,* Vol.5, No.5, pp. 1107-1113

Okada, M.; Saio, M.; Kito, Y.; Ohe, N.; Yano, H.; Yoshimura, S.; Iwama, T. & Takami, T. (2009). Tumor-associated macrophage/microglia infiltration in human gliomas is correlated with MCP-3, but not MCP-1. *Int J Oncol,* Vol.34, No.6, pp. 1621-1627

Orr, A. G.; Orr, A. L.; Li, X. J.; Gross, R. E. & Traynelis, S. F. (2009). Adenosine A(2A) receptor mediates microglial process retraction. *Nat Neurosci,* Vol.12, No.7, pp. 872-878

Parney, I. F.; Waldron, J. S. & Parsa, A. T. (2009). Flow cytometry and in vitro analysis of human glioma-associated macrophages. Laboratory investigation. *J Neurosurg,* Vol.110, No.3, pp. 572-582

Platten, M.; Kretz, A.; Naumann, U.; Aulwurm, S.; Egashira, K.; Isenmann, S. & Weller, M. (2003). Monocyte chemoattractant protein-1 increases microglial infiltration and aggressiveness of gliomas. *Ann Neurol,* Vol.54, No.3, pp. 388-392

Platten, M. & Steinman, L. (2005). Multiple sclerosis: trapped in deadly glue. *Nat Med,* Vol.11, No.3, pp. 252-253

Plautz, G. E.; Mukai, S.; Cohen, P. A. & Shu, S. (2000). Cross-presentation of tumor antigens to effector T cells is sufficient to mediate effective immunotherapy of established intracranial tumors. *J Immunol,* Vol.165, No.7, pp. 3656-3662

Prins, R. M.; Scott, G. P.; Merchant, R. E. & Graf, M. R. (2002). Irradiated tumor cell vaccine for treatment of an established glioma. II. Expansion of myeloid suppressor cells that promote tumor progression. *Cancer Immunol Immunother,* Vol.51, No.4, pp. 190-199

Prinz, M. & Mildner, A. (2011). Microglia in the CNS: immigrants from another world. *Glia,* Vol.59, No.2, pp. 177-187

Ransohoff, R. M. & Cardona, A. E. (2010). The myeloid cells of the central nervous system parenchyma. *Nature,* Vol.468, No.7321, pp. 253-262

Raychaudhuri, B.; Rayman, P.; Ireland, J.; Ko, J.; Rini, B.; Borden, E. C.; Garcia, J.; Vogelbaum, M. A. & Finke, J. (2011). Myeloid-derived suppressor cell accumulation and function in patients with newly diagnosed glioblastoma. *Neuro Oncol,* Vol.13, No.6, pp. 591-599

Rempel, S. A.; Dudas, S.; Ge, S. & Gutierrez, J. A. (2000). Identification and localization of the cytokine SDF1 and its receptor, CXC chemokine receptor 4, to regions of necrosis and angiogenesis in human glioblastoma. *Clin Cancer Res,* Vol.6, No.1, pp. 102-111

Rodero, M.; Marie, Y.; Coudert, M.; Blondet, E.; Mokhtari, K.; Rousseau, A.; Raoul, W.; Carpentier, C.; Sennlaub, F.; Deterre, P.; Delattre, J. Y.; Debre, P.; Sanson, M. & Combadiere, C. (2008). Polymorphism in the microglial cell-mobilizing CX3CR1 gene is associated with survival in patients with glioblastoma. *J Clin Oncol,* Vol.26, No.36, pp. 5957-5964

Rodrigues, J. C.; Gonzalez, G. C.; Zhang, L.; Ibrahim, G.; Kelly, J. J.; Gustafson, M. P.; Lin, Y.; Dietz, A. B.; Forsyth, P. A.; Yong, V. W. & Parney, I. F. (2010). Normal human monocytes exposed to glioma cells acquire myeloid-derived suppressor cell-like properties. *Neuro Oncol,* Vol.12, No.4, pp. 351-365

Roessler, K.; Suchanek, G.; Breitschopf, H.; Kitz, K.; Matula, C.; Lassmann, H. & Koos, W. T. (1995). Detection of tumor necrosis factor-alpha protein and messenger RNA in human glial brain tumors: comparison of immunohistochemistry with in situ hybridization using molecular probes. *J Neurosurg,* Vol.83, No.2, pp. 291-297

Roggendorf, W.; Strupp, S. & Paulus, W. (1996). Distribution and characterization of microglia/macrophages in human brain tumors. *Acta Neuropathol,* Vol.92, No.3, pp. 288-293

Rosales, A. A., Roque, R.S. (1996). Microglia-derived cytotoxic factors. Part I: Inhibition of tumor cell growth in vitro, *Brain Res,* Vol.748, No.1-2, pp. 195_204

Rossi, M. L.; Cruz-Sanchez, F.; Hughes, J. T.; Esiri, M. M.; Coakham, H. B. & Moss, T. H. (1988). Mononuclear cell infiltrate and HLA-DR expression in low grade astrocytomas. An immunohistological study of 23 cases. *Acta Neuropathol,* Vol.76, No.3, pp. 281-286

Rossi, M. L.; Hughes, J. T.; Esiri, M. M.; Coakham, H. B. & Brownell, D. B. (1987). Immunohistological study of mononuclear cell infiltrate in malignant gliomas. *Acta Neuropathol,* Vol.74, No.3, pp. 269-277

Rossi, M. L.; Jones, N. R.; Candy, E.; Nicoll, J. A.; Compton, J. S.; Hughes, J. T.; Esiri, M. M.; Moss, T. H.; Cruz-Sanchez, F. F. & Coakham, H. B. (1989). The mononuclear cell infiltrate compared with survival in high-grade astrocytomas. *Acta Neuropathol,* Vol.78, No.2, pp. 189-193

Ryuto, M.; Ono, M.; Izumi, H.; Yoshida, S.; Weich, H. A.; Kohno, K. & Kuwano, M. (1996). Induction of vascular endothelial growth factor by tumor necrosis factor alpha in human glioma cells. Possible roles of SP-1. *J Biol Chem,* Vol.271, No.45, pp. 28220-28228

Santambrogio, L.; Belyanskaya, S. L.; Fischer, F. R.; Cipriani, B.; Brosnan, C. F.; Ricciardi-Castagnoli, P.; Stern, L. J.; Strominger, J. L. & Riese, R. (2001). Developmental plasticity of CNS microglia. *Proc Natl Acad Sci U S A,* Vol.98, No.11, pp. 6295-6300

Schmid, C. D.; Melchior, B.; Masek, K.; Puntambekar, S. S.; Danielson, P. E.; Lo, D. D.; Sutcliffe, J. G. & Carson, M. J. (2009). Differential gene expression in LPS/IFNgamma activated microglia and macrophages: in vitro versus in vivo. *J Neurochem,* Vol.109 Suppl 1, pp. 117-125

Schwartzbaum, J. A.; Fisher, J. L.; Aldape, K. D. & Wrensch, M. (2006). Epidemiology and molecular pathology of glioma. *Nat Clin Pract Neurol,* Vol.2, No.9, pp. 494-503

Serot, J. M.; Bene, M. C.; Foliguet, B. & Faure, G. C. (2000). Monocyte-derived IL-10-secreting dendritic cells in choroid plexus epithelium. *J Neuroimmunol,* Vol.105, No.2, pp. 115-119

Shannon, P.; Sabha, N.; Lau, N.; Kamnasaran, D.; Gutmann, D. H. & Guha, A. (2005). Pathological and molecular progression of astrocytomas in a GFAP:12 V-Ha-Ras mouse astrocytoma model. *Am J Pathol,* Vol.167, No.3, pp. 859-867

Shinonaga, M.; Chang, C. C.; Suzuki, N.; Sato, M. & Kuwabara, T. (1988). Immunohistological evaluation of macrophage infiltrates in brain tumors. Correlation with peritumoral edema. *J Neurosurg,* Vol.68, No.2, pp. 259-265

Simpson, J. E.; Newcombe, J.; Cuzner, M. L. & Woodroofe, M. N. (1998). Expression of monocyte chemoattractant protein-1 and other beta-chemokines by resident glia and inflammatory cells in multiple sclerosis lesions. *J Neuroimmunol,* Vol.84, No.2, pp. 238-249

Singh, S. K.; Hawkins, C.; Clarke, I. D.; Squire, J. A.; Bayani, J.; Hide, T.; Henkelman, R. M.; Cusimano, M. D. & Dirks, P. B. (2004). Identification of human brain tumour initiating cells. *Nature,* Vol.432, No.7015, pp. 396-401

Sliwa, M.; Markovic, D.; Gabrusiewicz, K.; Synowitz, M.; Glass, R.; Zawadzka, M.; Wesolowska, A.; Kettenmann, H. & Kaminska, B. (2007). The invasion promoting effect of microglia on glioblastoma cells is inhibited by cyclosporin A. *Brain,* Vol.130, No.Pt 2, pp. 476-489

Soulet, D. & Rivest, S. (2008). Bone-marrow-derived microglia: myth or reality? *Curr Opin Pharmacol,* Vol.8, No.4, pp. 508-518

Stupp, R.; Hegi, M. E.; Mason, W. P.; van den Bent, M. J.; Taphoorn, M. J.; Janzer, R. C.; Ludwin, S. K.; Allgeier, A.; Fisher, B.; Belanger, K.; Hau, P.; Brandes, A. A.; Gijtenbeek, J.; Marosi, C.; Vecht, C. J.; Mokhtari, K.; Wesseling, P.; Villa, S.; Eisenhauer, E.; Gorlia, T.; Weller, M.; Lacombe, D.; Cairncross, J. G. & Mirimanoff, R. O. (2009). Effects of radiotherapy with concomitant and adjuvant temozolomide versus radiotherapy alone on survival in glioblastoma in a randomised phase III study: 5-year analysis of the EORTC-NCIC trial. *Lancet Oncol,* Vol.10, No.5, pp. 459-466

Szatmari, T.; Lumniczky, K.; Desaknai, S.; Trajcevski, S.; Hidvegi, E. J.; Hamada, H. & Safrany, G. (2006). Detailed characterization of the mouse glioma 261 tumor model for experimental glioblastoma therapy. *Cancer Sci,* Vol.97, No.6, pp. 546-553

Tran Thang, N. N.; Derouazi, M.; Philippin, G.; Arcidiaco, S.; Di Berardino-Besson, W.; Masson, F.; Hoepner, S.; Riccadonna, C.; Burkhardt, K.; Guha, A.; Dietrich, P. Y. & Walker, P. R. (2010). Immune infiltration of spontaneous mouse astrocytomas is dominated by immunosuppressive cells from early stages of tumor development. *Cancer Res,* Vol.70, No.12, pp. 4829-4839

Ueda, R.; Fujita, M.; Zhu, X.; Sasaki, K.; Kastenhuber, E. R.; Kohanbash, G.; McDonald, H. A.; Harper, J.; Lonning, S. & Okada, H. (2009). Systemic inhibition of transforming growth factor-beta in glioma-bearing mice improves the therapeutic efficacy of glioma-associated antigen peptide vaccines. *Clin Cancer Res,* Vol.15, No.21, pp. 6551-6559

Uhl, M.; Aulwurm, S.; Wischhusen, J.; Weiler, M.; Ma, J. Y.; Almirez, R.; Mangadu, R.; Liu, Y. W.; Platten, M.; Herrlinger, U.; Murphy, A.; Wong, D. H.; Wick, W.; Higgins, L. S. & Weller, M. (2004). SD-208, a novel transforming growth factor beta receptor I kinase inhibitor, inhibits growth and invasiveness and enhances immunogenicity of murine and human glioma cells in vitro and in vivo. *Cancer Res,* Vol.64, No.21, pp. 7954-7961

Umemura, N.; Saio, M.; Suwa, T.; Kitoh, Y.; Bai, J.; Nonaka, K.; Ouyang, G. F.; Okada, M.; Balazs, M.; Adany, R.; Shibata, T. & Takami, T. (2008). Tumor-infiltrating myeloid-derived suppressor cells are pleiotropic-inflamed monocytes/macrophages that bear M1- and M2-type characteristics. *J Leukoc Biol,* Vol.83, No.5, pp. 1136-1144

Voisin, P.; Bouchaud, V.; Merle, M.; Diolez, P.; Duffy, L.; Flint, K.; Franconi, J. M. & Bouzier-Sore, A. K. (2010). Microglia in close vicinity of glioma cells: correlation between phenotype and metabolic alterations. *Front Neuroenergetics,* Vol.2, pp. 131

Walker, P.; Prins, R. M.; Dietrich, P.-Y. & Liau, L. M. (2009). Harnessing T-cell immunity to target brain tumors, In: *CNS Cancer: models, markers, prognostic factors, targets and therapeutic approaches,* E. Van Meir, pp. 1165-1218, Humana Press, New York

Walker, P. R.; Calzascia, T.; de Tribolet, N. & Dietrich P. Y. (2003). T-cell immune responses in the brain and their relevance for cerebral malignancies. *Brain Res Brain Res Rev,* Vol.42, No.2, pp. 97-122

Wang, X.; Li, C.; Chen, Y.; Hao, Y.; Zhou, W.; Chen, C. & Yu, Z. (2008). Hypoxia enhances CXCR4 expression favoring microglia migration via HIF-1alpha activation. *Biochem Biophys Res Commun,* Vol.371, No.2, pp. 283-288

Wang, X. B.; Tian, X. Y.; Li, Y.; Li, B. & Li, Z. (2011). Elevated expression of macrophage migration inhibitory factor correlates with tumor recurrence and poor prognosis of patients with gliomas. *J Neurooncol*

Watters, J. J.; Schartner, J. M. & Badie, B. (2005). Microglia function in brain tumors. *J Neurosci Res,* Vol.81, No.3, pp. 447-455

Wei, J.; Wu, A.; Kong, L. Y.; Wang, Y.; Fuller, G.; Fokt, I.; Melillo, G.; Priebe, W. & Heimberger, A. B. (2011). Hypoxia potentiates glioma-mediated immunosuppression. *PLoS One,* Vol.6, No.1, pp. e16195

Wesolowska, A.; Kwiatkowska, A.; Slomnicki, L.; Dembinski, M.; Master, A.; Sliwa, M.; Franciszkiewicz, K.; Chouaib, S. & Kaminska, B. (2008). Microglia-derived TGF-beta as an important regulator of glioblastoma invasion--an inhibition of TGF-beta-dependent effects by shRNA against human TGF-beta type II receptor. *Oncogene,* Vol.27, No.7, pp. 918-930

Wood, G. W. & Morantz, R. A. (1979). Immunohistologic evaluation of the lymphoreticular infiltrate of human central nervous system tumors. *J Natl Cancer Inst,* Vol.62, No.3, pp. 485-491

Wu, A.; Wei, J.; Kong, L. Y.; Wang, Y.; Priebe, W.; Qiao, W.; Sawaya, R. & Heimberger, A. B. (2010). Glioma cancer stem cells induce immunosuppressive macrophages /microglia. *Neuro Oncol,* Vol.12, No.11, pp. 1113-1125

Yi, L.; Xiao, H.; Xu, M.; Ye, X.; Hu, J.; Li, F.; Li, M.; Luo, C.; Yu, S.; Bian, X. & Feng, H. (2011). Glioma-initiating cells: a predominant role in microglia/macrophages tropism to glioma. *J Neuroimmunol,* Vol.232, No.1-2, pp. 75-82

Zhai, H.; Heppner, F. L. & Tsirka, S. E. (2011). Microglia/macrophages promote glioma progression. *Glia,* Vol.59, No.3, pp. 472-485

Zhang, L.; Alizadeh, D.; Van Handel, M.; Kortylewski, M.; Yu, H. & Badie, B. (2009). Stat3 inhibition activates tumor macrophages and abrogates glioma growth in mice. *Glia,* Vol.57, No.13, pp. 1458-1467

Zhao, D.; Alizadeh, D.; Zhang, L.; Liu, W.; Farrukh, O.; Manuel, E.; Diamond, D. J. & Badie, B. (2010). Carbon nanotubes enhance CpG uptake and potentiate antiglioma immunity. *Clin Cancer Res,* Vol.17, No.4, pp. 771-782

Zhu, X.; Fujita, M.; Snyder, L. A. & Okada, H. (2010). Systemic delivery of neutralizing antibody targeting CCL2 for glioma therapy. *J Neurooncol,* Vol.104, No.1, pp. 83-92

10

The Role of Tumor Microenvironment in Oral Cancer

Masakatsu Fukuda[1], Yoshihiro Ohmori[2] and Hideaki Sakashita[1]
[1]Second Division of Oral and Maxillofacial Surgery,
Department of Diagnostic and Therapeutic Sciences,
[2]Division of Microbiology and Immunology,
Department of Oral Biology and Tissue Engineering,
Meikai University School of Dentistry, Keyakidai, Sakado, Saitama,
Japan

1. Introduction

Human oral squamous cell carcinoma (HOSCC) is the most common malignant neoplasm arising in the mucosa of the upper aerodigestive tract. It is an aggressive tumor that is difficult to treat with conventional therapies, including chemotherapy, radiation, and surgery. Because surgical treatment often affects profoundly the quality of life and activities of daily living of the affected patients with HOSCC, and thus new therapeutic strategies are necessary along with the other conventional therapy.

In recent years considerable progress has been made in understanding the genetic basis of the development of HOSCC. It is well established that an accumulation of genetic alterations is the basis for the progression from a normal cell to a cancer cell, referred to as multi-step carcinogenesis (Califano et al., 1996). Progression is enabled by the increasingly more aberrant function of genes that positively or negatively regulate aspects of proliferation, apoptosis, genome stability, angiogenesis, invasion and metastasis (Hanahan et al., 2000). Gene function can be altered in different ways: tumor suppressor genes may be inactivated by mutation, deletion or methylation and oncogenes can be activated by mutation or amplification. A description of these alterations and how these are detected has previously been described (van Houten et al., 2000, Reid et al., 1997, Braakhuis et al., 2002). Oral cancers are characterized by a multitude of these genetic alterations and ongoing research is focusing on identifying the critical genetic events and the order in which they occur during carcinogenesis. Frequently occurring genomic alterations are supposed to contain the genes that are the most important for the development of a certain type of cancer (Albertson et al., 2003). Common alterations for oral cancer are inactivation of TP53 (located at 17p13), gain of chromosomal material at 3q26 and 11q13, and losses at 3p21, 13q21 and 14q32 (Gollin, 2001, Forastiere et al., 2001). For most of these regions the putative tumor suppressor genes or oncogenes still need to be identified. In general, loss of chromosomal material (allelic losses) at 3p, 9q and 17p was observed in a relatively high proportion of dysplastic lesions and therefore these alterations were interpreted to be early markers of carcinogenesis. Several studies suggest, however, that early genetic changes do not necessarily correlate with altered morphology.

Although recent improvements in the diagnosis and treatment of malignant tumors have extended the average length of patients' lives, the incidence of multiple primary malignant tumors is increasing (Licciardello et al., 1989). In particular, it has been reported that patients with head and neck cancer often develop multiple primary neoplasms (Sakashita et al., 1996). This phenomenon has been attributed to 'field cancerization', a concept based in the hypothesis that prolonged exposure to certain risk factors, such as tobacco products, leads to the independent transformation of multiple epithelial cells at several distinct anatomic sites (Slaughter et al., 1953). In addition, it is now becoming clear that the tumor microenvironment, which is largely orchestrated by inflammatory cells, is an indispensable participant in the neoplastic process, fostering proliferation, survival and migration. Recent data have expanded the concept that tumor microenvironments including hypoxia, and inflammation that are the critical components of tumor progression. Many cancers arise from sites of infection, chronic irritation and inflammation. Many tumors also contain hypoxic microenvironments, a condition that is associated with poor prognosis and resistance to treatment (Helmlinger et al., 1997).

On the other hand, as is obvious, host has defense mechanisms against various carcinogenesis events like above. Host professional antigen-presenting cells (APCs) appear to play an important role in the presentation of tumor antigens and the induction of specific immune responses to tumors, a role that was initially attributed entirely to the tumor cells themselves (Huang 1994, Rock et al., 1993). However, despite their expression of these distinct APCs, attempts by the immune system to eliminate a tumor are often ineffective. It has recently been reported that in cancer patients the tumor cells themselves may also evade immune attack by expressing immunosuppressive cytokines.

Thus, oral carcinogenesis is a highly complex multifactorial process that takes place when epithelial cells are affected by several genetic alterations. The use of molecular biology techniques to diagnose oral cancerous lesion might be markedly improved the detection of alterations that are invisible under the microscope.

This chapter presents up-to-date evidence on molecular markers into the tumor microenvironment that have involved in the proliferation and progression mechanisms of the oral cancer.

2. Role of myelomonocytic cells in tumor microenvironment

Myeloid cells including monocytes and macrophages are key elements which regulate tissue homeostasis and local inflammation/immunity, differentiating into various cell types in response to provocative stimuli (Zeh et al., 2005, Demaria et al., 2010).

Monocytes exist as the second recruited effectors of the acute inflammatory response after neutrophils and also migrate to the site of tumor microenvironment, guided by chemotactic factors. It is known that monocytes, in the presence of granulocyte-macrophage colony stimulating factor (GM-CSF) and interleukin (IL)-4, differentiate into immature dendritic cells (DCs) (Talmor et al., 1998). DCs migrate into inflamed peripheral tissue where they capture antigens and, after maturation, migrate to lymph nodes to stimulate T-lymphocyte activation. Soluble factors such as IL-6 and M-CSF, derived from neoplastic cells, push myeloid precursors towards a macrophage-like phenotype (Allavena et al., 2000).

DCs are the most effective APCs in the induction of primary immune responses (Steinman 1991, Knight et al., 1993) and are considered to be the best vehicle for the delivery of tumor-specific antigens in cancer immunotherapy (Austin 1993, Zitvogel et al., 1996, Mayordomo et al., 1995, Hsu et al., 1996). The existence of DCs in cancer-bearing hosts has attracted a great deal of interest because of their potential significance for tumor immunity. However, despite their expression of these distinct APCs, attempts by the immune system to eliminate a tumor are often ineffective. It has recently been reported that in cancer patients the tumor cells themselves may also evade immune attack by expressing immunosuppressive cytokines such as interleukin IL-10, transforming growth factor (TGF)-β1, receptor-binding cancer antigen expressed on SiSo cells (RCAS1), IL-23, and vascular endothelial growth factor (VEGF), which induce defective immune cell function and a defective host immune response (Gabrilovich et al., 1996, Gabrilovich et al., 1998, Buelens et al., 1995, Mitra et al., 1995, Brooks et al., 1998). Several studies have also described the defective function of APCs, including macrophages, DCs, and B cells, in tumor-bearing hosts (Tan et al., 1994, Watson et al., 1995, Alcalay et al., 1991, Erroi et al., 1989). A proposed mechanism for the inhibition of the activation of high-potency DCs ex vivo is represented in **Fig. 1**.

Monocytes, which also differentiate into macrophages in tissues, are next to migrate to the site of tissue injury, guided by chemotactic factors. Once activated, macrophages are the main source of growth factors and cytokines, which profoundly affect endothelial, epithelial and mesenchymal cells in the local microenvironment.

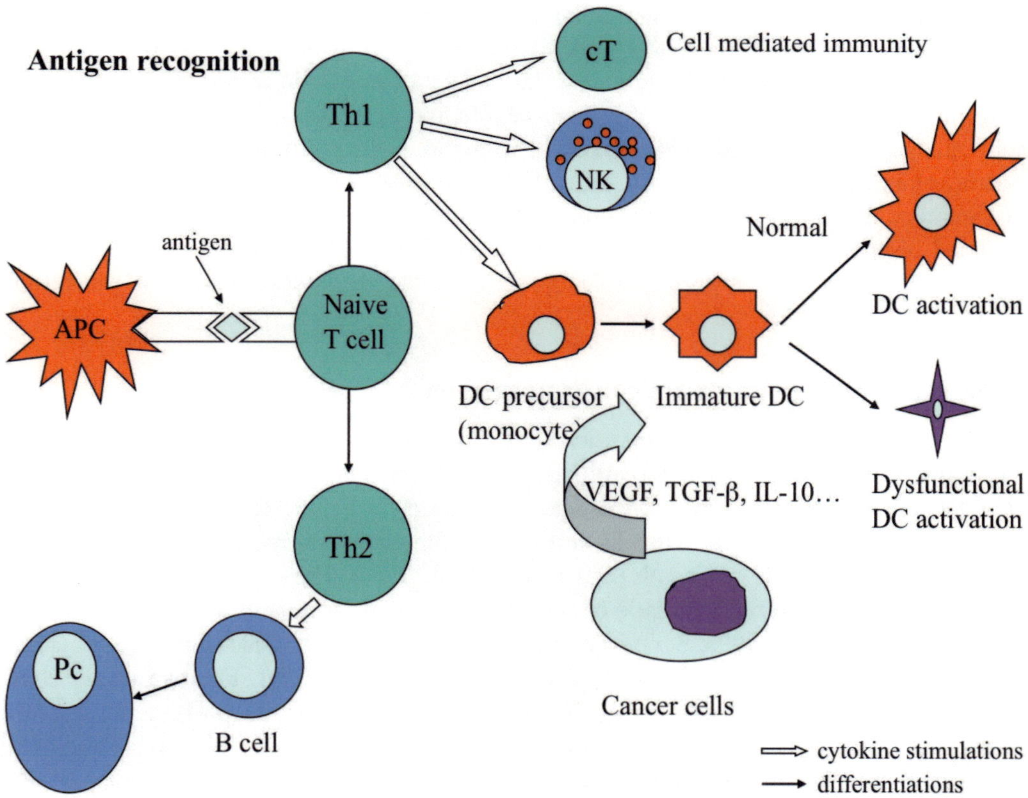

Fig. 1. A proposed mechanism for the DC activation and dysfunctional DC activation during the ex vivo. APC: antigen presenting cells, Th: helper T cell, cT: cytotoxic T cell, NK: Natural killer cell, DC: dendritic cell, Pc: plasma cell.

3. Role of cytokines in tumor microenvironment

The reciprocal interactions between tumor cells and their microenvironment – extracellular matrix (ECM), growth factors, fibroblasts, immune and endothelial cells – play an essential role in the earliest stages of transformation to malignant progression and metastasis (Nyberg et al., 2008). Particularly, fibroblasts have many prominent roles in the cancer progression. In fact, in many carcinomas, the majority of the stromal cells are fibroblasts that possess myofibroblastic characteristics and are called cancer-associated fibroblasts. They produce ECM molecules, proteases, growth factors, and chemokines that crucially affect the carcinoma cell behavior (Kalluri et al., 2006, Orimo et al., 2006). Furthermore, the causal relationship between chronic inflammation, innate immunity and cancer is now widely accepted, and the similarities in the regulatory mechanisms have been suggested for more than a century. Many cancers arise at the site of chronic inflammation and inflammatory mediators are often produced in tumors. The frequent use of anti-inflammatory drugs reduces the incidence of a variety of human tumors. Although blockading some of these mediators has been shown to be efficacious in experimental settings, it is still unclear whether the inflammatory reaction at the tumor site promotes tumor growth or simply implies the failed attempt of the immune system to eliminate the rising malignancy.

Neutrophils (and sometimes eosinophils) are the first recruited effectors of the acute inflammatory response. Monocytes, which differentiate into macrophages in tissues, are next to migrate to the site of tissue injury, guided by chemotactic factors. Once activated, macrophages are the main source of growth factors and cytokines, which profoundly affect endothelial, epithelial and mesenchymal cells in the local microenvironment. Mast cells are also important in acute inflammation owing to their release of stored and newly synthesized inflammatory mediators, such as histamine, cytokines and proteases complexed to highly sulphated proteoglycans, as well as lipid mediators. Thus, we have considered that various cytokines play the very important role by forming the cytokine cascades in the tumor microenvironment of the oral cancer.

3.1 Receptor-binding Cancer Antigen expressed on SiSo cells (RCAS1)

RCAS1 is a type II membrane protein isolated as a human tumor-associated antigen by a mouse monoclonal antibody (22-1-1 antibody) against a human uterine adenocarcinoma cell line, SiSo (Sonoda et al., 1995). RCAS1 acts as a ligand for a putative receptor present on immune cells such as T, B and NK cells and inhibits the growth of receptor-expressing cells, further induces apoptotic cell death (Nakashima et al., 1999). These observations suggest a role of RCAS1 in the immune escape of tumor cells. A variety of cancer tissues have been screened (Sonoda et al., 1996, Sonoda et al., 1998, Iwasaki et al., 2000, Izumi et al., 2001, Kubokawa et al., 2001, Noguchi et al., 2001, Takahashi et al., 2001, Hiraoka et al., 2002, Nakakubo et al., 2002, Fukuda et al., 2004) and were found to be positive for RCAS1 expression, including human uterine, ovarian, esophageal SCCs, pancreatic adenocarcinomas, hepatocarcinomas, skin SCCs, gastric adenocarcinomas, lung cancer cells and HOSCCs, but not in normal tissues.

We investigated whether tumor cells which are expressing RCAS1, induce apoptosis in its receptor-positive cells, PBLs. The apoptotic index (AI) of TILs was also examined in HOSCC tissues. The correlations between RCAS1 expressions and clinicopathological variables in HOSCC and adenoid cystic carcinoma (ACC) tissues were examined, respectively. As the results, it was demonstrated that RCAS1 was frequently expressed both in HOSCC and ACC, *in vitro and vivo,* and its function on KB cells clearly led apoptosis to PBLs *in vitro* (Fukuda et al., 2004). Our results indicated that RCAS1 expression plays a key role in the immune escape mechanism of oral cancer, thus that RCAS1 expression could be used as a predictor of poor prognosis in patients with oral cancer. Further investigation of the role of RCAS1 will be required to clarify RCAS1-mediated tumor survival and to establish a strategy of RCAS1-based oral cancer therapy.

3.2 Interleukin (IL)-12 & IL-23

The causal relationship between chronic inflammation, innate immunity and cancer is now widely accepted, and the similarities in the regulatory mechanisms have been suggested for more than a century (Balkwill et al., 2001, Coussens et al., 2002). Many cancers arise at the site of chronic inflammation and inflammatory mediators are often produced in tumors (Coussens et al., 2002, Balkwill et al., 2005). The frequent use of anti-inflammatory drugs reduces the incidence of a variety of human tumors (Zha et al., 2004). Although blockading some of these mediators has been shown to be efficacious in experimental settings, it is still unclear whether the inflammatory reaction at the tumor site promotes tumor growth or simply implies the failed attempt of the immune system to eliminate the rising malignancy.

IL-23, a heterodimeric cytokine with many similarities to IL-12, has recently been identified as a factor linking tumor-associated inflammation and a lack of tumor immune surveillance (Langowski et al., 2006). IL-23 comprises a p19 subunit that associates with the IL-12p40 subunit (Oppmann et al., 2000), whereas IL-12 is a combination of IL-12p35 and the same IL-12p40 subunit (Sospedra et al., 2005). Although p19 is expressed in various tissues and cell types, it lacks biological activity and only becomes biologically active when complexed with p40, which is normally secreted by activated macrophages and DCs (Oppmann et al., 2000). IL-23 uses many of the same signal-transduction components as IL-12, including the IL-12 receptor (R) β1 subunit (IL-12Rβ1), Janus kinase (Jak)2, Tyk2, signal transducer and activator of transcription (Stat)1, Stat3, Stat4, and Stat5 (Oppmann et al., 2000, Parham et al., 2002). IL-23R, composed of the IL-12Rβ1 and the IL-23R subunit, is also expressed in DCs, macrophages, and T cells (Parham et al., 2002). Consistent with the structural and biological similarities of IL-12 and IL-23, the IL-23R complex shares a subunit with that of IL-12 (IL-12Rβ1), however, it does not use or detectably bind to IL-12Rβ2 (Oppmann et al., 2000). The ability of cells to respond to either IL-12 or IL-23 is determined by expression of IL-12Rβ2 or IL-23R, respectively (Parham et al., 2002). Upon engaging IL-23, IL-12Rβ1 and IL-23R associate, marking the beginning of the IL-23 signal-transduction cascade, many of whose components are now known (**Fig. 2**).

Additionally, both cytokines promote the T helper cell type 1 (Th1) costimulatory function of antigen-presenting cells (Lankford et al., 2003) (**Fig. 3**).

However, IL-23 does differ from IL-12 in the T cell subsets that it targets. IL-12 acts on naive $CD4^+$ T cells, whereas IL-23 preferentially acts on memory $CD4^+$ T cells (Lankford et al., 2003). It has been reported that IL-12 has potent antitumor activity in a variety of murine

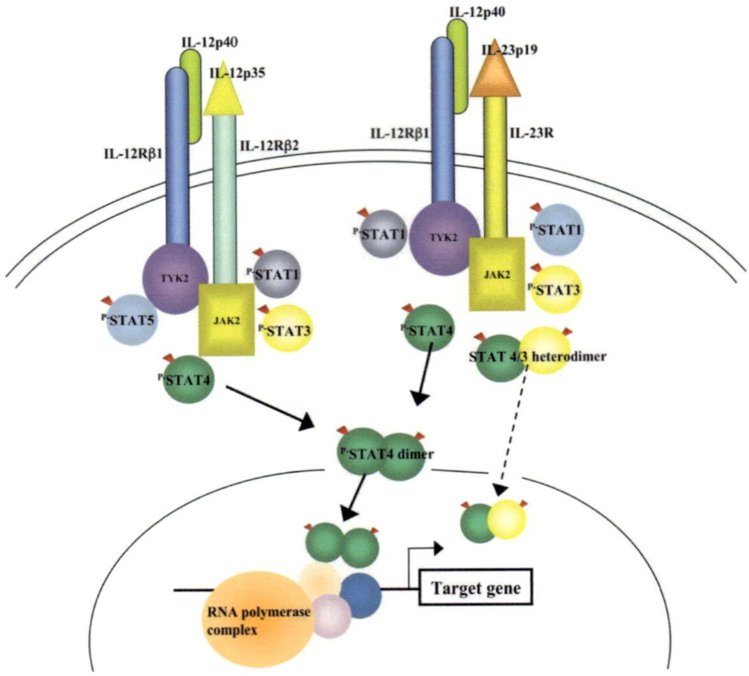

Fig. 2. Stat4 activation is a common feature of IL-23 and IL-12 signal-transduction pathways. IL-23 signal transduction is very similar to that of IL-12, they both use IL-12Rβ1, Jak2, Tyk2, Stat1, Stat3, Stat4, and Stat5. This common feature may explain similarities in TH1 function among IL-12 and IL-23.

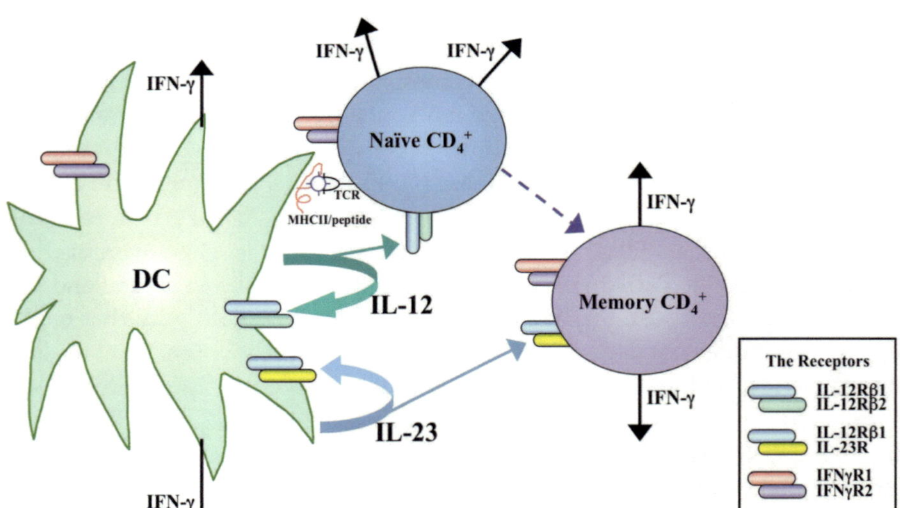

Fig. 3. IL-23 acts on memory CD4+ T cells and DC. IL-23 stimulation leads to IFN-γ production and proliferative response in memory but not naive CD4+ T cells. IL-23 differs from IL-12, which acts on naive cells but has negligible effects on murine memory cells. IL-23 and IL-12 share a similar function in promoting TH1 costimulation by inducing IL-12 and IFN-γ production by DC. MHCII, major histocompatibility complex class II.

tumor models, causing regression of established tumors (Brunda et al., 1993, Nastala et al., 1994, Cua et al., 2003) and inhibiting the formation of experimental metastases (Brunda et al., 1993, Nastala et al., 1994) and spontaneous metastases (Murphy et al., 2003, Becher et al., 2003). On the other hand, it has recently been reported that genetic deletion or antibody-mediated elimination of IL-23 in mice leads to increased infiltration of cytotoxic T cells into the transformed tissue, rendering a protective effect against chemically-induced carcinogenesis (Langowski et al., 2006). So far, it has been reported that expression of IL-23 and its receptors is detectable in activated macrophages, DCs, and keratinocytes in healthy skin (Piskin et al., 2006). We have previously reported that IL-23 is a potent and specific promoter of nuclear factor-kappaB (NF-κB) activation in HOSCC cells, *in vitro* and *in vivo* (Fukuda et al., 2010). Finally, we noted that IL-23 was secreted not only by DCs and macrophages, as shown in previous studies (Sospedra et al., 2005), but also by autologous cancer cells. Consequently, we consider the existence of an autocrine mechanism, in which tumor growth is promoted by IL-23 produced by autologous cancer cells. From these combined data, we believe that IL-23 plays a significant role in the growth and proliferation of oral cancer. Thus, IL-23 could be used as a predictor of poor prognosis in patients with oral cancer, and its antibody might be able to use as an inhibitor of oral cancer progression. Identification of the signaling pathways underlying these events might provide the key to elucidating the mechanism of development of oral cancer. Further investigations into the role of IL-23 will be required to fully understand IL-23-mediated tumor proliferation and to establish an IL-23-based oral cancer therapeutic strategy.

3.3 Vascular Endothelial Growth Factor (VEGF)

Oral cancer is an important cause of worldwide morbidity and mortality, with substantial economic, physiological, and psychosocial impacts due to its treatment modality and a great risk for recurrences and second primary OSCC development. Therefore, it is very important to understand the underlying cell biology of such tumors. It is now a well-accepted fact that angiogenesis is essential for the growth and metastasis of solid tumors, including oral squamous cell carcinoma. The main factor responsible for angiogenesis is VEGF and its receptors. The expression of VEGF protein has been found in a wide variety of cancer tissues, including human prostate cancer, head and neck squamous cell carcinomas, skin squamous cell carcinomas, gastric adenocarcinomas, and lung cancer cells (Weidne et al., 1993, Gasparini et al., 1993, Srivastava et al., 1998, Maeda et al., 1996, Kajita et al., 2001). It has also been shown that VEGF influences the differentiation, maturation, and function of DCs as an immunosuppressive cytokine (Gabrilovich et al., 1996, Banchereau et al., 1998). Interestingly, dendritic cells found in neoplastic infiltrates are frequently immature and defective in T-cell stimulatory capacity. It has been demonstrated that VEGFRs are also present on tumor cells themselves and other cells from the tumor microenvironment, in addition to tumoral endothelial cells (ECs) (Fukuda et al., 2010).

Therefore between these cells take place numerous and different interactions mediated via paracrine/autocrine pathways that promote angiogenesis, uncontrolled tumor proliferation and metastasis. In consequence, estimation of VEGF expression and its receptors became a reliable prognostic tool in OSCCS, predicting the poor disease-free survival, poor overall survival, and metastatic disease.

Furthermore, Saito et al. (1998, 1999) reported that the expression of VEGF is inversely related to the density of DCs in gastric adenocarcinoma tissue. In our study, it was found that VEGF in the primary oral tumor is expressed more strongly in PN^+ cases than in PN^- cases, thus demonstrating that VEGF is associated with the metastasis to RLNs in oral cancer. We also found that in oral cancer the expression of VEGF is inversely related to the density of S-100$^+$ and CD1a$^+$ DCs, although it is also positively correlated with the density of CD83$^+$ DCs (Kusama et al., 2005). Understanding the distribution and role of VEGF and its receptors in the progression of OSCC will be essential to the development and design of new therapeutic strategies.

4. Role of transcriptional factors in tumor microenvironment

The ancient stress response is the innate immune response, regulated by several transcription factors, among which NF-kappaB plays a central role. The hypoxic response is also ancient stress response triggered by low ambient oxygen (O_2) and controlled by hypoxia inducible transcription factor-1, whose a subunit is rapidly degraded under normoxia but stabilized when O_2-dependent prolylhydroxylases (PHDs) that target its O_2-dependent degradation domain are inhibited. Thus, the amount of HIF-1alpha, which controls genes involved in energy metabolism and angiogenesis, is regulated post-translationally. So, NF-kappaB and hypoxia-inducible factor-1 were selected as the typical transcriptional factors in this section.

4.1 Nuclear Factor (NF)-kappaB

Transcription factor NF-κB has key roles in inflammation, immune response, tumorigenesis and protection against apoptosis (Li et al., 2002, Karin et al., 2002, Orlowski et al., 2002). In most cells, NF-κB is kept inactive in the cytoplasm as a heterodimeric complex composed of p50 and p65 (RelA) subunits bound to the inhibitory protein, inhibitor of κB (IκBα) (Baeuerle et al., 1988, Baeuerle et al., 1989, Haskill et al., 1991). Insight into the signaling mechanisms that lead to IκBα phosphorylation have identified a high-molecular weight protein complex known collectively as the IκB kinase (IKK) signalosome and including IKKα, IKKβ and IKKγ also known as NF-κB essential modulator (NEMO) (Karin, 1999, Mercurio et al., 1997). IKKα and IKKβ have been identified as catalytic subunits, whereas IKKγ is a regulatory subunit (Karin, 1999, May et al., 1999). Generally, after stimulation by various reagents, IκBα is phosphorylated at serine residues 32 and 36 by IKKα and IKKβ, together with the scaffold protein NEMO/IKKγ (Karin, 1999). Serine phosphorylation results in polyubiquitination of IκB and its subsequent degradation by the proteasome, allowing NF-κB to translocate to the nucleus and activate its target gene (Karin et al., 2002, Karin, 1999, Smahi et al., 2002).

4.2 Hypoxia Inducible Factor (HIF)-1alpha

Protection against hypoxia in solid tumors is an important step in tumor development and progression. One system in hypoxia protection of tumor cells is represented by the hypoxia-inducible factor 1 (HIF-1) system which plays a crucial role in biologic processes under hypoxic conditions, especially in angiogenesis and carcinogenesis (Maxwell et al., 1997, Ryan et al., 1998).

HIF-1 is a heterodimer, composed of HIF-1α (120 kDa) and HIF-1β (91, 93, 94 kDa) (Wang et al., 1995). HIF-1α subunit, is a transcription factor in response to cellular hypoxia, plays an important role in tumor growth and metastasis by regulating energy metabolism and inducing angiogenesis (Seagroves et al., 2001). However, under normoxic conditions, HIF-1α is maintained at low levels due to continuous degradation via the ubiquitin-dependent proteosome pathway, and this pathway is inhibited by hypoxia and by p53 or von Hippel-Lindau tumor-suppressor gene defects, leading to stabilization of the HIF-1α protein (Huang et al., 1996, Ravi et al., 2000, Maxwell et al., 1999, Stroka et al., 2001). Therefore, hypoxia can lead to a rapid increase in HIF-1α protein levels (Huang et al., 1996, Stroka et al., 2001, Wang et al., 1993, Wang et al., 1995). Furthermore, HIF-1α up-regulates a number of important factors for tumor expansion, including VEGF, a key factor in tumor angiogenesis (Akakura et al., 2001, Carmeliet et al., 1998, An et al., 1998). In several cancers, overexpression of HIF-1α protein has been found to be associated with tumor aggressiveness and with an unfavorable prognosis (Maxwell et al., 1997, Birner et al., 2000, Kuwai et al., 2003). Hypoxia has also been reported to induce wild-type p53 via a different pathway than DNA-damaging agents (Graeber et al., 1994). The hypoxic/anoxic induction of p53 selects for tumor cells that lack functional p53, and hence evidence diminished apoptotic potential (Graeber et al., 1996). Elevated levels of HIF-1α are noted in various malignant tumors (Maxwell et al., 1997), but it is unclear whether this is so in oral carcinoma. Therefore, we have examined the implications of HIF-1α expression in HOSCC, *in vitro* and *in vivo*. NanoCulture plate system was used to duplicate hypoxic condition within tumor mass of living organisms by the three-dimensional cell culture. As the results, we found that HIF-1α regulates the expression of VEGF, and that HIF-1α may be regulated by p53 in SCC of the oral cavity (Fukuda et al., 2010).

4.3 p53

The p53 gene is a highly characterized tumor suppressor that encodes a protein with a molecular weight of 53 kilo Daltons. The p53 gene is also known as a transcription factor that can arrest the cell cycle at the late G1 phase in cells with sub-lethal damage in their genome until their complete repair, or induce apoptosis in cases of irreparable injury, and further activate the transcription of specific genes (El-Deiry et al., 1992, Cordon-Cardo, 1995). Hence, among the genetic changes involved, inactivation of the *p53* tumor suppressor gene by point mutation and allele loss is considered to be the most common event underlying malignancies of every organ (Hollstein et al., 1991). These alterations also seem to be related to the multi-step processes of oral carcinogenesis (Crosthwaite et al., 1996, Stoll et al., 1998). Mutations of *p53* must occur during early stages in the development of head and neck SCCs because they are already present in premalignant lesions (Shin et al., 1994). Mutations of *p53* gene are not necessarily the critical, sole, nor the consistent culprit in oral SCCs patients, however, between 30% and 50% of SCCs of this region have been reported to harbor *p53* gene alterations (Somers et al., 1992, Caamano et al., 1993, Nylander et al., 2000). By contrast, other markers are less suitable due to their lack of stability, variability, or difficulties with technical requirements for their detection. The genes that occur high frequent alterations more than *p53* have not been found so far. Furthermore, it has been described that cancer with the mutated *p53* gene is resistant to radio-/chemotherapy and the patient has poor prognosis than cancer patient with the wild-type *p53* gene (Obata et al., 2000). Therefore, analysis of mutations in this particular gene gives a good indication of clonal expansion of malignancies and important prognostic information. Because the wild-type form of p53 has a half-life of only 6 to 30 minutes, the protein cannot be generally detected by immunohistochemistry; however, if the DNA is damaged, p53 protein accumulates and

NO.	Age	Gender	Locaion	Differentiation	pTNM	Stage	immunohistochemistry	*p53* gene alteration
							p53	
1	87	M	Oral floor	well	T2N2bM0	IVA	+	Exon 7 codon 258: GAA → CAA Glu → Gln
2	48	F	Gingiva	well	T4N0M0	IVA	—	—
3	56	F	Buccal mucosa	well	T2N0M0	II	—	—
4	75	M	Tongue	well	T4N2cM0	IVA	+	Exon 7 codon 244: GGC → GGA (silent)
5	55	M	Oral floor	well	T2N0M0	II	—	—
6	54	M	Tongue	well	T4N2bM0	IVA	—	—
7	54	M	Oral floor	well	T2N2aM0	IVA	+	—
8	70	M	Tongue	well	T2N0M0	II	—	Sequencing failed
9	67	M	Maxillary gingiva	well	T4N3M0	IVB	4+	Exon 5 codon 151: CCC → CCA (silent)
10	92	M	Soft palate	well	T2N0M0	II	+	Sequencing failed
11	66	M	Tongue	well	T2N0M0	II	+	Exon 7 codon 244: GGC → AGC Gly → Ser
12	87	M	Tongue	well	T2N0M0	II	+	Exon 5 codon 154: 1 bp insertion (Frameshift)
13	48	F	Tongue	well	T1N0M0	I	+	—
14	85	M	Tongue	well	T2N1M0	III	—	—
15	56	F	Tongue	well	T1N2bM0	IVA	—	—
16	67	M	Mandibular gingiva	well	T1N2bM0	IVA	+	Sequencing failed
17	55	M	Tongue	well	T1N0M0	I	—	—
18	85	M	Buccal mucosa	well	T1N0M0	I	+	—
19	50	M	Mandibular gingiva	well	T3N1M0	III	—	—
20	67	M	Mandibular gingiva	well	T4N0M0	IVA	+	—
21	79	M	Buccal mucosa	well	T2N0M0	II	+	—
22	54	M	Buccal mucosa	well	T1N0M0	I	—	Exon 8 codon 282: C(T)GG (insertion) (Arg → Trp)
23	54	M	Mandibular gingiva	well	T4N1M0	IVA	+	Not amplified
24	62	M	Mandibular gingiva	well	T1N0M0	I	—	Exon 8 codon 274: G(C)TT (insertion) (Val → Leu)
25	60	M	Maxillary gingiva	well	T1N0M0	I	+	—
26	79	M	Mandibular gingiva	moderately	T4N2cM0	IVA	4+	—
27	85	F	Tongue	moderately	T2N1M0	III	—	Not amplified
28	54	M	Tongue	moderately	T1N0M0	I	+	—
29	54	M	Tongue	moderately	T4N2bM0	IVA	—	Exon 8 codon 282: CGG → CGC (silent)
30	75	M	Mandibular gingiva	moderately	T1N0M0	I	+	—
31	66	F	Mandibular gingiva	moderately	T1N0M0	I	4+	—
32	65	M	Mandibular gingiva	moderately	T2N0M0	II	—	Exon 8 codon 274: GTT → GCT Val → Ala
33	88	M	Mandibular gingiva	moderately	T2N0M0	II	—	Exon 8 codon 282: CGG → CGC (silent)
34	79	M	Mandibular gingiva	moderately	T2N0M0	II	+	Exon 6 codon 222: CCG → CCA (silent)
35	54	M	Buccal mucosa	moderately	T2N0M0	II	—	Exon 8 codon 274: GTT → CTT Val → Leu
36	64	M	Buccal mucosa	poorly	T2N0M0	II	4+	Sequencing failed
37	62	M	Tongue	poorly	T2N1M0	III	+	Exon 8 codon 274: GTT → CTT Val → Leu
38	60	M	Tongue	poorly	T2N1M0	III	—	—
39	60	M	Tongue	poorly	T1N0M0	I	+	Exon 8 codon 273: CGT → CCT Arg → Pro
40	68	M	Maxillary gingiva	poorly	T3N0M0	III	—	Not amplified

p53 gene alteration: 14/33 cases (42.4%)

Table 1. The correlations between p53 expression, *p53* gene alteration and clinicopathological variables in 40 cases of oral squamous cell carcinomas.

becomes detectable (Langdon et al., 1992). So, to assess the frequency of *p53* mutations in HOSCCs and the correlations between p53 immunohistochemical detections and *p53* gene alterations, we examined them by use of the formalin-fixed, paraffin-embedded specimens from 40 patients with oral SCC treated in the Department of Oral and Maxillofacial Surgery, Meikai University Hospital, Saitama, Japan, from 1970 to 2001. Diagnosis of oral lesions was based on histological examination of hematoxylin and eosin-stained slides. Of the 40 SCC patients, there were 34 men and 6 women, whose ages ranged from 48 to 92 years, with a mean age of 66.2 years. A majority of the patients were over 50 years of age. All specimens were obtained from surgical biopsies that no patients had undergone chemotherapy or radiotherapy preoperatively. As the results of immunohistochemistry using MAb p53 antibody, 22 of 40 cases (55%) were positive. Then the alterations in exons 5 to exon 8 of the *p53* gene were analyzed by PCR-SSCP and direct sequencing. The *p53* point mutations were detected in 14 of 33 cases (42.4 %) **(Table 1)**. However, it had no correlations between p53 immunoreactivity, the detection of *p53* gene alterations and clinico-pathological variables. These findings support those of previous reports (Kärjä et al., 1997).

It has recently been reported that in combination with an overexpression of p53 protein, HIF-1α protein overexpression tends to indicate a dismal prognosis (Sumiyoshi et al., 2006). In addition, it has also described that p53 inhibits expression of the p65 subunit of NF-κB and its gene product Bcl-2 (Amin et al., 2009). For these reasons, it has been suggested that there is close relationship between p53 and tumor microenvironment.

5. Conclusions

The efficient elimination of cancer cells via immunodefense mechanisms remains the most ideal therapy. However, it is important to recognize that the dysfunctional immune state that exists in cancer patients will result in a poor response to vaccination procedures. Therefore, in order to enable an immunotherapy challenge, it is necessary to restore the increased levels of immunosuppressive factors, such as IL-10, IL-23, RCAS1, VEGF and/or TGF-β1, in the tumor microenvironment of cancer patients to normal levels. In addition, whether DCs function normally and efficiently remains an important key for the induction of anticancer immunity.

Further investigation will be required to establish a strategy of basic molecular-mechanism-based and clinical studies to determine the most effective oral cancer therapy, which should be tailor-made for the individual patient.

6. References

Akakura, N., Kobayashi, M., Horiuchi, I., Suzuki, A., Wang, J., Chen, J., et al. (2001). Constitutive expression of hypoxia-inducible factor-1alpha renders pancreatic cancer cells resistant to apoptosis induced by hypoxia and nutrient deprivation. *Cancer Res* 61(17): 6548-6554.

Albertson, D.G., Collins, C., Mccormick, F. and Gray, J.W. (2003). Chromosome aberrations in solid tumors. *Nat Genet* 34: 369–376.

Alcalay, J. and Kripke, M.L. (1991). Antigen-presenting activity of draining lymph node cells from mice painted with a contact allergen during ultraviolet carcinogenesis. *J Immunol* 146: 1717-1721.

Allavena, P., Sica, A., Vecchi, A., Locati, M., Sozzani, S. and Mantovani, A. (2000). The chemokine receptor switch paradigm and dendritic cell migration: its significance in tumor tissues. *Immunol Rev* 177: 141–149.

Amin, A.R., Khuri, F.R., Chen, Z.G. and Shin, D.M. (2009). Synergistic Growth Inhibition of Squamous Cell Carcinoma of the Head and Neck by Erlotinib and Epigallocatechin-3-Gallate: The Role of p53-Dependent Inhibition of Nuclear Factor-κB. *Cancer Prevention Research* 2: 538-545.

An, W.G., Kanekal, M., Simon, M.C., Maltepe, E., Blagosklonny, M.V. and Neckers, L.M. (1998). Stabilization of wild-type p53 by hypoxia-inducible factor 1α. *Nature* 392: 405-408.

Austin, J.M. (1993). The dendritic cell system and anti-tumor immunity. *In Vivo* 7: 193-202.

Baeuerle, P.A. and Baltimore, D. (1988). I kappa B: a specific inhibitor of the NF-kappa B transcription factor. *Science* 242: 540-546.

Baeuerle, P.A. and Baltimore, D. (1989). A 65-kappaD subunit of active NF-kappaB is required for inhibition of NF-kappaB by I kappaB. *Genes Dev* 3: 1689-1698.

Balkwill, F. and Mantovani A. (2001). Inflammation and cancer: back to Virchow? *Lancet* 357: 539-545.

Balkwill, F., Charles, K.A. and Mantovani, A. (2005). Smoldering and polarized inflammation in the initiation and promotion of malignant disease. *Cancer Cell* 7: 211-217.

Banchereau, J. and Steinman, R.M. (1998). Dendritic cells and the control of immunity. *Nature* 392: 245-252.

Becher, B., Durell, B.G. and Noelle, R.J. (2003). IL-23 produced by CNS resident cells controls T cell encephalitogenicity during the effector phase of experimental autoimmune encephalomyelitis. *J Clin Invest* 112: 1186-1191.

Birner, P., Schindl, M., Obermair, A., Plank, C., Breitenecker, G. and Oberhuber, G. (2000). Overexpression of hypoxia-inducible factor 1α is a marker for an unfavorable prognosis in early-stage invasive cervical cancer. *Cancer Res* 60: 4693-4696.

Braakhuis, B.J.M., Tabor, M.P., Leemans, C.R., van der Waal, I., Snow, G.B. and Brakenhoff, R.H. (2002). Second primary tumors and field cancerization in oral and oropharyngeal cancer: molecular techniques provide new insights and definitions. *Head Neck* 24: 198–206.

Brooks, S.P., Bernstein, Z.P., Schneider, S.L., Gollnick, S.O. and Tomasi, T.B. (1998). Role of transforming growth factor-beta1 in the suppressed allostimulatory function of AIDS patients. *AIDS* 12: 481-487.

Brunda, M.J., Luistro, L., Warrier, R.R., Wright, R.B., Hubbard, B.R., Murphy, M., et al. (1993). Antitumor and antimetastatic activity of interleukin 12 against murine tumors. *J Exp Med* 178: 1223-1230.

Buelens, C., Willems, F., Delvaux, A., Pierard, G., Delville, J.P., Velu, T. and Goldman, M. (1995). Interleukin-10 differentially regulates B7-1 (CD80) and B7-2 (CD86) expression on human peripheral blood dendritic cells. *Eur J Immunol* 25: 2668-2672.

Caamano, J., Zhang, S.Y., Rosvold, E.A., Bauer, B. and Klein-Szanto, A.J. (1993). p53 alterations in human squamous cell carcinomas and carcinoma cell lines. *Am J Pathol* 142: 1131-1139.

Califano, J., van der Riet, P., Westra, W., Nawroz, H., Clayman, G., Piantadosi, S., et al. (1996). Genetic progression model for head and neck cancer: implications for field cancerization. *Cancer Res* 56: 2488–2492.

Carmeliet, P., Dor, Y., Herbert, J.M., Fukumura, D., Brusselmans, K., Dewerchin, M., et al. (1998). Role of HIF-1α in hypoxia-mediated apoptosis, cell proliferation and tumour angiogenesis. *Nature* 394: 485-490.

Cordon-Cardo C. (1995). Mutation of cell cycle regulators. Biological and clinical implications for human neoplasia. *Am J Pathol* 147: 545–560.

Coussens, L.M. and Werb, Z. (2002). Inflammation and cancer. *Nature* 420: 860-867.

Crosthwaite, N., Teale, D., Franklin, C., Foster, G.A. and Stringer, B. (1996). p53 protein expression in malignant, premalignant and non-malignant lesions of the lip. *J Clin Pathol* 49: 648–653.

Cua, D.J., Sherlock, J., Chen, Y., Murphy, C.A., Joyce, B., Seymour, B., et al. (2003). Interleukin-23 rather than interleukin-12 is the critical cytokine for autoimmune inflammation of the brain. *Nature* 421: 744-748.

Demaria, S., Pikarsky, E., Karin, M., Coussens, L.M., Chen, Y-C., El-Omar, E.M., Trinchieri, G., Dubinett, S.M., Mao, J.T., Szabo, E., Krieg, A., Weiner, G.J., Fox, B.A., Coukos, G., Wang, E., Abraham, R.T., Carbone, M., and Lotze, M.T. (2010). Cancer and inflammation: promise for biological therapy. *J Immunother* 33: 335–351.

El-Deiry, W.S., Kern, S.E., Pietenpol, J.A., Kinzler, K.W. and Vogelstein, B. (1992). Definition of a consensus binding site for p53. *Nature Genet* 1: 45-49.

Erroi, A., Sironi, M., Chiaffarino, F., Chen, Z.G., Mengozzi, M. and Mantovani, A. (1989). IL-1 and IL-6 release by tumor-associated macrophages from human ovarian carcinoma. *Int J Cancer* 44: 795-801.

Forastiere, A., Koch, W., Trotti, A. and Sidransky, D. (2001). Medical progress - head and neck cancer. *N Engl J Med* 345: 1890–1900.

Fukuda, M. and Sakashita, H. (2010). Expression of hypoxia-inducible factor-1α in squamous cell carcinoma of the oral cavity. *Hosp Dent (Tokyo)* 21 (2): 85-90.

Fukuda, M., Ehara, M., Suzuki, S. and Sakashita, H. (2010). Expression of interleukin-23 and its receptors in human squamous cell carcinoma of the oral cavity. *Mol Med Rep* 3: 89-93.

Fukuda, M., Ehara, M., Suzuki, S., Ohmori, Y. and Sakashita, H. (2010). IL-23 promotes growth and proliferation in human squamous cell carcinoma of the oral cavity. *Int J Oncol* 36: 1355-1365.

Fukuda, M., Tanaka, A., Hamao, A., Suzuki, S., Kusama, K. and Sakashita, H. (2004). Expression of RCAS1 and its function in human squamous cell carcinoma of the oral cavity. *Oncol Rep* 12: 259-267.

Gabrilovich, D.I., Chen, H.L., Girgis, K.R., Cunningham, H.T., Meny, G.M., Nadaf, S., Kavanaugh, D. and Carbone, D.P.: Production of vascular endothelial growth factor by human tumors inhibits the functional maturation of dendritic cells. Nat. Med. 2: 1096-1103, 1996.

Gabrilovich, J. and Steinman, R.M. (1998). Dendritic cells and the control of immunity. *Nature* 392: 245-252.

Gasparini, G., Weidner, N., Maluta, S., Pozza, F., Boracchi, P., Mezzetti, M., et al. (1993). Intratumoral microvessel density and p53 protein: correlation with metastasis in head-and-neck squamous-cell carcinoma. *Int J Cancer* 55: 739-744.

Gollin, S.M. (2001). Chromosomal alterations in squamous cell carcinomas of the head and neck: window to the biology of disease. *Head Neck* 23: 238–253.

Graeber, T.G., Osmanian, C., Jacks, T., Housman, D.E., Koch, C.J., Lowe, S.W., et al. (1996) Hypoxia-mediated selection of cells with diminshed apoptotic potential in solid tumours. *Nature* 379(6560): 88-91.

Graeber, T.G., Peterson, J.F., Tsai, M., Monica, K., Fornace, A.J. Jr and Giaccia, A.J. (1994). Hypoxia induces accumulation of p53 protein, but activation of a G1-phase checkpoint by low-oxygen conditions is independent of p53 status. *Mol Cell Biol* 14(9): 6264-6277.

Hanahan, D. and Weinberg, R.A. (2000). The hallmarks of cancer. *Cell* 100: 57–70.

Haskill, S., Beg, A.A., Tompkins, S.M., Morris, J.S., Yurochko, A.D., Sampson-Johannes, A., et al. (1991). Characterization of an immediate-early gene induced in adherent monocytes that encodes I kappa B-like activity. *Cell* 65: 1281-1289.

Helmlinger, G., Yuan, F., Dellian, M. and Jain, R.K. (1997). Interstitial pH and *p*O2 gradients in solid tumors *in vivo*: high-resolution measurements reveal a lack of correlation. *Nature Med* 3: 177–182.

Hiraoka, K., Hida, Y., Miyamoto, M., Oshikiri, T., Suzuoki, M., Nakakubo, Y., et al. (2002). High expression of tumor-associated antigen RCAS1 in pancreatic ductal adenocarcinoma is an unfavorable prognostic marker. *Int J Cancer* 99: 418-423.

Hollstein, M., Sidransky, D., Vogelstein, B. and Harris, C.C. (1991). *p53* mutations in human cancers. *Science* 253: 49-53.

Hsu, F.J., Benike, C., Fagnoni, F., Liles, T.M., Czerwinski, D., Taidi, B., Engleman, E.G. and Levy, R. (1996). Vaccination of patients with B-cell lymphoma using autologous antigen-pulsed dendritic cells. *Nat Med* 2: 52-58.

Huang, A.Y.C. (1994). Role of bone marrow-derived cells in presenting MHC class I-restricted tumor antigens. *Science* 264: 961-965.

Huang, L.E., Arany, Z., Livingston, D.M. and Bunn, H.F. (1996). Activation of hypoxia-inducible transcription factor depends primarily upon redox-sensitive stabilization of its alpha subunit. *J Biol Chem* 271: 32253-32259.

Iwasaki, T., Nakashima, M., Watanabe, T., Yamamoto, S., Inoue, Y., Yamanaka, H., et al. (2000). Expression and prognostic significance in lung cancer of human tumor-associated antigen RCAS1. *Int J Cancer* 89: 488-493.

Izumi, M., Nakanishi, Y., Yoshino, I., Nakashima, M., Watanabe, T. and Hara, N. (2001). Expression of tumor-associated antigen RCAS1 correlates significantly with poor prognosis in nonsmall cell lung carcinoma. *Cancer* 92: 446-451.

Kajita, T., Ohta, Y., Kimura, K., Tamura, M., Tanaka, Y., Tsunezuka, Y., et al. (2001). The expression of vascular endothelial growth factor C and its receptors in non-small cell lung cancer. *Br J Cancer* 85: 255-260.

Kalluri, R. and Zeisberg, M. (2006). Fibroblasts in cancer. *Nat Rev Cancer* 6: 392- 401.

Karin, M. (1999). How NF-κB is activated: the role of the IκB kinase (IKK) complex. *Oncogene* 18: 6867-6874.

Karin, M. (1999). The beginning of the end: IkappaB kinase (IKK) and NF-kappaB activation. *J Biol Chem* 274: 27339-27342.

Karin, M., Cao, Y., Greten, F.R. and Li, Z.W. (2002). NF-κB in cancer: from innocent bystander to major culprit. *Nat Rev Cancer* 2: 301-310.

Knight, S.C. and Stagg, A.J. (1993). Antigen-presenting cell types. *Curr Opin Immunol* 5: 374-382.

Kubokawa, M., Nakashima, M., Yao, T., Ito, K.I., Harada, N., Nawata, H., et al. (2001). Aberrant intracellular localization of RCAS1 is associated with tumor progression of gastric cancer. *Int J Oncol* 19: 695-700.

Kusama, K., Fukuda, M., Kikuchi, K., Ishikawa, M., Sakashita, H. and Nemoto, N. (2005). Dendritic Cells and Oral Cancer (Review). *J Oral Biosci* 47 (1): 42-51.

Kuwai, T., Kitadai, Y., Tanaka, S., Onogawa, S., Matsutani, N., Kaio, E., et al. (2003). Expression of hypoxia-inducible factor-1α is associated with tumor vascularization in human colorectal carcinoma. *Int J Cancer* 105(2): 176-181.

Kärjä, V.J., Syrjänen, K.J., Kurvinen, A-K. and Syrjänen, S.M. (1997). Expression and mutations of p53 in salivary gland tumors. *J Oral Pathol Med* 26: 217-223.

Langdon, J.D. and Partridge, M. (1992). Expression of the tumor suppressor gene p53 in oral cancer. *Br J Oral Maxillofac Surg* 30: 214-220.

Langowski, J.L., Zhang, X., Wu, L., Mattson, J.D., Chen, T., Smith, K., et al. (2006). IL-23 promotes tumour incidence and growth. *Nature* 27: 461-465.

Lankford, C.S.R. and Frucht, D.M. (2003). A unique role for IL-23 in promoting cellular immunity. *J Leukocyte Biol* 73: 49-56.

Li, Q. and Verma, I.M. (2002). NF-kappaB regulation in the immune system. *Nat Rev Immunol* 2: 725-734.

Licciardello, J.T., Spitz, M.R. and Hong, W.K. (1989). Multiple primary cancer in patients with cancer of the head and neck: second cancer of the head and neck, esophagus, and lung. *Int J Radiat Oncol Biol Phys* 17: 467-476.

Loercher, A., Lee, T.L., Ricker, J.L., Howard, A., Geoghegen, J., Chen, Z., et al. (2004). Nuclear factor-κB is an important modulator of the altered gene expression profile and malignant phenotype in squamous cell carcinoma. *Cancer Res* 64, 6511- 6523.

Maeda, K., Chung, Y.S., Ogawa, Y., Takatsuka, S., Kang, S.M., Ogawa, M., et al. (1996). Prognostic value of vascular endothelial growth factor expression in gastric carcinoma. *Cancer* 77: 858-863.

Maxwell, P.H., Dachs, G.U., Gleadle, J.M., Nicholls, L.G., Harris, A.L., Stratford, I.J., et al. (1997). Hypoxia-inducible factor-1 modulates gene expression in solid tumors and influences both angiogenesis and tumor growth. *Proc Natl Acad Sci USA* 94: 8104-8109.

Maxwell, P.H., Wiesener, M.S., Chang, G.W., Clifford, S.C., Vaux, E.C., Cockman, M.E., et al. (1999). The tumour suppressor protein VHL targets hypoxia-inducible factors for oxygen-dependent proteolysis. *Nature* 399: 271-275.

May, M.J. and Ghosh, S. (1999). IkappaB kinases: kinsmen with different crafts. *Science* 284: 271-273.

Mayordomo, J.I., Zorina, T., Storkus, W.J., Zitvogel, L., Celluzzi, C., Falo, L.D., Melief, C.J., Ildstad, S.T., Kast, W.M. and Deleo, A.B. (1995). Bone marrow-derived dendritic cells pulsed with synthetic tumour peptides elicit protective and therapeutic antitumour immunity. *Nat Med* 1: 1297-1302.

Mercurio, F., Zhu, H., Murray, B.W., Shevchenko, A., Bennett, B.L., Li, J., Young, D.B., Barbosa, M., Mann, M., Manning, A. and Rao, A. (1997). IKK-1 and IKK-2: cytokine-activated IkappaB kinases essential for NF-kappaB activation. *Science* 278: 860-866.

Mitra, R.S., Judge, T.A., Nestle, F.O., Turka, L.A. and Nickoloff, B.J. (1995). Psoriatic skin-derived dendritic cell function is inhibited by exogenous IL-10. Differential modulation of B7-1 (CD80) and B7-2 (CD86) expression. *J Immunol* 154: 2668-2677.

Murphy, C.A., Langrish, C.L., Chen, Y., Blumenschein, W., McClanahan, T., Kastelein, R.A., Sedgwick, J.D. and Cua, D.J. (2003). Divergent pro- and anti-inflammatory roles for IL-23 and IL-12 in joint auto-immune inflammation. *J Exp Med* 198: 1951-1957.

Nakakubo, Y., Hida, Y., Miyamoto, M., Hashida, H., Oshikiri, T., Kato, K., Suzuoki, M., Hiraoka, K., Ito, T., Morikawa, T., Okushiba, S., Kondo, S. and Katoh, H. (2002). The prognostic significance of RCAS1 expression in squamous cell carcinoma of the oesophagus. *Cancer Lett* 177: 101-105.

Nakashima, M., Sonoda, K. and Watanabe, T. (1999). Inhibition of cell growth and induction of apoptotic cell death by the human tumor-associated antigen RCAS1. *Nat Med* 5: 938-942.

Nastala, C.L., Edington, H.D., McKinney, T.G., Tahara, H., Nalesnik, M.A., Brunda, M.J., et al. (1994). Recombinant IL-12 administration induces tumor regression in association with IFN-production. *J Immunol* 153: 1697-1706.

Noguchi, K., Enjoji, M., Nakamuta, M., Nakashima, M., Nishi, H., Choi, I., Taguchi, K., Kotoh, K., Shimada, M., Sugimachi, K., Tsuneyoshi, M., Nawata, H. and Watanabe, T. (2001). Expression of tumor-associated antigen RCAS1 in hepatocellular carcinoma. *Cancer Lett* 168: 197-202.

Nyberg, P., Salo, T. and Kalluri. R. (2008). Tumor microenvironment and angiogenesis. *Front Biosci* 13: 6537–6553.

Nylander, K., Dabelsteen, E. and Hall, P.A. (2000). The p53 molecule and its prognostic role in squamous cell carcinomas of the head and neck. *J Oral Pathol Med* 29: 413-425.

Obata, A., Eura, M., Sasaki, J., Saya, H., Chikamatsu, K., Tada, M., Iggo, R.D. and Yumoto, E. (2000). Clinical significance of p53 functional loss in squamous cell carcinoma of the oropharynx. *Int J Cancer* 89: 187-193.

Oppmann, B., Lesley, R., Blom, B., Timans, J.C., Xu, Y., Hunte, B., et al. (2000). Novel p19 protein engages IL-12p40 to form a cytokine, IL-23, with biological activities similar as well as distinct from IL-12. *Immunity* 13: 715-725.

Orimo A, Weinberg RA: Stromal fibroblasts in cancer: a novel tumor- promoting cell type. Cell Cycle 2006, 5:1597–1601.

Orlowski, R.Z. and Baldwin, A.S. Jr. (2002). NF-kappaB as a therapeutic target in cancer. *Trends Mol Med* 8: 385-389.

Parham, C., Chirica, M., Timans, J., Vaisberg, E., Travis, M., Cheung, J., et al. (2002). A receptor for the heterodimeric cytokine IL-23 is composed of IL-12Rbeta1 and a novel cytokine receptor subunit, IL-23R. *J Immunol* 168: 5699-5708.

Piskin, G., Sylva-Steenland, R.M.R., Bos, J.D. and Teunissen, M.B.M. (2006). In vitro and in situ expression of IL-23 by keratinocytes in healthy skin and psoriasis lesions: enhanced expression in psoriatic skin. *J Immunol* 176: 1908-1915.

Ravi, R., Mookerjee, B., Bhujwalla, Z.M., Sutter, C.H., Artemov, D., Zeng, Q., et al. (2000). Regulation of tumor angiogenesis by p53-induced degradation of hypoxia-inducible factor 1 alpha. *Genes Dev* 14: 34-44.

Reid, C.B., Snow, G.B., Brakenhoff, R.H. and Braakhuis, B.J. (1997). Biologic implications of genetic changes in head and neck squamous cell carcinogenesis. *Aust N Z J Surg* 67: 410–416.

Rock, K.L., Rothstein, L., Gamble, S. and Fleischacker, C. (1993). Characterization of antigen-presenting cells that present exogenous antigens in association with class I MHC molecules. *J Immunol* 150: 438-446.

Ryan, H.E., Lo, J. and Johnson, R.S. (1998). HIF-1α is required for solid tumor formation and embryonic vascularization. *EMBO J* 17: 3005-3015.

Saito, H., Tsujitani, S., Ikeguchi, M., Maeta, M. and Kaibara, N. (1998). Relationship between the expression of vascular endothelial growth factor and the density of dendritic cells in gastric adenocarcinoma tissue. *Br J Cancer* 78: 1573-1577.

Saito, H., Tsujitani, S., Kondo, A., Ikeguchi, M., Maeta, M. and Kaibara, N. (1999). Combined analysis of tumour neoangiogenesis and local immune response in advanced gastric carcinoma. *Oncol Rep* 6: 459-463.

Sakashita, H., Miyata, M., Miyamoto, H. and Kurumaya, H. (1996). A case of quadruple cancer, including triple cancers in the head and neck region. *J Oral Maxillofac Surg* 54: 501-505.

Seagroves, T.N., Ryan, H.E., Lu, H., Wouters, B.G., Knapp, M., Thibault, P., et al. (2001). Transcription factor HIF-1 is a necessary mediator of the pasteur effect in mammalian cells. *Mol Cell Biol* 21(10): 3436-3444.

Slaughter, D.P., Southwick, H.W. and Smejkal, W. (1953). Field cancerization in oral stratified squamous epithelium, clinical implications of multicentric origin. *Cancer* 6: 963-968.

Smahi, A., Courtois, G., Rabia, S.H., Döffinger, R., Bodemer, C., Munnich, A., et al. (2002). The NF-kappaB signalling pathway in human diseases: from incontinentia pigmenti to ectodermal dysplasias and immune-deficiency syndromes. *Hum Mol Genet* 11: 2371-2375.

Somers, K.D., Merrick, M.A., Lopez, M.E., Incognito, L.S., Schechter, G.L. and Casey, G. (1992). Frequent p53 mutations in head and neck cancer. *Cancer Res* 52: 5997-6000.

Sonoda, K., Kaku, T., Kamura, T., Nakashima, M., Watanabe, T. and Nakano H. (1998). Tumor-associated antigen 22-1-1 expression in the uterine cervical squamous neoplasias. *Clin Cancer Res* 4: 1517-1520.

Sonoda, K., Nakashima, M., Kaku, T., Kamura, T., Nakano, H. and Watanabe, T. (1996). A novel tumor-associated antigen expressed in human uterine and ovarian carcinomas. *Cancer* 77: 1501-1509.

Sonoda, K., Nakashima, M., Saito, T., Amada, S., Kamura, T., Nakano, H., et al. (1995). Establishment of a new human uterine cervical adenocarcinoma cell line, SiSo, and its reactivity to anti-cancer reagents. *Int J Oncol* 6: 1099-1104.

Sospedra, M. and Martin, R. (2005). Immunology of multiple sclerosis. *Annu Rev Immunol* 23: 683-747.

Srivastava, A., Laidler, P., Davies, R.P., Horgan, K. and Hughes, L.E., et al. (1988). The prognostic significance of tumor vascularity in intermediate-thickness (0.76-4.0 mm thick) skin melanoma. A quantitative histologic study. *Am J Pathol* 133: 419-423.

Steinman, R.M. (1991). The dendritic cell system and its role in immunogenicity. *Annu Rev Immunol* 9: 271-296.

Stoll, C., Baretton, G. and Lohrs, U. (1998). The influence of p53 and associated factors on the outcome of patients with oral squamous cell carcinoma. *Virchows Arch* 433: 427–433.

Stroka, D.M., Burkhardt, T., Desbaillets, I., Wenger, R.H., Neil, D.A., Bauer, C., et al. (2001). HIF-1 is expressed in normoxic tissue and displays an organ-specific regulation under systemic hypoxia. *FASEB J* 15: 2445-2453.

Sumiyoshi, Y., Kakeji, Y., Egashira, A., Mizokami, K., Orita, H. and Maehara, Y. (2006). Overexpression of Hypoxia-inducible factor 1α and p53 is a marker for an unfavorable prognosis in gastric cancer. *Clin Cancer Res* 12: 5112-5117.

Takahashi, H., Iizuka, H., Nakashima, M., Wada, T., Asano, K., Ishida-Yamamoto, A., et al. (2001). RCAS1 antigen is highly expressed in extramammary Paget's disease and in advanced stage squamous cell carcinoma of the skin. *J Dermatol Sci* 26: 140-144.

Talmor, M., Mirza, A., Turley, S., Mellman, I., Hoffman, L.A. and Steinman, R.M. (1998). Generation of large numbers of immature and mature dendritic cells from rat bone marrow cultures. *Eur J Immunol* 28: 811–817.

Tan, K.C., Hosoi, J., Grabbe, S., Asahina, A. and Granstein, R.D. (1994). Epidermal cell presentation of tumor-associated antigens for induction of tolerance. *J Immunol* 153: 760-767.

Wang, G.L. and Semenza, G.L. (1993). General involvement of hypoxia-inducible factor 1 in transcriptional response to hypoxia. *Proc Natl Acad Sci USA* 90: 4304-4308.

Wang, G.L. and Semenza, G.L. (1995). Purification and characterization of hypoxia-inducible factor 1. *J Biol Chem* 270: 1230-1237.

Wang, G.L., Jiang, B.H., Rue, E.A. and Semenza, G.L. (1995). Hypoxia-inducible factor-1 is a basic-helix-loop-helix-PAS heterodimer regulated by cellular O_2 tension. *Proc Natl Acad Sci USA* 92: 5510-5514.

Watson, G.A. and Lopez, D.M. (1995). Aberrant antigen presentation by macrophages from tumor-bearing mice is involved in the down-regulation of their T cell responses. *J Immunol* 155: 3124-3134.

Weidner, N., Carroll, P.R., Flax, J., Blumenfeld, W. and Folkman, J. (1993). Tumor angiogenesis correlates with metastasis in invasive prostate carcinoma. *Am J Pathol* 143: 401-409.

Zeh, H.J. and Lotze, M.T. (2005). Addicted to death: invasive cancer and the immune response to unscheduled cell death. *J Immunother* 28: 1–9.

Zha, S., Yegnasubramanian, V., Nelson, W.G., Isaacs, W.B. and De Marzo, A.M. (2004). Cyclooxygenases in cancer: progress and perspective. *Cancer Lett* 215: 1-20.

Zitvogel, L., Mayordomo, J.I., Tjandrawan, T., DeLeo, A.B., Clarke, M.R., Lotze, M.T. and Storkus, W.J. (1996). Therapy of murine tumors with tumor peptide-pulsed dendritic cells: dependence on T cells, B7 costimulation, and T helper cell 1-associated cytokines. *J Exp Med* 183: 87-97.

van Houten, V.M., Tabor, M.P., van den Brekel, M.W., Denkers, F., Wishaupt, R.G., Kummer, J.A., et al. (2000). Molecular assays for the diagnosis of minimal residual head-and-neck cancer: Methods, reliability, pitfalls, and solutions. *Clin Cancer Res* 6: 3803–3816.

Part 3

Regulation of Tumor Microenvironment – New Players and Approaches

11

Modulation of Cancer Progression by Tumor Microenvironmental Leukocyte-Expressed microRNAs

Lorenzo F. Sempere[1] and Jose R. Conejo-Garcia[2]
[1]*Department of Medicine, Dartmouth Medical School,*
[2]*Immunology Program, Wistar Institute,*
USA

1. Introduction

microRNAs (miRNAs) have rapidly emerged as a widespread and important regulatory layer of gene expression (Ambros, 2004; Bartel & Chen, 2004). miRNAs can coordinately modulate the expression of hundreds of target genes, mainly by negatively affecting mRNA stability and/or protein output (Baek et al., 2008; Bentwich et al., 2005; Kozomara & Griffiths-Jones, 2011; Lim et al., 2005; Selbach et al., 2008). With this mode of gene expression control, a single miRNA can concomitantly influence multiple cellular programs under physiological and pathological conditions. Examples abound in which perturbation of miRNA functions can have catastrophic consequences for proper execution of developmental programs, for maintenance of cellular homeostasis, and for optimal performance of cellular processes (De Smaele et al., 2010; Garzon et al., 2010; Saba & Schratt, 2010; Sempere & Kauppinen, 2009; Ventura & Jacks, 2009).

Only one year after the discovery of miRNAs in 2001, Croce and colleagues found the first association between miRNAs and cancer when they noted the frequent occurrence of chromosomal deletion and the concurrent downregulation of two miRNA genes, miR-15a and miR-16-1, in B-cell chronic lymphocytic leukemia patients (Calin et al., 2002). Since that time, progress towards understanding the basic molecular and biological mechanisms of miRNA biogenesis, their normal patterns of temporal and spatial expression, and their roles in development and physiology has unfolded slowly compared to the rapid path towards translational and clinical applications of miRNAs, especially in cancer.

A particular active area of research has been high-throughput expression profiling of miRNAs in a variety of cancer types (Barbarotto et al., 2008; Sempere, 2011). The general interpretation of these expression profiling experiments has been to assign altered miRNA expression to the cancer cells and promptly labelled the implicated miRNA as having tumor suppressive or oncogenic properties depending on whether miRNA levels were detected a lower or higher levels, respectively, in tumor tissues compared to normal. However, the cancer cell compartment of many of the most aggressive types of solid tumors represents a minority of the variety of cell types in cancer lesions (Sempere, 2011). A tumor microenvironmental (TME) cell type invariably associated with cancer progression is the leukocyte. Immune cells are the site of cancer origin in leukemias and lymphomas, whereas epithelial cells are the site of cancer origin in carcinomas and the immune cells constitute the inflammatory component of TME. Thus, inflammation and infiltrating leukocytes present as co-disease or co-morbidity in solid tumors and are a major confounding factor to correctly interpret expression profiling experiments. A salient example to illustrate this dichotomy between cancer cell and immune cell infiltrate is miR-155 in solid tumors. miR-155 resides in non-protein coding B-cell integration cluster (*BIC*) gene (Faraoni et al., 2009; Tili et al., 2009). miR-155 is frequently detected at high levels in leukemias, lymphomas and solid tumors (e.g., carcinomas) and overexpression of miR-155 causes rapid and aggressive disease progression in a mouse model of B cell lymphoma (Faraoni et al., 2009; Tili et al., 2009). Thus, miR-155 has been regarded as a master oncogenic miRNA in hematological and solid tumors. However, a large body of evidence also attributes important roles to miR-155 as a mediator of lymphoid and myeloid cell responses to infection and inflammation, which is further supported by immunological deficiency exhibited by mir-155 knockout mouse models (Faraoni et al., 2009; Tili et al., 2009). We recently showed that expression of miR-155 was confined to a subpopulation of infiltrating immune cells in breast, colorectal, lung, pancreas and prostate tumor lesions (Sempere et al., 2010). Importantly, these results indicated that the majority of miR-155 signal detected by RT-PCR assays in whole tissue biopsies or blood samples likely emanates from TME cells, drawing into question whether miR-155 plays any role within the cancer cells in these carcinomas. In the light of these findings, we revisit here altered expression of miR-155 and other leukocyte-expressed miRNAs (e.g., miR-17-5p, miR-20a, miR-21, miR-25, miR-29a, miR-142-3p, miR-146a, miR-150, miR-181a, miR-221, miR-223) in solid tumors, which are likely to reflect, at least in part, immune cell responses in the TME rather than molecular aberrations within the cancer cells per se. We review the emerging roles of these leukocyte-expressed miRNAs in the immune system with an especial emphasis on myelomonocytic-derived cells, and discuss their implications in the modulation of cancer initiation and progression in the context of a reactive and/or permissive TME.

2. Physiological roles of microRNAs in the immune system

In the bone marrow, pluripotent hematopoietic stem cells give rise to common progenitors of the lymphoid and myeloid lineages. In the blood, these progenitors will continue distinct differentiation paths to produce the principal cell types of the immune system: B and T lymphocytes and natural killer (NK) cells in the lymphoid branch, and basophils, neutrophils, eosinophils, mast cells and monocytes in the myeloid branch; other non-immune cell types such as erythrocytes and thrombocytes are also produced in the myeloid branch. In tissues, further maturation awaits for lymphoid and myeloid lineages to mount innate and adaptive responses against bacterial, viral and other pathogens as well as against cancer cells and other aberrant cells not recognized as self. These differentiation programs are crucial to establish a fully functional immune system. Expression profiling and functional studies have implicated miRNAs as key regulators of specific stages of differentiation and maturation of specific immune cell lineages, which in general have overt deleterious consequences at the organismal level.

Mature and biologically active miRNAs, ~21-23 nucleotides-long, function as guides to recognize and bind partially complementary elements (miRNA recognition element; MRE) on the 3′ untranslated region (UTR) of target mRNAs. miRNA biogenesis and processing determine the total levels of mature miRNA and to a large extent miRNA function (however see these reviews for cooperative and competitive effects of RNA binding proteins (Van Kouwenhove et al., 2011) and competing endogenous RNAs (Salmena et al., 2011) on miRNA activity). Most miRNA genes are transcribed by RNA polymerase II, which produces a long primary transcript (pri-miRNA) with a 5′ cap and a 3′ poly(A) tail (Ketting, 2011; van et al., 2011). In the nucleus the pri-miRNA is recognized by the microprocessor, a multiprotein complex that cleaves off a 70 nts-long precursor miRNA hairpin (pre-miRNA). The catalyzes this cleavage as DGCR8 recognizes structural features of the hairpin and accordingly position the pre-miRNA for cleavage by RNAse III endonuclease Drosha. The pre-miRNA is exported to the cytoplasm by Exportin-5 in a RAN-GTP dependent manner. Then, the pre-miRNA is cleaved by another RNAse III endonuclease Dicer in association with TARBP2 or PACT and the mature miRNA strand (guide) is loaded in Argonaute-containing RNA-induced silencing complexes (Ketting, 2011; van et al., 2011).

The expression of key components of the miRNA processing machinery such Dicer can be inhibited under physiological stress and disease states, including cancer (Tomasi et al., 2010). Moreover, Dicer expression is affected by cortisone, interferon and other pharmacological agents prescribed for the treatment of immune disorders (Tomasi et al., 2010). Thus, perturbation of global miRNA activity can have undesirable clinical implications. In mouse models, deleterious effects of global miRNA impairment by conditional removal of Dicer or DGCR8 in specific immune cell lineage using the Cre/LoxP system has pinpointed important roles of miRNAs in production of antibody diversity, terminal differentiation and survival of B cells (Belver et al., 2010; Koralov et al., 2008), function of regulatory T (Treg) cells and Treg-mediated control of autoimmunity (Liston et al., 2008; Zhou et al., 2008), the development and function of invariant natural killer T cells (Bezman et al., 2010; Seo et al., 2010; Zhou et al., 2009), and terminal differentiation, activation, migration and survival of CD8+ T cell (Muljo et al., 2005; Zhang & Bevan, 2010). Subsequent studies have uncovered a major role of a single or small subset of miRNAs for immunological phenotypes observed in animals deficient in miRNA processing machinery (see below). As we describe in the next subsections, high-throughput expression profiling has been a useful discovery tool to correlate expression with function and thereby highlight specific miRNAs for further mechanistic characterization.

2.1 Dynamic expression of microRNAs during hematopoietic lineage differentiation

Using primarily the mouse as a model system, several groups have characterized in detail changes of miRNA expression during immune cell lineage differentiation as a means to infer from this a functional involvement of specific miRNAs at key steps of these processes (Malumbres & Lossos, 2010; O'Connell et al., 2010b; O'Neill et al., 2011).

2.1.1 microRNA expression in granulocyte differentiation and maturation

There are several well-defined differentiation stages that mature granulocytes (PB-N) undergo from a common myeloid progenitor (CMP): granulocyte-monocyte progenitor (GMP), immature bone marrow neutrophils (BM-N). Expression of miR-223 gradually increases from CMP to BM-N stages, reaching the highest level of expression in PB-N cells

(Johnnidis et al., 2008). This differentiation pathway is crucial for the mobilization of the massive amount of immature myeloid leukocytes typically found in cancer patients.

2.1.2 microRNA expression in monocytic-macrophage differentiation and maturation

There are several well-defined differentiation stages that mature macrophages (Mϕs) undergo from a CMP cell: GMP, monocyte. Using similar strategies, several groups independently profiled miRNA expression in *in vitro* cell culture systems that induce monocytic differentiation and maturation into Mϕs (Fontana et al., 2007; Ghani et al., 2011). Expression of miR-17-5p, miR-20a, miR-106a was downregulated during differentiation and maturation of unilineage monocytic cell culture (Fontana et al., 2007). Expression of miR-99, miR-146a, miR-155, miR-342 and others was upregulated and that of miR-20a, miR-25, miR-26a, miR-223 and others was downregulated during differentiation and maturation of PU.1-expressing PUER cells (Ghani et al., 2011). Downregualtion of miR-223 in monoctyes had been previously noticed (Johnnidis et al., 2008).

2.1.3 microRNA expression in dendritic cell differentiation and maturation

There are several well-defined differentiation stages that mature dendritic cells (DCs) undergo from a CMP cell: GMP, monocyte. Expression of miR-99a, miR-193b was exclusively upregulated during induced differentiation and maturation into DC of *ex vivo* culture of human blood-derived monocytes, whereas upregulation of miR-34a, miR-125a-5p, miR-99b, miR-511 expression was observed in both DC and Mϕs (Tserel et al., 2011). These results are in good, but not in complete, agreement with similar studies in which relative miRNA expression levels were compared between monocytes, immature and mature DCs (Hashimi et al., 2009; Lu et al., 2011a). Upregulation of miR-21, miR-342 expression and downregulation of miR-17-5p, miR-25, miR-93, miR-106a expression in immature and/or mature DCs was observed in both studies (Hashimi et al., 2009; Lu et al., 2011a). Upregulation of miR-146a and miR-155 expression in mature DC upon activation by various pro-inflammatory stimuli, including bacterial lipopolysaccharide (LPS) and interleukin (IL) 1β, has been consistently observed by independent groups (Turner et al., 2011).

2.1.4 microRNA expression in B cell differentiation and maturation

There are several well-defined differentiation stages that mature memory B cell or plasma cells undergo from a common lymphoid progenitor cell (CLP): Pro-B, Pre-B, IM-B, Naive B and germinal center (GC) cell. When comparing relative expression levels between pro-B and naive B cells (Monticelli et al., 2005), expression of the following miRNAs was enriched at a specific stage: miR-24, miR-93, miR-101, miR-107, miR-324 in pro-B cells; miR-26, miR-29a, miR-142-3p, miR-142-5p, miR-150 in naive B cells. When comparing relative expression levels between naive, GC and memory B cells (Malumbres et al., 2009; Tan et al., 2009), expression of the following miRNAs was enriched at a specific stage: let-7a, miR-92, miR-95, miR-142-3p, miR-142-5p, miR-193 and others in naive cells; miR-15b, miR-16, miR-17-3p, miR-17-5p, miR-20, miR-25, miR-93, miR-106a, miR-181a, miR-181b and others in GC cells; miR-21, miR-23a, miR-24, miR-29c, miR-30b, miR-146, miR-150 and others in memory cells.

2.1.5 microRNA expression in T cell differentiation and maturation

There are several well-defined differentiation stages that naive CD4+ or CD8+ T cells undergo from a CLP cell: double negative (DN) 1, DN2, DN3, DN4, double positive (DP). When comparing relative expression levels between DN1-DP to CD4+ or CD8+ cells (Neilson et al., 2007), expression of the following miRNAs was enriched at a specific stage: miR-21, miR-29b, miR-221, miR-223, miR-342 in DN1 cells; miR-191 in DN3 cells, miR-16, miR-20a miR-128b, miR142-5p in DN4; miR-92, miR-181a, miR-181b, miR-350 in DP cells; miR-297 and miR-669c in CD4+ cells; and miR-15b, mir-24, miR-27a, miR-150 in CD8+ cells. When comparing relative expression levels between antigen-specific naive, effector and memory CD8+ T cells (Wu et al., 2007), expression of the following miRNAs was enriched at a specific stage: let-7f, miR-16, miR-142-3p, miR-142-5p, miR-150 in naive cells; miR-21, miR-221, miR-222 in both effector and memory cells; miR-18, miR-31, miR-146a, miR-146b in memory cells.

2.2 Roles of microRNAs in cellular components of the innate immune system

Inflammation is now recognized as a hallmark of established tumors (Hanahan & Weinberg, 2011). Over the last years, multiple independent lines of research have identified inflammation as a promoter of both cancer initiation and malignant progression. The secretion of inflammatory cytokines and chemokines that drive inflammatory responses by cells of the innate immune system are primarily elicited by the recognition of common structures shared by many microorganisms by receptors that activate complex transcriptional programs. Toll-like receptors (TLR) are an important component of inflammatory responses in this context. They are present in various myeloid cell lineages and serve as sensor to pathogenic RNA and other molecules from parasites. However, TLRs can also recognize certain cellular components and promote inflammation under sterile conditions. For instance, HMGB1 (Tang et al., 2010) and several S100 proteins (Ehrchen et al., 2009; Hiratsuka et al., 2008) have been associated with TLR-dependent carcinogenic inflammation. TLRs have also been shown to regulate expression of specific miRNAs in Mϕs, DCs and other myeloid-derived cell types (O'Neill et al., 2011). Transcription and expression of miR-21, miR-146a and miR-155 among other miRNAs is regulated by several TLRs in different cellular contexts that we discuss in more detail below. In turn, miRNAs regulate TLR-dependent signalling by targeting mRNAs of TRLs, of downstream signalling proteins and/or of effector transcriptional factors (O'Neill et al., 2011).

2.2.1 microRNA-mediated neutrophil responses

Transcriptional repression of miR-21 and miR-196a expression by zinc finger factor independent-1 (Ggi1) is required for granulocytic development and differentiation as persistent high levels of these miRNAs in CMP cells block this program (Velu et al., 2009). Similarly, overexpression of miR-125b blocks granulocytic differentiation induced by granulocyte colony stimulating factor (G-CSF) in 32D cell lines (Surdziel et al., 2011). Conversely, upregulation of miR-27 expression by G-CSF3-induced C/EBPα transcriptional factor enhances granulocytic differentiation (Feng et al., 2009). High levels of miR-27 post-transcriptionally repress expression of Runx1 transcriptional factor, which antagonizes differentiation of CMPs or myoblast cell lines into granulocytes (Feng et al., 2009).

Unlike these previous examples of miRNA-mediated granulocyte differentiation which primarily affect the overall number, but not function, of available neutrophils, miR-223 controls differentiation and activation of neutrophils (Johnnidis et al., 2008). *mir-223* knockout mice have an increased number of neutrophils as a result of an abnormal expansion of the GMP cells due to dysregulation of transcriptional factor Mef2c (Johnnidis et al., 2008). Moreover, these miR-223-deficient neutrophils are hypermature and hyperactive causing spontaneous pulmonary inflammation and excessive tissue damage upon endotoxin challenge (Johnnidis et al., 2008).

2.2.2 microRNA-mediated Mϕ responses

Several pro-inflammatory mediators such as LPS, polyriboinosinic–polyribocytidylic acid (poly IC), Tumor Necrosis Factor (TNF) α, interferon (IFN) β, have been shown to induce miR-155 expression in monocyte and/or Mϕs (Faraoni et al., 2009). miR-155 enhances type I IFN signaling-mediated Mϕ responses against viral infection, mainly by downregulating expression of suppressor of cytokine signaling 1 (SOCS1) (Wang et al., 2010). miR-155 is also an important player in the interleukin (IL) 13-dependent fate determination between M1 (classical, pro-Th1, tumoricidal) and M2 (alternative, pro-Th2, tumorigenic) Mϕs. As IL-13 signalling via its cognate receptor IL13Rα1 and consequent phosphorylation of STAT6 favors M2 programs, miR-155 antagonizes this process by directly repressing expression of IL13Rα1 mRNA as well as by repressing expression of IL-13 responsive genes such as SOCS1, DC-SIGN, CCL18, CD23, and SERPINE (Martinez-Nunez et al., 2011).

Induction of miR-146a/b expression by IL-1β, LPS, TNF-α in monocytes is an NF-κB-dependent process (Taganov et al., 2006). miR-146 is engaged in a negative feedback loop with TLR and cytokine signalling via downregulation of IL-1 receptor-associated kinase 1 (IRAK1) and TNF receptor-associated factor 6 (TRAF6) mRNA levels, which are transducers of these signals (Taganov et al., 2006). Several studies indicate the importance of miR-146 regulatory role in Mϕs. *mir-146a* knockout mice develop lymphoid and myeloid malignancies as well as myeoloproliferation and myelofibrosis; dysregulated and increased activation of NF-κB-mediated transcription is a major contributing factor to the observed phenotypes (Zhao et al., 2011). Some viruses such as vesicular stomatitis virus (VSV) can disrupt the miR-146 regulatory loop as a means to dampen IFN-β (Hou et al., 2009). Mice infected with VSV upregulate miR-146 expression in Mϕs in a TRL-independent, but NF-κB-dependent manner, and thereby triggers miR-146-mediated downregulation of TRAF6, IRAK1 and IRAK2 target genes (Hou et al., 2009).

In contrast, high levels of miR-125b expression potentiate IFN-γ-mediated Mϕ responses (Chaudhuri et al., 2011). Enforced miR-125b expression enhances Mϕ activation and antigen presentation to T cells (Chaudhuri et al., 2011). miR-125b-mediated downregulation of IFN regulatory factor 4 (IRF4) explained in great part the observed phenotypes and the enhanced ability of miR-125b-overexpressing Mϕs to elicit more effective cancer cell rejection (Chaudhuri et al., 2011).

2.2.3 microRNA-mediated DC responses

mir-155 knockout mice exhibit impaired B cell, T cell, and DC immune responses (Rodriguez et al., 2007; Thai et al., 2007). Several evidences indicate that impaired B cell responses result from disruption of intrinsic miR-155-mediated processes (Turner & Vigorito, 2008; Vigorito et al., 2007). However, impaired T cell responses may reflect functional defects in miR-155-deficient DCs, which have a decreased capacity to present antigens to T cells (Rodriguez et al., 2007), rather than intrinsic T cell proceses. Intriguingly, *in vitro* studies suggest that high levels of miR-155 interfere with antigen binding ability of DC, and therery antigen presentation to and activation of T cells (Mao et al., 2011; Martinez-Nunez et al., 2009). miR-155 has been shown to promote pro-inflammatory or anti-inflammatory responses in DCs via downregulation, along with other targets genes, of SH2-containing inositol 5-phosphatase (SHIP) and SOCS1 or IL-1β and TAK1-binding protein 2 (TAB2), respectively (Ceppi et al., 2009; Lu et al., 2008; O'Connell et al., 2008; O'Connell et al., 2009). Thus, miR-155 may exert different roles in DCs that are context-dependent such as physiological resolution of viral infection or pathological interaction with cancer cells in solid tumors.

As miR-146a/b and miR-155, expression of miR-148 family members (miR-148a, miR-148b, miR-152) is induced by TLR signalling in DCs (Liu et al., 2010b). By targeting expression of calcium/calmodulin-dependent protein kinase II (CaMKII), these miRNAs diminished antigen presenting capacity of DCs (Liu et al., 2010b).

2.2.4 microRNA-mediated NK cell reponses

NK mediate contact-dependent cytotoxicity and produce immunostimulatory cytokines that activate other immune cells. Cytotoxic granules contain perforin (Prf1) and granzymes (Gmzs), which are delivered by exocytosis into the target cells. miR-27a* modulates cytotoxic NK cell responses by regulating expression levels of both Prf1 and GzmB in resting and activated NK cells (Kim et al., 2011). Similarly, miR-29 dampens interferon (IFN) γ-mediate responses in NK and other lymphocyte lineages as observed in animals infected with intracellular bacterial pathogens such as *Listeria monocytogenes* (Ma et al., 2011).

2.3 Roles of microRNAs in cellular components of the adaptive immune system

The adaptive immune system comprises lymphocytes and their products (e.g., antibodies). Although the role of innate immune cells (e.g., NK cells) may be crucial to prevent tumor initiation, adaptive immune responses, particularly those mediated by effector T cells, are responsible for exerting spontaneous (and clinically relevant) immune pressure against the progression of many established cancers (Dunn et al., 2005; Yu & Fu, 2006). While the role of miRNAs in the development and functions of T and B cells has only started emerging very recently, it is becoming increasingly clear that B and T cell responses are tightly regulated by a network of miRNAs (O'Connell et al., 2010b).

2.3.1 microRNA-mediated B cell responses

Genetic manipulation of miR-150 expression and activity indicate an important role of this miRNA in B cell development and function (Malumbres & Lossos, 2010). Unimmunized *mir-150* knockout mice exhibit an expansion in splenic and peritoneal B1 cells and enhanced humoral responses as determined by increased serum immunoglobulin levels (Xiao et al., 2007). Conversely, enforced expression of miR-150 in B cell lineages caused arrested development at the pro-B to pre-B transition. miR-150-mediated processes largely impinge on negative regulation of c-Myb transcriptional factor involved at multiple steps of lymphocyte development (Xiao et al., 2007).

Similar to miR-150 enforced expression, mice deficient in the *mir-17~mir-92* gene cluster (miR-17-5p, miR-18a, miR-19a, miR-19b-1 miR-20a, miR-92-1) also exhibit a disrupted B cell development at the pro-B to pre-B transition (Ventura et al., 2008). Dysregulated and increased levels of pro-apoptotic protein Bim are a key molecular alteration responsible for this defect (Ventura et al., 2008).

2.3.2 microRNA-mediated T cell responses

The importance of miRNAs in controlling T cell-mediated responses was first illustrated by the demonstration that specific deletion of Dicer in the T cell lineage resulted in impaired T cell development and aberrant T helper cell differentiation and cytokine production (Muljo et al., 2005). Subsequent studies have confirmed that Dicer controls CD8+ T-cell activation, migration, and survival (Zhang & Bevan, 2010). More recently, a unique signature of 71 miRNAs has been identified in activated T cells (Grigoryev et al., 2011). In an independent study, seven miRNAs (let-7f, miR-15b, miR-16, miR-21, miR-142-3p, miR-142-5p, miR-150) alone were shown to account for approximately 60% of all miRNAs in naive, effector and memory $CD8^+$ T cells. Among the multiple miRNAs modulated by T cell activation, miR-155 appears to be particularly important. miR-155 enhances inflammatory T cell development (O'Connell et al., 2010a), and it is known to be essential for the T cell-mediated control of *Helicobacter pylori* infection and for the induction of chronic gastritis and colitis (Oertli et al., 2011). miR-155 is also crucial for T helper cell differentiation and generating optimal T cell-dependent antibody responses (Thai et al., 2007).

Robust T cell responses require the up-regulation of anti-apoptotic pathways, accelerated cell cycle progression, and efficient antigen presentation. miR-181a modulates these processes by regulating expression levels of anti-apoptotic protein BCL2, transmembrane C-type lectin protein CD69 and T cell receptor (TCR) α during T cell binding to an antigen (Neilson et al., 2007). miR-181a exerts an important role for antigen sensitivity and selection during T cell development imparted by downregulation of TCR and phosphatases relaying TCR signalling (Li et al., 2007). These effects, however, have been mainly investigated in thymocytes, and further studies are needed to conclusively extend these results to peripheral T lymphocytes.

CD69 is upregulated by antigen-specific T cells following acute infection, but CD69 expression returns to basal levels after 72 hrs. CD69 regulates sphingosine 1-phosphate (S1P1) and controls the release and migration of activated T cell from central lymphoid organs (lymph nodes and spleen) to infection site (Shiow et al., 2006). Expression of miR-130 and miR-301 is dramatically upregulated following CD8+ T cells activation *in vitro* by TCR stimuli. miR-130 and miR-301, in addition to miR-181a, inhibit CD69 expression via binding to an MRE in the 3'UTR of CD69 mRNA (Zhang & Bevan, 2010). These results suggest that this miR-130/mir-301-mediated process is important to establish the timing of activated T cells into circulation.

Finally, miR-182 has been recently found to be induced by IL-2 to promote clonal expansion of activated helper T lymphocytes (Stittrich et al., 2010).

3. Pathological roles of microRNAs in cancer-related inflammation and immunity

Twenty-five years ago Dvorak compared tumors with wounds that do not heal for the first time in a seminal paper (Dvorak, 1986). As in wounds, inflammatory cells are present in the microenvironment of virtually all solid tumors. In addition, chronic inflammation increases the risk of developing cancers in certain organs (e.g., in the digestive tract). Most importantly, inflammation is a hallmark of cancer (Hanahan & Weinberg, 2011), including those tumors that are not associated with chronic inflammatory conditions (Colotta et al., 2009). Over the last years, the crucial role of TME inflammatory cells such as MDSCs, Mϕs and Tregs to the survival and proliferation of cancer cells, angiogenesis, metastasis, and, especially, immnosuppression, has been progressively unveiled.

miRNA-mediated regulation is required for optimal functioning of the immune system. Impairment of global or specific miRNA activity in leukocyte subsets can lead a broad spectrum of diseases and pathological conditions from autoimmune disorders (destruction of normal self cells) to cancer (protection of abnormal non-self cells). We focus here on the emerging roles in initiation and progression of cancer of leukocyte-expressed miRNAs in the TME of most solid tumors.

3.1 microRNA roles in anti-tumor immune surveillance and modulation of cancer progression

The crucial role of immune surveillance in the prevention of cancer is today beyond question among immunologists (Zitvogel et al., 2006). However, we cannot detect the tumors that are rejected by the immune system during the course of our lives. This implies that tumors that become clinically noticeable are the result of failure of the immune system. Multiple mechanisms cooperate in the TME and at distal locations in tumor-bearing hosts to prevent the rejection of established cancers. Independent work from several laboratories has recently demonstrated that tolerance to tumor antigens in advanced malignancies is not a merely passive event but, rather, an active process whereby multiple immunosuppressive cell types confer immune privilege to tumors (Zou, 2005). How the phenotype and mobilization of these immunosuppressive leukocytes are regulated by miRNAs is only starting to be understood.

3.1.1 Role of microRNAs in Myeloid-Derived Suppressor Cell (MDSC)-mediated immunosuppression

MDSCs are one of the major components of the immune suppressive networks operating in cancer-bearing hosts (Gabrilovich & Nagaraj, 2009). Tumor-derived factors (e.g., S100, proteins) induce excessive myelopoiesis, resulting in the massive mobilization of immature myelomonocytic cells in virtually all solid tumor-bearing hosts (Sinha et al., 2008). These myeloid cells correspond to precursors of both monocytes and granulocytes, but are influenced by tumor-derived inflammatory signals that multiply their regular numbers and transform them into crucial contributors to immunosuppression. The specific abrogation of anti-tumor T cells in the absence of global immunosuppression in cancer patients has been elegantly explained via a mechanism of nitration of the T cell receptor on the T-cell surface (Nagaraj et al., 2007). How MDSCs specifically take up tumor antigen (thereby preventing cancer patients from being severely immunodeficient) remains to be clarified, but this mechanism provides a framework to explain the unresponsiveness of tumor-specific T cells in established tumors. In addition, other mechanisms such as production of Arginase are relevant for T cell tolerogenic function.

These immature leukocytes migrate from the bone marrow where they are produced to the periphery, and differentiate into immunosuppressive Mϕs or regulatory DCs at tumor sites. This primarily occurs from cells of the monocytic lineage, as granulocytic MDSCs tend to disappear in the periphery. However, many tumors accumulate myeloid cells that, at least in terms of light scatter properties and phenotypic markers, show attributes of classical neutrophils (Rodriguez et al., 2009). A great deal of phenotypic overlap and heterogeneity among myeloid leukocytes is therefore typically found in the microenvironment of different tumors, and even within the same tumor specimen. What these cells have in common is a strong immunosuppressive activity and the production of angiogenic factors that are crucial for tumor neovascularization (Ahn & Brown, 2008; Conejo-Garcia et al., 2004; Huarte et al., 2008; Mantovani, 2010; Mazzieri et al., 2011). Together, this heterogeneous mix of MDSCs, Mϕs, regulatory DCs and monocytes also contributes to the promotion of tumor growth and metastasis.

Very little is known about how miRNAs regulate the mobilization and activities of this crucial and abundant tolerogenic population. The most compelling evidence for the contribution of miRNAs to MDSC-mediated immune suppression has recently arised from the demonstration that the expression of STAT3, which promotes the suppressive activity of MDSCs, is silenced by the combined activity of miR-17-5p and miR-20a. Correspondingly, ectopic expression of miR-17-5p or miR-20a significantly reduced the capacity of MDSCs to suppress antigen-specific CD4 and CD8 T cells, both *in vitro* and *in vivo* (Zhang et al., 2011). Further research is needed to understand the contribution of miRNAs to the activity of MDSCs, as well as to design potential therapeutic interventions based on delivery of miRNA mimetics to promote their differentiation into immunocompetent (or at least less immunosuppressive) cells types.

3.1.2 Role of microRNAs in the function of Antigen-Presenting Cells (APCs)

Another hallmark of adaptive immune responses against tumor antigens is the abrogation of the capacity of APCs to elicit strong T cell activation. Among the miRNAs that participate in this process, miR-155 appears to be particularly important, because miR-155-defficient DCs simply fail to activate T cells (Rodriguez et al., 2007). In addition, miR-155 expression in bone marrow-derived DCs increases upon LPS-induced maturation and miR-155 is the only miRNA substantially up-regulated in primary Mϕs stimulated with a TLR3 agonist plus IFN-β (O'Connell et al., 2007; Rodriguez et al., 2007). Furthermore, our results indicate that tumor-derived regulatory DCs express very low levels of miR-155, and that delivery of miR-155 mimetics (see **Section 5**) to these cells promotes their capacity to effectively present tumor antigens and elicit protective anti-tumor immunity (manuscript under consideration). Interestingly, DCs matured in the absence of miR-155 express levels of MHC–II and co-stimulatory molecules similar to those seen on identically treated matured wild-type DCs, but they fail to present antigens or co-stimulate T cells.

In contrast to miR-155, expression of miR-21 decreases Th1 responses by preventing IL-12 secretion in activated DCs (Lu et al., 2011b).

3.1.3 Role of microRNAs in Treg-mediated immunosuppression

One of the crucial cell players actively suppressing the anti-tumor activity of effector anti-tumor T cells are Foxp3+ regulatory T cells (Treg). Treg are essential to prevent autoimmunity in healthy hosts by suppressing autoreactive T cells. Because most epitopes recognized by tumor-reactive T cells are self-antigens, advanced tumors co-opt their regulatory functions to suppress anti-tumor T cell responses, which specifically occurs in the TME (Curiel et al., 2004). Correspondingly, Treg infiltration is associated with accelerated tumor progression and reduced survival. Several miRNAs have been reported to contribute to the tolerogenic function of Treg, and therefore can only be important for immunosuppression in the TME. Among them, miR-146a, typically overexpressed in Treg, is critical for their suppressor function by controlling the expression of Stat1 (Lu et al., 2010). In addition, miR-155, miR-21 and miR-7, which are all targets of Foxp3, silence Satb1 and are also collectively required for the suppressive function of Treg (Beyer et al., 2011).

3.1.4 Tumor-infiltrating T cells

Infiltration of tumor islets by T cells has been associated with significantly improved outcomes in multiple histological types of cancer (Dunn et al., 2005; Yu & Fu, 2006). As many tumor-specific antigens have been identified and shown to induce the production of specific antibodies in cancer patients, the protective activity of these lymphocytes has provided a rationale for using them to treat cancer (Ertl et al., 2011). Over the last years, some authors have restricted the protective role of T cells to the activity of cytotoxic (CD8+) lymphocytes (Hamanishi et al., 2007; Sato et al., 2005), primarily because CD4+ T cells include significant proportions of Treg. The considerations about the immunostimulatory and immunosuppressive roles of the miRNAs described above are extensive to tumor-associated lymphocytes. Other miRNAs that deserve further investigation specifically in tumor-associated T cells are miR-29, which suppresses immune responses by targeting IFN-γ (Ma et al., 2011); and miR-125b, which prevents differentiation of naive lymphocytes into effector T cells (Rossi et al., 2011).

3.1.5 Antibody-mediated B cell/mast cell carcinogenic interactions

B cells are another leukocyte subset crucially associated with the progression of at least certain epithelial cancer models through the production of antibodies with the collaboration of CD4+ T cells (Andreu et al., 2010). These antibodies against extracellular matrix components engage mast cells via Fc receptors and trigger secretion of pro-angiogenic factors and chemokines by mast cells. This induces the recruitment of myelomonocytic cells, including alternatively activated Mϕs (M2). Then, these M2 cells promote tumorigenicity in a completely Fc-dependent fashion (Andreu et al., 2010). The observation that mast cells, which are known to accumulate in the periphery of tumors, can contribute to immunosuppression has been solidly documented by elegant studies (de Vries et al., 2011; Lu et al., 2006; Wasiuk et al., 2009). The role of miRNAs in mast cells is particularly important in this context because mast cells actively release microparticles that transfer miRNAs and mRNAs to other cells (Valadi et al., 2007). This exosome-mediated exchange of genetic materials between tumor-infiltrating leukocytes and cancer cells in the TME, remains a poorly understood mechanism (Brase et al., 2010; Mostert et al., 2011; Scholer et al., 2010; Schwarzenbach et al., 2011).

3.1.6 Role of microRNAs in immunosuppression-driven metastasis

To be able to metastasize, sprouted cancer cells need to evade multiple mechanisms of immune surveillance. The role of miRNAs in this active process of immunosuppression has been recently illustrated by studies focused on miR-30b and miR-30d. Ectopic expression of miR-30b/d was shown to promote the metastatic behavior of melanoma cells by silencing the GalNAc transferase GALNT7 (Gaziel-Sovran et al., 2011). This resulted in the up-regulation of the immunosuppressive cytokine IL-10, which impaired anti-tumor immunity and promote metastatic spreading at these locations.

4. microRNA signatures in cancer

Whole tissue profiling is a powerful discovery tool to identify differential expression of miRNAs in cancerous tissues. Changes of miRNA expression in tumor samples compared to normal samples or between groups of tumor samples with a favourable and poor clinical outcome have been used to generate miRNA signatures with potential prognostic and/or predictive value. Differential miRNA expression in tumor samples has also been used to infer molecular alterations in miRNA-mediated processes within cancer cells, but without carefully considering the contribution of other cellular components of the TME to these changes of miRNA levels.

Similar experimental designs, approaches, statistical analyses and data interpretations have been applied to the study of leukemias and lymphomas, in which immune cells are the site of cancer, and solid tumors such as carcinomas (e.g. breast and lung cancer), in which immune cells are the inflammatory component of TME and epithelial cells are the site of cancer. The techniques employed in the majority of these profiling experiments did not allow to identify specific cell type(s) as the source of altered miRNA expression. Altered expression of leukocyte-expressed miRNAs likely reflects the recruitment of inflammatory cells to the TME in solid tumors rather than molecular aberrations within the cancer cell per se. Nonetheless, most of these leukocyte-expressed miRNAs are also expressed to some extent in other cell types (including in some instances cancer cells) and consequently total contribution of each individual cell and cell type(s) to the overall RNA levels of these miRNAs cannot be ascertained with these experiments (see **section 4.3**). We review below cancer-associated miRNA signatures in hematological and solid tumors. It is apparent that many of these signatures contain leukocyte-expressed miRNAs.

Consistent with its upregulation in several hematological cancers, including B cell lymphomas and acute myeloid leukemia, miR-155 is a contributor to malignant hematological progression when it is overexpressed in cancer cells (Xiao & Rajewsky, 2009). In mice, retroviral expression of miR-155 in bone marrow progenitors causes a myeloproliferative disorder (O'Connell et al., 2008) and constitutive overexpression of miR-155 in the B cell lineage results in pre-B cell proliferation and eventually B cell malignancy (Costinean et al., 2006). Deletions and certain polymorphisms in BRCA1 promote carcinogensis by preventing epigenetic repression of miR-155 expression (Chang et al., 2011). The paradoxical association between oncogenesis and effective immunity is not surprising, because robust adaptive immune responses require rapid expansion of leukocytes. For instance, T cell expansion requires the upregulation of anti-apoptotic mediators, including Bcl-x. Therefore, miR-155 plays a tumorigenic role when it is upregulated in cancer cells of hematological origin and a protective, anti-tumor function when it is expressed by certain immune cell types, including APCs, in the TME of solid tumors.

4.1 Altered microRNA expression in hematological tumors

Altered miRNA expression has been reported in all studied hematological malignancies, including chronic lymphocytic leukemia (CLL), B cell lymphomas, acute myeloid leukemia (AML), multiple myeloma, acute lymphoblastic leukemia, myeloproliferative neoplasms and others (Calvo et al., 2011; Fabbri et al., 2009; Fabbri & Croce, 2011; Kotani et al., 2010; Marcucci et al., 2011b; Schotte et al., 2011; Wieser et al., 2010; Williams et al., 2011). It is common for many of these hematological malignancies to harbor recurrent chromosomal abnormalities that: serve to classify types and subtypes; affect specific molecular pathways; and have different disease progression dynamics, response to treatment and outcome.

4.1.1 Altered microRNA expression in chronic lymphocytic leukemia

CLL is the most common type of leukemia in the United States (Parker & Strout, 2011). Risk of contracting this clonal malignancy of immature/mature B cells increases exponentially with age, especially after age 50 (Parker & Strout, 2011). This heterogeneous disease has an indolent and an aggressive presentation. Patients afflicted with indolent disease will not progress clinical for years, but patient afflicted with aggressive disease can have rapid disease progression. Standard of care consists of chemotherapy-based treatment for patients with progressive or aggressive disease, with no obvious benefit of early treatment in patients with indolent disease. miRNA expression profiling has been used to improve prognostics based on expression of zeta-chain (TCR)-associated protein kinase 70kDa (ZAP70) and T-cell leukemia/lymphoma 1 (TCL1) as well as recurrent chromosomal abnormalities (Parker & Strout, 2011). As a matter of fact, decreased expression of miR-15a and miR-16-1 gene cluster as a consequence of 13q14.3 chromosomal deletion was the first link between miRNAs and cancer (Calin et al., 2002). Similarly, decrease of miR-34b and miR-34c gene cluster and TP53 expression is due to 11q and 17 p chromosomal deletions, respectively (Fabbri et al., 2011). This association between decreased miRNA expression and chromosomal deletion has uncovered a regulatory feedback loop between p53 that transcriptionally activates expression of miR-15a~miR-16-1 and miR-34b~miR-34c which in turn regulate post-transcriptionally the expression of p53 and ZAP70, respectively (Fabbri et al., 2011). This provides a mechanistic understanding for indolent CLL that could be applied as a prognostic tool and therapeutic target. Expression profiling experiments have also highlighted miRNA signatures that could be useful to separate indolent and aggressive CLL cases. Along with miR-15a, miR16-1, miR-34b/c, differential expression of miR-17-5p, miR-21, miR-29b, miR-29c, miR-34a, miR-103, miR-155, miR-181a, miR-181b, miR-223, miR-342-3p has been shown to have diagnostic and/or prognostic value (Asslaber et al., 2010; Calin et al., 2005; Fabbri et al., 2011; Li et al., 2011; Merkel et al., 2010; Mraz et al., 2009; Pekarsky et al., 2006; Rossi et al., 2010; Sampath et al., 2011; Stamatopoulos et al., 2009, 2010; Zhu et al., 2011). Several mechanistic links have been proposed between these miRNAs and oncogenic pathways. Briefly, miR-15a and miR-16-1 inhibit expression of TP53, Bcl2, Mcl1 (Fabbri et al., 2011), miR-29 and miR-181 family members inhibit Tcl-1 expression (Pekarsky et al., 2006), miR-34 family member inhibit expression of B-Myb, E2F1 and ZAP70 (Fabbri et al., 2011; Zauli et al., 2011).

4.1.2 Altered microRNA expression in B cell lymphomas

B cell lymphomas are a heterogeneous group of diseases that more frequently present in older individuals and immunocompromised patients. These five types of B cell lymphomas accounts for more than 75% of all cases: Diffuse large B cell lymphoma (DLBCL), follicular lymphoma (FL), mucosa-associated lymphatic tissue lymphoma, small cell lymphocytic lymphoma and mantle cell lymphoma (MCL) (Jemal et al., 2010). A 10-miRNA signature (miR-17-5p, miR-92, miR-125b, miR-126, miR-135a, miR-150, miR-213, miR-301, miR-330, miR-338) and a 26-miRNA signature (including miR-34a, miR-92, miR-93, miR-150, miR-199a, miR-200c, miR-634, miR-638) separed cases from the most common types of B cell lymphoma, DLBCL and FL (Lawrie et al., 2009; Roehle et al., 2008). Moreover, miRNA signatures with prognostic and/or predictive value in all or specific (sub)types of B cell lymphomas have been reported. An 8-miRNA signature (let-7g, miR-19a, miR-21, miR-23a, miR-27a, miR-34a, miR-127, miR-195) was associated with outcome in DLBCL cases (Roehle et al., 2008), a 21-miRNA signature (including miR-21, miR-23, miR-27a, miR-30e, miR-199b, miR-330) with outcome in *de novo* DLBCL cases (Lawrie et al., 2009), and a 23-miRNA signature (including let-7a, let-7f, miR-20a, miR-20b, miR-30b, miR-96, miR-195, miR-221*, miR-1260, miR-1274a) with treatment response to chemotherapy in FL cases (Wang et al., 2011b). Differential expression of individual miRNAs has enough power to predict outcome as is the case for miR-18a, miR181a and miR-222 in DLBCL (Alencar et al., 2011), for miR-29 family members in MCL (Zhao et al., 2010) and for miR-92a in plasma of patients afflicted with different types of non-Hodgkin's B cell lymphomas (Ohyashiki et al., 2011). Several mechanistic links have been proposed between these miRNAs and oncogenic pathways. Briefly, miR-29 family members inhibit CDK6 expression in MCL (Zhao et al., 2010), and miR-34a inhibits FoxP1 expression in DLBCL (Craig et al., 2011).

4.1.3 Altered microRNA expression in acute myeloid leukemia

AML is the most common acute leukemia affecting adults in the United States (Jemal et al., 2010). AML is a very heterogenous disease and different types have been tradictionally classified based on cytological and cytogenetic characteristics. Molecular studies have provided clinical useful prognostic and functional factors, including gene mutations in c-KIT, Fms-like tyrosine kinase 3 (FLT3), nucleophosmin 1 (NPM1), and CCAAT enhancer-binding protein-α (CEBPα) (Foran, 2010). A 27-miRNA signature (including let-7a, miR-21, miR-23a, miR-27a, miR-125a, miR-128a, miR-199b, miR-210, miR-221, miR-222, miR-223) separed AML cases from acute lymphoblastic leukemia (Mi et al., 2007). Moreover, miRNA signatures with diagnostic, prognostic and/or predictive value in all or specific (sub)types of AML have been reported (Marcucci et al., 2009, 2011a). A 57-miRNA signature (including let-7a, miR-29a, miR-15a, miR-16-1, miR-17-5p, miR-20a, miR-25, miR-92a) correlated with mutation status of NPM1 (Garzon et al., 2008a), a 3-miRNA signature (miR-1331a, miR-155, miR-302a) with mutation status of FTL3 (Garzon et al., 2008a), a 5-miRNA signature (miR-20a, miR-25, miR-191, miR-199a, miR-199b) and a 2-miRNA signature (miR-29a, miR-142-3p) were associated with outcome in AML cases (Garzon et al., 2008b; Wang et al., 2011a). Differenntial expression of individual miRNAs has enough power to predict outcome as is the case for miR-181a, miR-191 and miR-199a (Garzon et al., 2008b; Schwind et al., 2010), to predict response to decitabine treatment as is the case for miR-29b (Blum et al., 2010). Several mechanistic links have been proposed between these miRNAs and oncogenic pathways. Briefly, CEBPα-induced miR-29 family members inhibit expression of Mcl-1 and

Ski (Eyholzer et al., 2010; Garzon et al., 2009; Teichler et al., 2011; Xiong et al., 2011), CEBPα-induced miR-34a inhibits E2F3 (Pulikkan et al., 2010), miR-193b, miR-221 and miR-222 inhibit c-KIT expression (Gao et al., 2011; Isken et al., 2008).

4.2 Altered microRNA expression in solid tumors

Altered miRNA expression has been reported in all studied solid tumors, including breast, brain, colorectal, gastric, lung, ovarian, pancreatic, prostate, skin, and thyroid cancers (Barbarotto et al., 2008; Fabbri, 2010; Li et al., 2010; Liu et al., 2011; Pallante et al., 2010; Sempere, 2011). Carcinomas of the breast, colon and lung collectively account for more than 247,000 cancer-related deaths per year in the United States (Jemal et al., 2010). We will use these solid tumors to exemplify the etiological contribution of TME leukoctyes and to expose the enrichment of leukocyte-expressed miRNAs in reported diagnostic and prognostic miRNA-based signatures.

Immunohistochemical (IHC) characterization of cell type(s) present in the immune cell infiltrate in the TME can also be indicative of response to treatment. In breast cancer, the ratio of CD4+ T cells, CD8+ T cells and CD68+ monocytes/Mϕs is an independent prognostic indicator of recurrence-free and overall survival (DeNardo et al., 2011). A high number of infiltrating CD68+ cells, presumably with M2 attributes, in the TME is thought to decrease treatment response to chemotherapy (DeNardo et al., 2011). Recent gene ontology-annotated mRNA signatures has uncovered the important contribution and prognostic value of immune cell signatures in breast, colorectal and lung cancer (Finak et al., 2008; Kristensen et al., 2011; Roepman et al., 2009).

4.2.1 Altered microRNA expression in breast cancer

Breast cancer is the most prevalent and second most common cause for cancer-related death of women in the United States (Jemal et al., 2010). There are four major intrinsic subtypes based on mRNA expression profiles (Sims et al., 2006; Sorlie, 2004) which closely correlate with expression status of estrogen receptor (ER), progesterone (PR) and Human Epidermal growth factor Receptor-like 2 (HER2) (Carey et al., 2006). Targeted therapies exist to interfere with ER and HER2 oncogenic signalling pathways (Caskey, 2010). Several groups have reported prognostic miRNA signatures, which include multiple leukocyte-expressed miRNAs (miR-7, miR-21, miR-150, miR-221, miR-222, miR-342). A 4-miRNA signature (miR-7, miR-128a, miR-210, miR-516-3p), a 3-miRNA signature (miR-30a-3p, miR-30c, miR-182), and a 4-miRNA signature (miR-128a, miR-135a, miR-767-3p, miR-769-3p) were associated with outcome in ER+ cases (Buffa et al., 2011; Foekens et al., 2008; Rodriguez-Gonzalez et al., 2011), a 6-miRNA signature (miR-27b, miR-30c, miR-144, miR-150, miR-210, miR-342) with outcome in ER- cases (Buffa et al., 2011), a 4-miRNA signature (miR-21, miR-210, miR-221, miR-222) with outcome in ER-PR-HER2- cases (Radojicic et al., 2011), and a 2-miRNA signature (miR-21, miR-181a) with outcome in all comers (Ota et al., 2011).

4.2.2 Altered microRNA expression in colorectal cancer

Colorectal cancer is the third leading cause of cancer-related death for both men and women in the United States (Jemal et al., 2010). There are two major molecular subtypes: microsatellite stable (MSS) and microsatellite instable (MSI). MSI phenotype is observed in about 15% of cases, is associated with a better prognosis and exhibits a different chemosensitivity profile to therapeutic agents (Pino & Chung, 2011; Vilar & Gruber, 2010). Several groups have reported diagnostic and prognostic miRNA signatures, which include multiple leukocyte-expressed miRNAs (miR-17-5p, miR-20, miR-25, miR-142-3p, miR-155, miR-223). A 8-miRNA signature (miR-92, miR-93, miR-106a, miR-125a, miR-142-3p, miR-144, miR-151, miR-212) and a 14-miRNA signature (miR-17-5p, miR-20, miR-25, miR-32, miR-92, miR-93, miR-106a, miR-125a, miR-155, miR-191, miR-192, miR-203, miR-215, miR-223) separated MSS and MSI cases (Lanza et al., 2007; Schepeler et al., 2008), a 2-miRNA signature (miR-320, miR-498) was associated with outcome in stage II MSS cases (Schepeler et al., 2008).

4.2.3 Altered microRNA expression in lung cancer

Lung cancer is the leading cause of cancer-related death for men and women in the United States (Jemal et al., 2010). There are two major histological subtypes: small-cell (SCLC) and non-small cell (NSCLC). NSCLC represent about 80% of all lung cancer cases and can be further divided in three histological groups: large cell carcinoma, squamous cell (SCC), adenocarcinoma (AdCa) (Wistuba & Gazdar, 2006). Several groups have reported diagnostic and prognostic miRNA signatures, which include multiple leukocyte-expressed miRNAs (miR-16, miR-17-5p, miR-20a, miR-20b, miR-29a, miR-29b, miR-29c, miR-106a, miR-106b, miR-146-5p, miR-146b, miR-155, miR-181a, miR-221). A 34-miRNA signature (including let-7a, let-7e, miR-16, miR-17-5p, miR-19b, miR-20a, miR-29a, miR-29b, miR-29c, miR-30b, miR-106a, miR-106b, miR-146-5p, miR-181a, miR-191, miR-195, miR-491-5p, miR-663) separated AdCa and SCC subtypes in male smokers (Landi et al., 2010), a 6-miRNA signature (let-7a, miR-221, miR-137, miR-182*, miR-372) was associated with outcome in NSCLC (Yu et al., 2008), a 19-miRNA signature (let-7e, miR-17-5p, miR-20a, miR-20b, miR-21, miR-93, miR-106a, miR-106b, miR-126, miR-146b, miR-155, miR-182, miR-183, miR-191, miR-200a, miR-200c, miR-210, miR-224) with outcome in SCC cases (Raponi et al., 2009), and a 5-miRNA signature (let-7e, miR-34a, miR-34-5p, miR-25, miR-191) with outcome in male smoker SCC cases (Landi et al., 2010).

4.3 Characterization of miRNA expression at single cell resolution in the TME

Solid tumor tissues are a complex and heterogeneous mixture of different cell types, in which cancer cell interact and intermingle with other cellular components of the TME. We and others have implemented similar *in situ* hybridization (ISH) methods to identify the cellular compartment(s) of altered miRNA expression in a variety of solid tumors, including brain, breast, colorectal, lung, pancreatic, and prostate cancer (Dillhoff et al., 2008; Donnem et al., 2011; Gupta & Mo, 2011; Habbe et al., 2009; Jorgensen et al., 2010; Liu et al., 2010a; Nelson et al., 2006, 2010; Nelson & Wilfred, 2009; Nielsen et al., 2011; Preis et al., 2011; Qian et al., 2011; Rask et al., 2011; Schepeler et al., 2008; Schneider et al., 2011; Sempere et al., 2007, 2010; Yamamichi et al., 2009). miR-21 and miR-155 are frequently detected at higher levels in solid tumors and their differential expression correlates with outcome (Barbarotto et al., 2008; Sempere, 2011). Using a combined ISH/IHC multiplex assay, we determined that miR-21 and miR-155 are expressed in different cellular compartments of the TME (Sempere et al., 2010). miR-21 was predominantly expressed within reactive stroma (tumor associated fibroblasts) in breast and colorectal tumors, and within cancer cells in lung, pancreatic and prostate tumors. Cellular co-localization of miR-155 and CD45 (leukocyte marker) signals, but not that of CK19 (epithelial cell marker) indicated a predominant expression of miR-155 within a subset of immune cells in the TME (Sempere et al. 2010). Our unpublished observations suggest that miR-155 is predominantly expressed in a subset of myeloid-derived immune cells (MPO+CD68-) in the TME of breast and colorectal tumors as determined by co-staining with cell type-specific and functional markers of major immune cell types (e.g., CD4, CD8, CD19). Further contextual characterization to identify the immune cells that upregulate or downregulate miR-155 and other leukocyte-expressed miRNAs in the TME should shed light on their etiological contribution to modulate cancer aggressiveness and progression.

5. Manipulation of microRNA activity in the tumor microenvironment by non-viral synthetic compounds as a novel approach for cancer therapy

The crucial role of miRNAs in the immunobiology of cancer makes them attractive targets for the design of novel interventions to modulate their activity. Delivery of miRNAs that are lost in cancer cells has been accomplished using viral vectors, which results in impressive therapeutic benefits (Kota et al., 2009). However, direct administration of viral vectors to cancer patients represents a major challenge in terms of clinical implementation. Alternatively, synthetic miRNA oligonucleotides or antagonistic compounds could be delivered through nanoparticles or microparticles, complexed to polymers or liposomes. The caveat of this approach is that, as commented above, a myriad of phagocytic cells with enhanced endocytic pathways are present in the microenvironment of virtually all solid tumors. Overcoming endocytosis by these abundant leukocytes and reaching cancer cells represents a barrier that, at least in our hands, has proven impossible (Cubillos-Ruiz et al., 2009a, 2009b; Cubillos-Ruiz et al., 2010). Nevertheless, the myeloid leukocytes that spontaneously take up particulate materials are also optimal targets for miRNA mimetics-based interventions. Thus, the crucial role of these cells in promoting the survival and proliferation of cancer cells, angiogenesis, metastasis and immnosuppression, as well as their plasticity and preferential homing to tumor sites facilitates their targeting as "Trojan Horses". In proof-of-concept experiments, we have been able to deliver double-stranded RNA oligonucleotides specifically to myeloid leukocytes in TME of ovarian cancer mouse models, which transformed these myeloid leukocytes from an immunosuppressive to an immunostimulatory cell type, resulting in significant therapeutic activity (Cubillos-Ruiz et al., 2009a). More recently, taking advantage of this established delivery system, we have been able to deliver synthetic miRNAs to the same cells, which transformed more than a third of their transcriptional profile and turned them into effective antigen-presenting cells that elicit protective anti-tumor immunity (manuscript under consideration). Furthermore, synthetic miRNA mimetics, as double-stranded oligonucleotides, are recognized by TLR3 and TLR7, which results in an additional non-specific activation stimulus. Because TLR agonists are known to synergize with CD40 activating reagents (Scarlett et al., 2009), which have demonstrated impressive effectiveness against pancreatic cancer (Beatty et al., 2011), their combined activity could be even stronger. Consequently, the abundance of natural phagocytic cells that avidly take up nanoparticles, which has been traditionally a major hurdle for targeted delivery of systemically administered nanoparticles, represents an advantage for effectively reaching this immunological-based therapeutic target.

6. Conclusion

We have reviewed evidences of miRNA-mediated processes that modulate immune responses. The effects of miRNA-mediated regulation are cell type-, stage- and context-dependent. Thus, cautions should be exercised when observed effects of miRNAs on clearly demarcated and controlled set of experiments in animal models are to be extrapolated from a physiological to a pathological context such as cancer and are to be generalized to human physiology and disease. This is of great importance when fragmentary knowledge of altered miRNA expression in whole tumor tissue biopsies is used to infer etiological roles and functional consequences of this presumed miRNA dysregulation in cancer cells.

As commented above, hematological cells are the site of cancer origin in leukemias and lymphomas. Therefore, it is reasonable to assume that dysregulation of leukocyte-expressed miRNA-mediated developmental and differentiation programs can be exploited by the cancer cells to become malignantly transformed. However, immune cells are an inescapable and important component of the TME in solid tumors, in which epithelial cells or mesenchymal cells are the site of cancer origin, in carcinomas or sarcomas, respectively. Although it is possible that cancer cells dysregulate within themselves the activity of leukocyte-expressed miRNAs to hijack and stimulate tumorigenic immune responses in the TME of solid tumors, it is more parsimonious that cancer cells via cellular interactions and paracrine signals interfere with immunomodulatory properties of leukocyte expressed-miRNAs such as miR-29 and miR-155 within specific subsets of infiltrating immune cells.

Further investigations are needed to understand the role that miRNAs play in cancer, both in hematological and solid tumors. We hope that our reflections here serve to inform the experimental design of future pre-clinical and clinical studies, namely, that cell type-specific and context-dependent effects of miRNA-mediated immunomodulation are appropriately considered and distinguished from miRNA-mediated processes within cancer cells and other cellular compartments of the TME. This could have important clinical implications and applications since reprogramming a subset of immune cells to elicit anti-tumor responses is an appealing and potentially feasible approach for therapeutic intervention.

7. Acknowledgment

This work was supported, in part, by National Institutes of Health (NIH) and National Cancer Institute (NCI) grants: R03 CA141564 and R21 CA141017 (LFS), CA124515, CA124515S, CA132026 and P30CA010815 (JRC), and by DoD grant OC100059 (JRC).

8. References

Ahn, G. O. & Brown, J. M. Matrix metalloproteinase-9 is required for tumor vasculogenesis but not for angiogenesis: role of bone marrow-derived myelomonocytic cells. Cancer Cell 13[3], 193-205. 2008.

Alencar, A. J., Malumbres, R., Kozloski, G. A., Advani, R., Talreja, N., Chinichian, S., Briones, J., Natkunam, Y., Sehn, L. H., Gascoyne, R. D., Tibshirani, R., & Lossos, I. S. MicroRNAs are independent predictors of outcome in diffuse large B-cell lymphoma patients treated with R-CHOP. Clin.Cancer Res. 17[12], 4125-4135. 6-15-2011.

Ambros, V. The functions of animal microRNAs. Nature 431[7006], 350-355. 9-16-2004.

Andreu, P., Johansson, M., Affara, N. I., Pucci, F., Tan, T., Junankar, S., Korets, L., Lam, J., Tawfik, D., DeNardo, D. G., Naldini, L., de Visser, K. E., De, Palma M., & Coussens, L. M. FcRgamma activation regulates inflammation-associated squamous carcinogenesis. Cancer Cell 17[2], 121-134. 2-17-2010.

Asslaber, D., Pinon, J. D., Seyfried, I., Desch, P., Stocher, M., Tinhofer, I., Egle, A., Merkel, O., & Greil, R. microRNA-34a expression correlates with MDM2 SNP309 polymorphism and treatment-free survival in chronic lymphocytic leukemia. Blood 115[21], 4191-4197. 5-27-2010.

Baek, D., Villen, J., Shin, C., Camargo, F. D., Gygi, S. P., & Bartel, D. P. The impact of microRNAs on protein output. Nature 455[7209], 64-71. 9-4-2008.

Barbarotto, E., Schmittgen, T. D., & Calin, G. A. MicroRNAs and cancer: profile, profile, profile. Int.J.Cancer 122[5], 969-977. 3-1-2008.

Bartel, D. P. & Chen, C. Z. Micromanagers of gene expression: the potentially widespread influence of metazoan microRNAs. Nat.Rev.Genet. 5[5], 396-400. 2004.

Beatty, G. L., Chiorean, E. G., Fishman, M. P., Saboury, B., Teitelbaum, U. R., Sun, W., Huhn, R. D., Song, W., Li, D., Sharp, L. L., Torigian, D. A., O'Dwyer, P. J., & Vonderheide, R. H. CD40 agonists alter tumor stroma and show efficacy against pancreatic carcinoma in mice and humans. Science 331[6024], 1612-1616. 3-25-2011.

Belver, L., de, Yebenes, V, & Ramiro, A. R. MicroRNAs prevent the generation of autoreactive antibodies. Immunity. 33[5], 713-722. 11-24-2010.

Bentwich, I., Avniel, A., Karov, Y., Aharonov, R., Gilad, S., Barad, O., Barzilai, A., Einat, P., Einav, U., Meiri, E., Sharon, E., Spector, Y., & Bentwich, Z. Identification of hundreds of conserved and nonconserved human microRNAs. Nat.Genet. 37[7], 766-770. 2005.

Beyer, M., Thabet, Y., Muller, R. U., Sadlon, T., Classen, S., Lahl, K., Basu, S., Zhou, X., Bailey-Bucktrout, S. L., Krebs, W., Schonfeld, E. A., Bottcher, J., Golovina, T., Mayer, C. T., Hofmann, A., Sommer, D., bey-Pascher, S., Endl, E., Limmer, A., Hippen, K. L., Blazar, B. R., Balderas, R., Quast, T., Waha, A., Mayer, G., Famulok, M., Knolle, P. A., Wickenhauser, C., Kolanus, W., Schermer, B., Bluestone, J. A., Barry, S. C., Sparwasser, T., Riley, J. L., & Schultze, J. L. Repression of the genome organizer SATB1 in regulatory T cells is required for suppressive function and inhibition of effector differentiation. Nat.Immunol. 12[9], 898-907. 2011.

Bezman, N. A., Cedars, E., Steiner, D. F., Blelloch, R., Hesslein, D. G., & Lanier, L. L. Distinct requirements of microRNAs in NK cell activation, survival, and function. J.Immunol. 185[7], 3835-3846. 10-1-2010.

Blum, W., Garzon, R., Klisovic, R. B., Schwind, S., Walker, A., Geyer, S., Liu, S., Havelange, V., Becker, H., Schaaf, L., Mickle, J., Devine, H., Kefauver, C., Devine, S. M., Chan, K. K., Heerema, N. A., Bloomfield, C. D., Grever, M. R., Byrd, J. C., Villalona-Calero, M., Croce, C. M., & Marcucci, G. Clinical response and miR-29b predictive significance in older AML patients treated with a 10-day schedule of decitabine. Proc.Natl.Acad.Sci.U.S.A 107[16], 7473-7478. 4-20-2010.

Brase, J. C., Wuttig, D., Kuner, R., & Sultmann, H. Serum microRNAs as non-invasive biomarkers for cancer. Mol.Cancer 9, 306. 2010.

Buffa, F. M., Camps, C., Winchester, L., Snell, C. E., Gee, H. E., Sheldon, H., Taylor, M., Harris, A. L., & Ragoussis, J. microRNA associated progression pathways and potential therapeutic targets identified by integrated mRNA and microRNA expression profiling in breast cancer. Cancer Res. 7-7-2011.

Calin, G. A., Dumitru, C. D., Shimizu, M., Bichi, R., Zupo, S., Noch, E., Aldler, H., Rattan, S., Keating, M., Rai, K., Rassenti, L., Kipps, T., Negrini, M., Bullrich, F., & Croce, C. M. Frequent deletions and down-regulation of micro- RNA genes miR15 and miR16 at 13q14 in chronic lymphocytic leukemia. Proc.Natl.Acad.Sci.U.S.A 99[24], 15524-15529. 11-26-2002.

Calin, G. A., Ferracin, M., Cimmino, A., Di, Leva G., Shimizu, M., Wojcik, S. E., Iorio, M. V., Visone, R., Sever, N. I., Fabbri, M., Iuliano, R., Palumbo, T., Pichiorri, F., Roldo, C., Garzon, R., Sevignani, C., Rassenti, L., Alder, H., Volinia, S., Liu, C. G., Kipps, T. J., Negrini, M., & Croce, C. M. A MicroRNA signature associated with prognosis and progression in chronic lymphocytic leukemia. N.Engl.J.Med. 353[17], 1793-1801. 10-27-2005.

Calvo, K. R., Landgren, O., Roccaro, A. M., & Ghobrial, I. M. Role of microRNAs from monoclonal gammopathy of undetermined significance to multiple myeloma. Semin.Hematol. 48[1], 39-45. 2011.

Carey, L. A., Perou, C. M., Livasy, C. A., Dressler, L. G., Cowan, D., Conway, K., Karaca, G., Troester, M. A., Tse, C. K., Edmiston, S., Deming, S. L., Geradts, J., Cheang, M. C., Nielsen, T. O., Moorman, P. G., Earp, H. S., & Millikan, R. C. Race, breast cancer subtypes, and survival in the Carolina Breast Cancer Study. JAMA 295[21], 2492-2502. 6-7-2006.

Caskey, C. T. Using genetic diagnosis to determine individual therapeutic utility. Annu.Rev.Med. 61, 1-15. 2010.

Ceppi, M., Pereira, P. M., Dunand-Sauthier, I., Barras, E., Reith, W., Santos, M. A., & Pierre, P. MicroRNA-155 modulates the interleukin-1 signaling pathway in activated human monocyte-derived dendritic cells. Proc.Natl.Acad.Sci.U.S.A 106[8], 2735-2740. 2-24-2009.

Chang, S., Wang, R. H., Akagi, K., Kim, K. A., Martin, B. K., Cavallone, L., Haines, D. C., Basik, M., Mai, P., Poggi, E., Isaacs, C., Looi, L. M., Mun, K. S., Greene, M. H., Byers, S. W., Teo, S. H., Deng, C. X., & Sharan, S. K. Tumor suppressor BRCA1 epigenetically controls oncogenic microRNA-155. Nat.Med. 17[10], 1275-1282. 2011.

Chaudhuri, A. A., So, A. Y., Sinha, N., Gibson, W. S., Taganov, K. D., O'Connell, R. M., & Baltimore, D. MicroRNA-125b Potentiates Macrophage Activation. J.Immunol. 187[10], 5062-5068. 11-15-2011.

Colotta, F., Allavena, P., Sica, A., Garlanda, C., & Mantovani, A. Cancer-related inflammation, the seventh hallmark of cancer: links to genetic instability. Carcinogenesis 30[7], 1073-1081. 2009.

Conejo-Garcia, J. R., Benencia, F., Courreges, M. C., Kang, E., Mohamed-Hadley, A., Buckanovich, R. J., Holtz, D. O., Jenkins, A., Na, H., Zhang, L., Wagner, D. S., Katsaros, D., Caroll, R., & Coukos, G. Tumor-infiltrating dendritic cell precursors recruited by a beta-defensin contribute to vasculogenesis under the influence of Vegf-A. Nat.Med. 10[9], 950-958. 2004.

Costinean, S., Zanesi, N., Pekarsky, Y., Tili, E., Volinia, S., Heerema, N., & Croce, C. M. Pre-B cell proliferation and lymphoblastic leukemia/high-grade lymphoma in E{micro}-miR155 transgenic mice. Proc.Natl.Acad.Sci.U.S.A. 103[18], 7024-7029. 5-2-2006.

Craig, V. J., Cogliatti, S. B., Imig, J., Renner, C., Neuenschwander, S., Rehrauer, H., Schlapbach, R., Dirnhofer, S., Tzankov, A., & Muller, A. Myc-mediated repression of microRNA-34a promotes high-grade transformation of B-cell lymphoma by dysregulation of FoxP1. Blood 117[23], 6227-6236. 6-9-2011.

Cubillos-Ruiz, J. R., Engle, X., Scarlett, U. K., Martinez, D., Barber, A., Elgueta, R., Wang, L., Nesbeth, Y., Durant, Y., Gewirtz, A. T., Sentman, C. L., Kedl, R., & Conejo-Garcia, J. R. Polyethylenimine-based siRNA nanocomplexes reprogram tumor-associated dendritic cells via TLR5 to elicit therapeutic antitumor immunity. J.Clin.Invest 119[8], 2231-2244. 2009a.

Cubillos-Ruiz, J. R., Fiering, S., & Conejo-Garcia, J. R. Nanomolecular targeting of dendritic cells for ovarian cancer therapy. Future.Oncol. 5[8], 1189-1192. 2009b.

Cubillos-Ruiz, J. R., Rutkowski, M., & Conejo-Garcia, J. R. Blocking ovarian cancer progression by targeting tumor microenvironmental leukocytes. Cell Cycle 9[2], 260-268. 1-15-2010.

Curiel, T. J., Coukos, G., Zou, L., Alvarez, X., Cheng, P., Mottram, P., Evdemon-Hogan, M., Conejo-Garcia, J. R., Zhang, L., Burow, M., Zhu, Y., Wei, S., Kryczek, I., Daniel, B., Gordon, A., Myers, L., Lackner, A., Disis, M. L., Knutson, K. L., Chen, L., & Zou, W. Specific recruitment of regulatory T cells in ovarian carcinoma fosters immune privilege and predicts reduced survival. Nat.Med. 10[9], 942-949. 2004.

De Smaele E., Ferretti, E., & Gulino, A. MicroRNAs as biomarkers for CNS cancer and other disorders. Brain Res. 1338, 100-111. 6-18-2010.

de Vries, V, Pino-Lagos, K., Nowak, E. C., Bennett, K. A., Oliva, C., & Noelle, R. J. Mast cells condition dendritic cells to mediate allograft tolerance. Immunity. 35[4], 550-561. 10-28-2011.

DeNardo, David G., Brennan, Donal J., Rexhepaj, Elton, Ruffell, Brian, Shiao, Stephen L., Madden, Stephen F., Gallagher, William M., Wadhwani, Nikhil, Keil, Scott D., Junaid, Sharfaa A., Rugo, Hope S., Hwang, E. Shelley, Jirstr+¦m, Karin, West, Brian L., & Coussens, Lisa M. Leukocyte Complexity Predicts Breast Cancer Survival and Functionally Regulates Response to Chemotherapy. Cancer Discovery . 4-3-2011.

Dillhoff, M., Liu, J., Frankel, W., Croce, C., & Bloomston, M. MicroRNA-21 is Overexpressed in Pancreatic Cancer and a Potential Predictor of Survival. J.Gastrointest.Surg. 12[12], 2171-2176. 7-19-2008.

Donnem, T., Eklo, K., Berg, T., Sorbye, S. W., Lonvik, K., Al-Saad, S., Al-Shibli, K., Andersen, S., Stenvold, H., Bremnes, R. M., & Busund, L. T. Prognostic impact of MiR-155 in non-small cell lung cancer evaluated by in situ hybridization. J.Transl.Med. 9, 6. 2011.

Dunn, G. P., Ikeda, H., Bruce, A. T., Koebel, C., Uppaluri, R., Bui, J., Chan, R., Diamond, M., White, J. M., Sheehan, K. C., & Schreiber, R. D. Interferon-gamma and cancer immunoediting. Immunol.Res. 32[1-3], 231-245. 2005.

Dvorak, H. F. Tumors: wounds that do not heal. Similarities between tumor stroma generation and wound healing. N.Engl.J.Med. 315[26], 1650-1659. 12-25-1986.

Ehrchen, J. M., Sunderkotter, C., Foell, D., Vogl, T., & Roth, J. The endogenous Toll-like receptor 4 agonist S100A8/S100A9 (calprotectin) as innate amplifier of infection, autoimmunity, and cancer. J.Leukoc.Biol. 86[3], 557-566. 2009.

Ertl, H. C., Zaia, J., Rosenberg, S. A., June, C. H., Dotti, G., Kahn, J., Cooper, L. J., Corrigan-Curay, J., & Strome, S. E. Considerations for the clinical application of chimeric antigen receptor T cells: observations from a recombinant DNA Advisory Committee Symposium held June 15, 2010. Cancer Res. 71[9], 3175-3181. 5-1-2011.

Eyholzer, M., Schmid, S., Wilkens, L., Mueller, B. U., & Pabst, T. The tumour-suppressive miR-29a/b1 cluster is regulated by CEBPA and blocked in human AML. Br.J.Cancer 103[2], 275-284. 7-13-2010.

Fabbri, M. miRNAs as molecular biomarkers of cancer. Expert.Rev.Mol.Diagn. 10[4], 435-444. 2010.

Fabbri, M., Bottoni, A., Shimizu, M., Spizzo, R., Nicoloso, M. S., Rossi, S., Barbarotto, E., Cimmino, A., Adair, B., Wojcik, S. E., Valeri, N., Calore, F., Sampath, D., Fanini, F., Vannini, I., Musuraca, G., Dell'Aquila, M., Alder, H., Davuluri, R. V., Rassenti, L. Z., Negrini, M., Nakamura, T., Amadori, D., Kay, N. E., Rai, K. R., Keating, M. J., Kipps, T. J., Calin, G. A., & Croce, C. M. Association of a microRNA/TP53 feedback circuitry with pathogenesis and outcome of B-cell chronic lymphocytic leukemia. JAMA 305[1], 59-67. 1-5-2011.

Fabbri, M. & Croce, C. M. Role of microRNAs in lymphoid biology and disease. Curr.Opin.Hematol. 18[4], 266-272. 2011.

Fabbri, M., Croce, C. M., & Calin, G. A. MicroRNAs in the ontogeny of leukemias and lymphomas. Leuk.Lymphoma 50[2], 160-170. 2009.

Faraoni, I., Antonetti, F. R., Cardone, J., & Bonmassar, E. miR-155 gene: a typical multifunctional microRNA. Biochim.Biophys.Acta 1792[6], 497-505. 2009.

Feng, J., Iwama, A., Satake, M., & Kohu, K. MicroRNA-27 enhances differentiation of myeloblasts into granulocytes by post-transcriptionally downregulating Runx1. Br.J.Haematol. 145[3], 412-423. 2009.

Finak, G., Bertos, N., Pepin, F., Sadekova, S., Souleimanova, M., Zhao, H., Chen, H., Omeroglu, G., Meterissian, S., Omeroglu, A., Hallett, M., & Park, M. Stromal gene expression predicts clinical outcome in breast cancer. Nat.Med. 14[5], 518-527. 2008.

Foekens, J. A., Sieuwerts, A. M., Smid, M., Look, M. P., de, Weerd, V, Boersma, A. W., Klijn, J. G., Wiemer, E. A., & Martens, J. W. Four miRNAs associated with aggressiveness of lymph node-negative, estrogen receptor-positive human breast cancer. Proc.Natl.Acad.Sci.U.S.A 105[35], 13021-13026. 9-2-2008.

Fontana, L., Pelosi, E., Greco, P., Racanicchi, S., Testa, U., Liuzzi, F., Croce, C. M., Brunetti, E., Grignani, F., & Peschle, C. MicroRNAs 17-5p-20a-106a control monocytopoiesis through AML1 targeting and M-CSF receptor upregulation. Nat.Cell Biol. 9[7], 775-787. 2007.

Foran, J. M. New prognostic markers in acute myeloid leukemia: perspective from the clinic. Hematology.Am.Soc.Hematol.Educ.Program. 2010, 47-55. 2010.

Gabrilovich, D. I. & Nagaraj, S. Myeloid-derived suppressor cells as regulators of the immune system. Nat.Rev.Immunol. 9[3], 162-174. 2009.

Gao, X. N., Lin, J., Gao, L., Li, Y. H., Wang, L. L., & Yu, L. MicroRNA-193b regulates c-Kit proto-oncogene and represses cell proliferation in acute myeloid leukemia. Leuk.Res. 35[9], 1226-1232. 2011.

Garzon, R., Garofalo, M., Martelli, M. P., Briesewitz, R., Wang, L., Fernandez-Cymering, C., Volinia, S., Liu, C. G., Schnittger, S., Haferlach, T., Liso, A., Diverio, D., Mancini, M., Meloni, G., Foa, R., Martelli, M. F., Mecucci, C., Croce, C. M., & Falini, B. Distinctive microRNA signature of acute myeloid leukemia bearing cytoplasmic mutated nucleophosmin. Proc.Natl.Acad.Sci.U.S.A 105[10], 3945-3950. 3-11-2008a.

Garzon, R., Heaphy, C. E., Havelange, V., Fabbri, M., Volinia, S., Tsao, T., Zanesi, N., Kornblau, S. M., Marcucci, G., Calin, G. A., Andreeff, M., & Croce, C. M. MicroRNA 29b functions in acute myeloid leukemia. Blood 114[26], 5331-5341. 12-17-2009.

Garzon, R., Marcucci, G., & Croce, C. M. Targeting microRNAs in cancer: rationale, strategies and challenges. Nat.Rev.Drug Discov. 9[10], 775-789. 2010.

Garzon, R., Volinia, S., Liu, C. G., Fernandez-Cymering, C., Palumbo, T., Pichiorri, F., Fabbri, M., Coombes, K., Alder, H., Nakamura, T., Flomenberg, N., Marcucci, G., Calin, G. A., Kornblau, S. M., Kantarjian, H., Bloomfield, C. D., Andreeff, M., & Croce, C. M. MicroRNA signatures associated with cytogenetics and prognosis in acute myeloid leukemia. Blood 111[6], 3183-3189. 3-15-2008b.

Gaziel-Sovran, A., Segura, M. F., Di, Micco R., Collins, M. K., Hanniford, D., Vega-Saenz de, Miera E., Rakus, J. F., Dankert, J. F., Shang, S., Kerbel, R. S., Bhardwaj, N., Shao, Y., Darvishian, F., Zavadil, J., Erlebacher, A., Mahal, L. K., Osman, I., & Hernando, E. miR-30b/30d regulation of GalNAc transferases enhances invasion and immunosuppression during metastasis. Cancer Cell 20[1], 104-118. 7-12-2011.

Ghani, S., Riemke, P., Schonheit, J., Lenze, D., Stumm, J., Hoogenkamp, M., Lagendijk, A., Heinz, S., Bonifer, C., Bakkers, J., bdelilah-Seyfried, S., Hummel, M., & Rosenbauer, F. Macrophage development from HSCs requires PU.1-coordinated microRNA expression. Blood 118[8], 2275-2284. 8-25-2011.

Grigoryev, Y. A., Kurian, S. M., Hart, T., Nakorchevsky, A. A., Chen, C., Campbell, D., Head, S. R., Yates, J. R., III, & Salomon, D. R. MicroRNA regulation of molecular networks mapped by global microRNA, mRNA, and protein expression in activated T lymphocytes. J.Immunol. 187[5], 2233-2243. 9-1-2011.

Gupta, A. & Mo, Y. Y. Detection of microRNAs in cultured cells and paraffin-embedded tissue specimens by in situ hybridization. Methods Mol.Biol. 676, 73-83. 2011.

Habbe, N., Koorstra, J. B., Mendell, J. T., Offerhaus, G. J., Ryu, J. K., Feldmann, G., Mullendore, M. E., Goggins, M. G., Hong, S. M., & Maitra, A. MicroRNA miR-155 is a biomarker of early pancreatic neoplasia. Cancer Biol.Ther. 8[4], 340-346. 2009.

Hamanishi, J., Mandai, M., Iwasaki, M., Okazaki, T., Tanaka, Y., Yamaguchi, K., Higuchi, T., Yagi, H., Takakura, K., Minato, N., Honjo, T., & Fujii, S. Programmed cell death 1 ligand 1 and tumor-infiltrating CD8+ T lymphocytes are prognostic factors of human ovarian cancer. Proc.Natl.Acad.Sci.U.S.A 104[9], 3360-3365. 2-27-2007.

Hanahan, D. & Weinberg, R. A. Hallmarks of cancer: the next generation. Cell 144[5], 646-674. 3-4-2011.

Hashimi, S. T., Fulcher, J. A., Chang, M. H., Gov, L., Wang, S., & Lee, B. MicroRNA profiling identifies miR-34a and miR-21 and their target genes JAG1 and WNT1 in the coordinate regulation of dendritic cell differentiation. Blood 114[2], 404-414. 7-9-2009.

Hiratsuka, S., Watanabe, A., Sakurai, Y., kashi-Takamura, S., Ishibashi, S., Miyake, K., Shibuya, M., Akira, S., Aburatani, H., & Maru, Y. The S100A8-serum amyloid A3-TLR4 paracrine cascade establishes a pre-metastatic phase. Nat.Cell Biol. 10[11], 1349-1355. 2008.

Hou, J., Wang, P., Lin, L., Liu, X., Ma, F., An, H., Wang, Z., & Cao, X. MicroRNA-146a feedback inhibits RIG-I-dependent Type I IFN production in macrophages by targeting TRAF6, IRAK1, and IRAK2. J.Immunol. 183[3], 2150-2158. 8-1-2009.

Huarte, E., Cubillos-Ruiz, J. R., Nesbeth, Y. C., Scarlett, U. K., Martinez, D. G., Buckanovich, R. J., Benencia, F., Stan, R. V., Keler, T., Sarobe, P., Sentman, C. L., & Conejo-Garcia, J. R. Depletion of dendritic cells delays ovarian cancer progression by boosting antitumor immunity. Cancer Res. 68[18], 7684-7691. 9-15-2008.

Isken, F., Steffen, B., Merk, S., Dugas, M., Markus, B., Tidow, N., Zuhlsdorf, M., Illmer, T., Thiede, C., Berdel, W. E., Serve, H., & Muller-Tidow, C. Identification of acute myeloid leukaemia associated microRNA expression patterns. Br.J.Haematol. 140[2], 153-161. 2008.

Jemal, A., Siegel, R., Xu, J., & Ward, E. Cancer statistics, 2010. CA Cancer J.Clin. 60[5], 277-300. 2010.

Johnnidis, J. B., Harris, M. H., Wheeler, R. T., Stehling-Sun, S., Lam, M. H., Kirak, O., Brummelkamp, T. R., Fleming, M. D., & Camargo, F. D. Regulation of progenitor cell proliferation and granulocyte function by microRNA-223. Nature 451[7182], 1125-1129. 2-28-2008.

Jorgensen, S., Baker, A., Moller, S., & Nielsen, B. S. Robust one-day in situ hybridization protocol for detection of microRNAs in paraffin samples using LNA probes. Methods 52[4], 375-381. 2010.

Ketting, R. F. microRNA Biogenesis and Function : An overview. Adv.Exp.Med.Biol. 700, 1-14. 2011.

Kim, T. D., Lee, S. U., Yun, S., Sun, H. N., Lee, S. H., Kim, J. W., Kim, H. M., Park, S. K., Lee, C. W., Yoon, S. R., Greenberg, P. D., & Choi, I. Human microRNA-27a* targets Prf1 and GzmBexpression to regulate NK cell cytotoxicity. Blood . 9-29-2011.

Koralov, S. B., Muljo, S. A., Galler, G. R., Krek, A., Chakraborty, T., Kanellopoulou, C., Jensen, K., Cobb, B. S., Merkenschlager, M., Rajewsky, N., & Rajewsky, K. Dicer ablation affects antibody diversity and cell survival in the B lymphocyte lineage. Cell 132[5], 860-874. 3-7-2008.

Kota, J., Chivukula, R. R., O'Donnell, K. A., Wentzel, E. A., Montgomery, C. L., Hwang, H. W., Chang, T. C., Vivekanandan, P., Torbenson, M., Clark, K. R., Mendell, J. R., & Mendell, J. T. Therapeutic microRNA delivery suppresses tumorigenesis in a murine liver cancer model. Cell 137[6], 1005-1017. 6-12-2009.

Kotani, A., Harnprasopwat, R., Toyoshima, T., Kawamata, T., & Tojo, A. miRNAs in normal and malignant B cells. Int.J.Hematol. 92[2], 255-261. 2010.

Kozomara, A. & Griffiths-Jones, S. miRBase: integrating microRNA annotation and deep-sequencing data. Nucleic Acids Res. 39[Database issue], D152-D157. 2011.

Kristensen, V. N., Vaske, C. J., Ursini-Siegel, J., Van, Loo P., Nordgard, S. H., Sachidanandam, R., Sorlie, T., Warnberg, F., Haakensen, V. D., Helland, A., Naume, B., Perou, C. M., Haussler, D., Troyanskaya, O. G., & Borresen-Dale, A. L. Integrated molecular profiles of invasive breast tumors and ductal carcinoma in situ (DCIS) reveal differential vascular and interleukin signaling. Proc.Natl.Acad.Sci.U.S.A . 9-9-2011.

Landi, M. T., Zhao, Y., Rotunno, M., Koshiol, J., Liu, H., Bergen, A. W., Rubagotti, M., Goldstein, A. M., Linnoila, I., Marincola, F. M., Tucker, M. A., Bertazzi, P. A., Pesatori, A. C., Caporaso, N. E., McShane, L. M., & Wang, E. MicroRNA expression differentiates histology and predicts survival of lung cancer. Clin.Cancer Res. 16[2], 430-441. 1-15-2010.

Lanza, G., Ferracin, M., Gafa, R., Veronese, A., Spizzo, R., Pichiorri, F., Liu, C. G., Calin, G. A., Croce, C. M., & Negrini, M. mRNA/microRNA gene expression profile in microsatellite unstable colorectal cancer. Mol.Cancer 6, 54. 2007.

Lawrie, C. H., Chi, J., Taylor, S., Tramonti, D., Ballabio, E., Palazzo, S., Saunders, N. J., Pezzella, F., Boultwood, J., Wainscoat, J. S., & Hatton, C. S. Expression of microRNAs in diffuse large B cell lymphoma is associated with immunophenotype, survival and transformation from follicular lymphoma. J.Cell Mol.Med. 13[7], 1248-1260. 2009.

Li, Q. J., Chau, J., Ebert, P. J., Sylvester, G., Min, H., Liu, G., Braich, R., Manoharan, M., Soutschek, J., Skare, P., Klein, L. O., Davis, M. M., & Chen, C. Z. miR-181a is an intrinsic modulator of T cell sensitivity and selection. Cell 129[1], 147-161. 4-6-2007.

Li, S., Moffett, H. F., Lu, J., Werner, L., Zhang, H., Ritz, J., Neuberg, D., Wucherpfennig, K. W., Brown, J. R., & Novina, C. D. MicroRNA expression profiling identifies activated B cell status in chronic lymphocytic leukemia cells. PLoS.ONE. 6[3], e16956. 2011.

Li, S. D., Zhang, J. R., Wang, Y. Q., & Wan, X. P. The role of microRNAs in ovarian cancer initiation and progression. J.Cell Mol.Med. 14[9], 2240-2249. 2010.

Lim, L. P., Lau, N. C., Garrett-Engele, P., Grimson, A., Schelter, J. M., Castle, J., Bartel, D. P., Linsley, P. S., & Johnson, J. M. Microarray analysis shows that some microRNAs downregulate large numbers of target mRNAs. Nature 433[7027], 769-773. 2-17-2005.

Liston, A., Lu, L. F., O'Carroll, D., Tarakhovsky, A., & Rudensky, A. Y. Dicer-dependent microRNA pathway safeguards regulatory T cell function. J.Exp.Med. 205[9], 1993-2004. 9-1-2008.

Liu, X., Sempere, L. F., Guo, Y., Korc, M., Kauppinen, S., Freemantle, S. J., & Dmitrovsky, E. Involvement of microRNAs in lung cancer biology and therapy. Transl.Res. 157[4], 200-208. 2011.

Liu, X., Sempere, L. F., Ouyang, H., Memoli, V. A., Andrew, A. S., Luo, Y., Demidenko, E., Korc, M., Shi, W., Preis, M., Dragnev, K. H., Li, H., DiRenzo, J., Bak, M., Freemantle, S. J., Kauppinen, S., & Dmitrovsky, E. MicroRNA-31 functions as an oncogenic microRNA in mouse and human lung cancer cells by repressing specific tumor suppressors. J.Clin.Invest 120[4], 1298-1309. 2010a.

Liu, X., Zhan, Z., Xu, L., Ma, F., Li, D., Guo, Z., Li, N., & Cao, X. MicroRNA-148/152 impair innate response and antigen presentation of TLR-triggered dendritic cells by targeting CaMKIIalpha. J.Immunol. 185[12], 7244-7251. 12-15-2010b.

Lu, C., Huang, X., Zhang, X., Roensch, K., Cao, Q., Nakayama, K. I., Blazar, B. R., Zeng, Y., & Zhou, X. miR-221 and miR-155 regulate human dendritic cell development, apoptosis, and IL-12 production through targeting of p27kip1, KPC1, and SOCS-1. Blood 117[16], 4293-4303. 4-21-2011a.

Lu, F., Weidmer, A., Liu, C. G., Volinia, S., Croce, C. M., & Lieberman, P. M. Epstein-Barr virus-induced miR-155 attenuates NF-kappaB signaling and stabilizes latent virus persistence. J.Virol. 82[21], 10436-10443. 2008.

Lu, L. F., Boldin, M. P., Chaudhry, A., Lin, L. L., Taganov, K. D., Hanada, T., Yoshimura, A., Baltimore, D., & Rudensky, A. Y. Function of miR-146a in controlling Treg cell-mediated regulation of Th1 responses. Cell 142[6], 914-929. 9-17-2010.

Lu, L. F., Lind, E. F., Gondek, D. C., Bennett, K. A., Gleeson, M. W., Pino-Lagos, K., Scott, Z. A., Coyle, A. J., Reed, J. L., Van, Snick J., Strom, T. B., Zheng, X. X., & Noelle, R. J. Mast cells are essential intermediaries in regulatory T-cell tolerance. Nature 442[7106], 997-1002. 8-31-2006.

Lu, T. X., Hartner, J., Lim, E. J., Fabry, V., Mingler, M. K., Cole, E. T., Orkin, S. H., Aronow, B. J., & Rothenberg, M. E. MicroRNA-21 limits in vivo immune response-mediated activation of the IL-12/IFN-gamma pathway, Th1 polarization, and the severity of delayed-type hypersensitivity. J.Immunol. 187[6], 3362-3373. 9-15-2011b.

Ma, F., Xu, S., Liu, X., Zhang, Q., Xu, X., Liu, M., Hua, M., Li, N., Yao, H., & Cao, X. The microRNA miR-29 controls innate and adaptive immune responses to intracellular bacterial infection by targeting interferon-gamma. Nat.Immunol. 12[9], 861-869. 2011.

Malumbres, R. & Lossos, I. S. Expression of miRNAs in lymphocytes: a review. Methods Mol.Biol. 667, 129-143. 2010.

Malumbres, R., Sarosiek, K. A., Cubedo, E., Ruiz, J. W., Jiang, X., Gascoyne, R. D., Tibshirani, R., & Lossos, I. S. Differentiation stage-specific expression of microRNAs in B lymphocytes and diffuse large B-cell lymphomas. Blood 113[16], 3754-3764. 4-16-2009.

Mantovani, A. La mala educacion of tumor-associated macrophages: Diverse pathways and new players. Cancer Cell 17[2], 111-112. 2-17-2010.

Mao, C. P., He, L., Tsai, Y. C., Peng, S., Kang, T. H., Pang, X., Monie, A., Hung, C. F., & Wu, T. C. In vivo microRNA-155 expression influences antigen-specific T cell-mediated immune responses generated by DNA vaccination. Cell Biosci. 1[1], 3. 2011.

Marcucci, G., Mrozek, K., Radmacher, M. D., Garzon, R., & Bloomfield, C. D. The prognostic and functional role of microRNAs in acute myeloid leukemia. Blood 117[4], 1121-1129. 1-27-2011b.

Marcucci, G., Mrozek, K., Radmacher, M. D., Garzon, R., & Bloomfield, C. D. The prognostic and functional role of microRNAs in acute myeloid leukemia. Blood 117[4], 1121-1129. 1-27-2011a.

Marcucci, G., Radmacher, M. D., Mrozek, K., & Bloomfield, C. D. MicroRNA expression in acute myeloid leukemia. Curr.Hematol.Malig.Rep. 4[2], 83-88. 2009.

Martinez-Nunez, R. T., Louafi, F., Friedmann, P. S., & Sanchez-Elsner, T. MicroRNA-155 modulates the pathogen binding ability of dendritic cells (DCs) by down-regulation of DC-specific intercellular adhesion molecule-3 grabbing non-integrin (DC-SIGN). J.Biol.Chem. 284[24], 16334-16342. 6-12-2009.

Martinez-Nunez, R. T., Louafi, F., & Sanchez-Elsner, T. The interleukin 13 (IL-13) pathway in human macrophages is modulated by microRNA-155 via direct targeting of interleukin 13 receptor alpha1 (IL13Ralpha1). J.Biol.Chem. 286[3], 1786-1794. 1-21-2011.

Mazzieri, R., Pucci, F., Moi, D., Zonari, E., Ranghetti, A., Berti, A., Politi, L. S., Gentner, B., Brown, J. L., Naldini, L., & De, Palma M. Targeting the ANG2/TIE2 axis inhibits tumor growth and metastasis by impairing angiogenesis and disabling rebounds of proangiogenic myeloid cells. Cancer Cell 19[4], 512-526. 4-12-2011.

Merkel, O., Asslaber, D., Pinon, J. D., Egle, A., & Greil, R. Interdependent regulation of p53 and miR-34a in chronic lymphocytic leukemia. Cell Cycle 9[14], 2764-2768. 7-15-2010.

Mi, S., Lu, J., Sun, M., Li, Z., Zhang, H., Neilly, M. B., Wang, Y., Qian, Z., Jin, J., Zhang, Y., Bohlander, S. K., Le Beau, M. M., Larson, R. A., Golub, T. R., Rowley, J. D., & Chen, J. MicroRNA expression signatures accurately discriminate acute lymphoblastic leukemia from acute myeloid leukemia. Proc.Natl.Acad.Sci.U.S.A 104[50], 19971-19976. 12-11-2007.

Monticelli, S., Ansel, K. M., Xiao, C., Socci, N. D., Krichevsky, A. M., Thai, T. H., Rajewsky, N., Marks, D. S., Sander, C., Rajewsky, K., Rao, A., & Kosik, K. S. MicroRNA profiling of the murine hematopoietic system. Genome Biol. 6[8], R71. 2005.

Mostert, B., Sieuwerts, A. M., Martens, J. W., & Sleijfer, S. Diagnostic applications of cell-free and circulating tumor cell-associated miRNAs in cancer patients. Expert.Rev.Mol.Diagn. 11[3], 259-275. 2011.

Mraz, M., Malinova, K., Kotaskova, J., Pavlova, S., Tichy, B., Malcikova, J., Stano, Kozubik K., Smardova, J., Brychtova, Y., Doubek, M., Trbusek, M., Mayer, J., & Pospisilova, S. miR-34a, miR-29c and miR-17-5p are downregulated in CLL patients with TP53 abnormalities. Leukemia 23[6], 1159-1163. 2009.

Muljo, S. A., Ansel, K. M., Kanellopoulou, C., Livingston, D. M., Rao, A., & Rajewsky, K. Aberrant T cell differentiation in the absence of Dicer. J.Exp.Med. 202[2], 261-269. 7-18-2005.

Nagaraj, S., Gupta, K., Pisarev, V., Kinarsky, L., Sherman, S., Kang, L., Herber, D. L., Schneck, J., & Gabrilovich, D. I. Altered recognition of antigen is a mechanism of CD8+ T cell tolerance in cancer. Nat.Med. 13[7], 828-835. 2007.

Neilson, J. R., Zheng, G. X., Burge, C. B., & Sharp, P. A. Dynamic regulation of miRNA expression in ordered stages of cellular development. Genes Dev. 21[5], 578-589. 3-1-2007.

Nelson, P. T., Baldwin, D. A., Kloosterman, W. P., Kauppinen, S., Plasterk, R. H., & Mourelatos, Z. RAKE and LNA-ISH reveal microRNA expression and localization in archival human brain. RNA. 12[2], 187-191. 2006.

Nelson, P. T., Dimayuga, J., & Wilfred, B. R. MicroRNA in Situ Hybridization in the Human Entorhinal and Transentorhinal Cortex. Front Hum.Neurosci. 4, 7. 2010.

Nelson, P. T. & Wilfred, B. R. In situ hybridization is a necessary experimental complement to microRNA (miRNA) expression profiling in the human brain. Neurosci.Lett. 466[2], 69-72. 4-23-2009.

Nielsen, B. S., Jorgensen, S., Fog, J. U., Sokilde, R., Christensen, I. J., Hansen, U., Brunner, N., Baker, A., Moller, S., & Nielsen, H. J. High levels of microRNA-21 in the stroma of colorectal cancers predict short disease-free survival in stage II colon cancer patients. Clin.Exp.Metastasis 28[1], 27-38. 2011.

O'Connell, R. M., Chaudhuri, A. A., Rao, D. S., & Baltimore, D. Inositol phosphatase SHIP1 is a primary target of miR-155. Proc.Natl.Acad.Sci.U.S.A 106[17], 7113-7118. 4-28-2009.

O'Connell, R. M., Kahn, D., Gibson, W. S., Round, J. L., Scholz, R. L., Chaudhuri, A. A., Kahn, M. E., Rao, D. S., & Baltimore, D. MicroRNA-155 promotes autoimmune inflammation by enhancing inflammatory T cell development. Immunity. 33[4], 607-619. 10-29-2010a.

O'Connell, R. M., Rao, D. S., Chaudhuri, A. A., & Baltimore, D. Physiological and pathological roles for microRNAs in the immune system. Nat.Rev.Immunol. 10[2], 111-122. 2010b.

O'Connell, R. M., Rao, D. S., Chaudhuri, A. A., Boldin, M. P., Taganov, K. D., Nicoll, J., Paquette, R. L., & Baltimore, D. Sustained expression of microRNA-155 in hematopoietic stem cells causes a myeloproliferative disorder. J.Exp.Med. 205[3], 585-594. 3-17-2008.

O'Connell, R. M., Taganov, K. D., Boldin, M. P., Cheng, G., & Baltimore, D. MicroRNA-155 is induced during the macrophage inflammatory response. Proc.Natl.Acad.Sci.U.S.A 104[5], 1604-1609. 1-30-2007.

O'Neill, L. A., Sheedy, F. J., & McCoy, C. E. MicroRNAs: the fine-tuners of Toll-like receptor signalling. Nat.Rev.Immunol. 11[3], 163-175. 2011.

Oertli, M., Engler, D. B., Kohler, E., Koch, M., Meyer, T. F., & Muller, A. MicroRNA-155 is essential for the T cell-mediated control of helicobacter pylori infection and for the induction of chronic Gastritis and Colitis. J.Immunol. 187[7], 3578-3586. 10-1-2011.

Ohyashiki, K., Umezu, T., Yoshizawa, S., Ito, Y., Ohyashiki, M., Kawashima, H., Tanaka, M., Kuroda, M., & Ohyashiki, J. H. Clinical impact of down-regulated plasma miR-92a levels in non-Hodgkin's lymphoma. PLoS.ONE. 6[2], e16408. 2011.

Ota, D., Mimori, K., Yokobori, T., Iwatsuki, M., Kataoka, A., Masuda, N., Ishii, H., Ohno, S., & Mori, M. Identification of recurrence-related microRNAs in the bone marrow of breast cancer patients. Int.J.Oncol. 38[4], 955-962. 2011.

Pallante, P., Visone, R., Croce, C. M., & Fusco, A. Deregulation of microRNA expression in follicular-cell-derived human thyroid carcinomas. Endocr.Relat Cancer 17[1], F91-104. 2010.

Parker, T. L. & Strout, M. P. Chronic lymphocytic leukemia: prognostic factors and impact on treatment. Discov.Med. 11[57], 115-123. 2011.

Pekarsky, Y., Santanam, U., Cimmino, A., Palamarchuk, A., Efanov, A., Maximov, V., Volinia, S., Alder, H., Liu, C. G., Rassenti, L., Calin, G. A., Hagan, J. P., Kipps, T., & Croce, C. M. Tcl1 expression in chronic lymphocytic leukemia is regulated by miR-29 and miR-181. Cancer Res. 66[24], 11590-11593. 12-15-2006.

Pino, M. S. & Chung, D. C. Microsatellite instability in the management of colorectal cancer. Expert.Rev.Gastroenterol.Hepatol. 5[3], 385-399. 2011.

Preis, M., Gardner, T. B., Gordon, S. R., Pipas, M. J., Mackenzie, T. A., Klein, E. E., Longnecker, D. S., Gutmann, E. J., Sempere, L. F., & Korc, M. microRNA-10b Expression Correlates with Response to Neoadjuvant Therapy and Survival in Pancreatic Ductal Adenocarcinoma. Clin.Cancer Res. 6-7-2011.

Pulikkan, J. A., Peramangalam, P. S., Dengler, V., Ho, P. A., Preudhomme, C., Meshinchi, S., Christopeit, M., Nibourel, O., Muller-Tidow, C., Bohlander, S. K., Tenen, D. G., & Behre, G. C/EBPalpha regulated microRNA-34a targets E2F3 during granulopoiesis and is down-regulated in AML with CEBPA mutations. Blood 116[25], 5638-5649. 12-16-2010.

Qian, P., Zuo, Z., Wu, Z., Meng, X., Li, G., Wu, Z., Zhang, W., Tan, S., Pandey, V., Yao, Y., Wang, P., Zhao, L., Wang, J., Wu, Q., Song, E., Lobie, P. E., Yin, Z., & Zhu, T. Pivotal role of reduced let-7g expression in breast cancer invasion and metastasis. Cancer Res. 71[20], 6463-6474. 10-15-2011.

Radojicic, J., Zaravinos, A., Vrekoussis, T., Kafousi, M., Spandidos, D. A., & Stathopoulos, E. N. MicroRNA expression analysis in triple-negative (ER, PR and Her2/neu) breast cancer. Cell Cycle 10[3], 507-517. 2-1-2011.

Raponi, M., Dossey, L., Jatkoe, T., Wu, X., Chen, G., Fan, H., & Beer, D. G. MicroRNA classifiers for predicting prognosis of squamous cell lung cancer. Cancer Res. 69[14], 5776-5783. 7-15-2009.

Rask, L., Balslev, E., Jorgensen, S., Eriksen, J., Flyger, H., Moller, S., Hogdall, E., Litman, T., & Schnack, Nielsen B. High expression of miR-21 in tumor stroma correlates with increased cancer cell proliferation in human breast cancer. APMIS 119[10], 663-673. 2011.

Rodriguez, A., Vigorito, E., Clare, S., Warren, M. V., Couttet, P., Soond, D. R., van, Dongen S., Grocock, R. J., Das, P. P., Miska, E. A., Vetrie, D., Okkenhaug, K., Enright, A. J., Dougan, G., Turner, M., & Bradley, A. Requirement of bic/microRNA-155 for normal immune function. Science 316[5824], 608-611. 4-27-2007.

Rodriguez, P. C., Ernstoff, M. S., Hernandez, C., Atkins, M., Zabaleta, J., Sierra, R., & Ochoa, A. C. Arginase I-producing myeloid-derived suppressor cells in renal cell carcinoma are a subpopulation of activated granulocytes. Cancer Res. 69[4], 1553-1560. 2-15-2009.

Rodriguez-Gonzalez, F. G., Sieuwerts, A. M., Smid, M., Look, M. P., Meijer-van Gelder, M. E., de, Weerd, V, Sleijfer, S., Martens, J. W., & Foekens, J. A. MicroRNA-30c expression level is an independent predictor of clinical benefit of endocrine therapy in advanced estrogen receptor positive breast cancer. Breast Cancer Res.Treat. 127[1], 43-51. 2011.

Roehle, A., Hoefig, K. P., Repsilber, D., Thorns, C., Ziepert, M., Wesche, K. O., Thiere, M., Loeffler, M., Klapper, W., Pfreundschuh, M., Matolcsy, A., Bernd, H. W., Reiniger, L., Merz, H., & Feller, A. C. MicroRNA signatures characterize diffuse large B-cell lymphomas and follicular lymphomas. Br.J.Haematol. 142[5], 732-744. 2008.

Roepman, P., Jassem, J., Smit, E. F., Muley, T., Niklinski, J., van, de, V, Witteveen, A. T., Rzyman, W., Floore, A., Burgers, S., Giaccone, G., Meister, M., Dienemann, H., Skrzypski, M., Kozlowski, M., Mooi, W. J., & van, Zandwijk N. An immune response enriched 72-gene prognostic profile for early-stage non-small-cell lung cancer. Clin.Cancer Res. 15[1], 284-290. 1-1-2009.

Rossi, R. L., Rossetti, G., Wenandy, L., Curti, S., Ripamonti, A., Bonnal, R. J., Birolo, R. S., Moro, M., Crosti, M. C., Gruarin, P., Maglie, S., Marabita, F., Mascheroni, D., Parente, V., Comelli, M., Trabucchi, E., De, Francesco R., Geginat, J., Abrignani, S., & Pagani, M. Distinct microRNA signatures in human lymphocyte subsets and enforcement of the naive state in CD4+ T cells by the microRNA miR-125b. Nat.Immunol. 12[8], 796-803. 2011.

Rossi, S., Shimizu, M., Barbarotto, E., Nicoloso, M. S., Dimitri, F., Sampath, D., Fabbri, M., Lerner, S., Barron, L. L., Rassenti, L. Z., Jiang, L., Xiao, L., Hu, J., Secchiero, P., Zauli, G., Volinia, S., Negrini, M., Wierda, W., Kipps, T. J., Plunkett, W., Coombes, K. R., Abruzzo, L. V., Keating, M. J., & Calin, G. A. microRNA fingerprinting of CLL patients with chromosome 17p deletion identify a miR-21 score that stratifies early survival. Blood 116[6], 945-952. 8-12-2010.

Saba, R. & Schratt, G. M. MicroRNAs in neuronal development, function and dysfunction. Brain Res. 1338, 3-13. 6-18-2010.

Salmena, L., Poliseno, L., Tay, Y., Kats, L., & Pandolfi, P. P. A ceRNA hypothesis: the Rosetta Stone of a hidden RNA language? Cell 146[3], 353-358. 8-5-2011.

Sampath, D., Liu, C., Vasan, K., Sulda, M., Puduvalli, V. K., Wierda, W. G., & Keating, M. J. Histone deacetylases mediate the silencing of miR-15a, miR-16 and miR-29b in chronic lymphocytic leukemia. Blood . 11-16-2011.

Sato, E., Olson, S. H., Ahn, J., Bundy, B., Nishikawa, H., Qian, F., Jungbluth, A. A., Frosina, D., Gnjatic, S., Ambrosone, C., Kepner, J., Odunsi, T., Ritter, G., Lele, S., Chen, Y. T., Ohtani, H., Old, L. J., & Odunsi, K. Intraepithelial CD8+ tumor-infiltrating lymphocytes and a high CD8+/regulatory T cell ratio are associated with favorable prognosis in ovarian cancer. Proc.Natl.Acad.Sci.U.S.A 102[51], 18538-18543. 12-20-2005.

Scarlett, U. K., Cubillos-Ruiz, J. R., Nesbeth, Y. C., Martinez, D. G., Engle, X., Gewirtz, A. T., Ahonen, C. L., & Conejo-Garcia, J. R. In situ stimulation of CD40 and Toll-like receptor 3 transforms ovarian cancer-infiltrating dendritic cells from immunosuppressive to immunostimulatory cells. Cancer Res. 69[18], 7329-7337. 9-15-2009.

Schepeler, T., Reinert, J. T., Ostenfeld, M. S., Christensen, L. L., Silahtaroglu, A. N., Dyrskjot, L., Wiuf, C., Sorensen, F. J., Kruhoffer, M., Laurberg, S., Kauppinen, S., Orntoft, T. F., & Andersen, C. L. Diagnostic and prognostic microRNAs in stage II colon cancer. Cancer Res. 68[15], 6416-6424. 8-1-2008.

Schneider, M., Andersen, D. C., Silahtaroglu, A., Lyngbaek, S., Kauppinen, S., Hansen, J. L., & Sheikh, S. P. Cell-specific detection of microRNA expression during cardiomyogenesis by combined in situ hybridization and immunohistochemistry. J.Mol.Histol. 42[4], 289-299. 2011.

Scholer, N., Langer, C., Dohner, H., Buske, C., & Kuchenbauer, F. Serum microRNAs as a novel class of biomarkers: a comprehensive review of the literature. Exp.Hematol. 38[12], 1126-1130. 2010.

Schotte, D., Moqadam, F. A., Lange-Turenhout, E. A., Chen, C., van Ijcken, W. F., Pieters, R., & den Boer, M. L. Discovery of new microRNAs by small RNAome deep sequencing in childhood acute lymphoblastic leukemia. Leukemia 25[9], 1389-1399. 2011.

Schwarzenbach, H., Hoon, D. S., & Pantel, K. Cell-free nucleic acids as biomarkers in cancer patients. Nat.Rev.Cancer 11[6], 426-437. 2011.

Schwind, S., Maharry, K., Radmacher, M. D., Mrozek, K., Holland, K. B., Margeson, D., Whitman, S. P., Hickey, C., Becker, H., Metzeler, K. H., Paschka, P., Baldus, C. D., Liu, S., Garzon, R., Powell, B. L., Kolitz, J. E., Carroll, A. J., Caligiuri, M. A., Larson, R. A., Marcucci, G., & Bloomfield, C. D. Prognostic significance of expression of a single microRNA, miR-181a, in cytogenetically normal acute myeloid leukemia: a Cancer and Leukemia Group B study. J.Clin.Oncol. 28[36], 5257-5264. 12-20-2010.

Selbach, M., Schwanhausser, B., Thierfelder, N., Fang, Z., Khanin, R., & Rajewsky, N. Widespread changes in protein synthesis induced by microRNAs. Nature 455[7209], 58-63. 9-4-2008.

Sempere, L. F. Integrating contextual miRNA and protein signatures for diagnostic and treatment decisions in cancer. Expert.Rev.Mol.Diagn. 11[8], 813-827. 2011.

Sempere, L. F., Christensen, M., Silahtaroglu, A., Bak, M., Heath, C. V., Schwartz, G., Wells, W., Kauppinen, S., & Cole, C. N. Altered MicroRNA expression confined to specific epithelial cell subpopulations in breast cancer. Cancer Res. 67[24], 11612-11620. 12-15-2007.

Sempere, L. F. & Kauppinen, S. Translational Implications of MicroRNAs in Clinical Diagnostics and Therapeutics. Bradshaw R.A. and Dennis E.A. Handbook of Cell Signaling. 2nd[340], 2965-2981 . 2009. Oxford, Academic Press. Ref Type: Book Chapter

Sempere, L. F., Preis, M., Yezefski, T., Ouyang, H., Suriawinata, A. A., Silahtaroglu, A., Conejo-Garcia, J. R., Kauppinen, S., Wells, W., & Korc, M. Fluorescence-based codetection with protein markers reveals distinct cellular compartments for altered MicroRNA expression in solid tumors. Clin.Cancer Res. 16[16], 4246-4255. 8-15-2010.

Seo, K. H., Zhou, L., Meng, D., Xu, J., Dong, Z., & Mi, Q. S. Loss of microRNAs in thymus perturbs invariant NKT cell development and function. Cell Mol.Immunol. 7[6], 447-453. 2010.

Shiow, L. R., Rosen, D. B., Brdickova, N., Xu, Y., An, J., Lanier, L. L., Cyster, J. G., & Matloubian, M. CD69 acts downstream of interferon-alpha/beta to inhibit S1P1 and lymphocyte egress from lymphoid organs. Nature 440[7083], 540-544. 3-23-2006.

Sims, A. H., Ong, K. R., Clarke, R. B., & Howell, A. High-throughput genomic technology in research and clinical management of breast cancer. Exploiting the potential of gene expression profiling: is it ready for the clinic? Breast Cancer Res. 8[5], 214. 2006.

Sinha, P., Okoro, C., Foell, D., Freeze, H. H., Ostrand-Rosenberg, S., & Srikrishna, G. Proinflammatory S100 proteins regulate the accumulation of myeloid-derived suppressor cells. J.Immunol. 181[7], 4666-4675. 10-1-2008.

Sorlie, T. Molecular portraits of breast cancer: tumour subtypes as distinct disease entities. Eur.J.Cancer 40[18], 2667-2675. 2004.

Stamatopoulos, B., Meuleman, N., De, Bruyn C., Pieters, K., Anthoine, G., Mineur, P., Bron, D., & Lagneaux, L. A molecular score by quantitative PCR as a new prognostic tool at diagnosis for chronic lymphocytic leukemia patients. PLoS.ONE. 5[9]. 2010.

Stamatopoulos, B., Meuleman, N., Haibe-Kains, B., Saussoy, P., Van Den, Neste E., Michaux, L., Heimann, P., Martiat, P., Bron, D., & Lagneaux, L. microRNA-29c and microRNA-223 down-regulation has in vivo significance in chronic lymphocytic leukemia and improves disease risk stratification. Blood 113[21], 5237-5245. 5-21-2009.

Stittrich, A. B., Haftmann, C., Sgouroudis, E., Kuhl, A. A., Hegazy, A. N., Panse, I., Riedel, R., Flossdorf, M., Dong, J., Fuhrmann, F., Heinz, G. A., Fang, Z., Li, N., Bissels, U., Hatam, F., Jahn, A., Hammoud, B., Matz, M., Schulze, F. M., Baumgrass, R., Bosio, A., Mollenkopf, H. J., Grun, J., Thiel, A., Chen, W., Hofer, T., Loddenkemper, C., Lohning, M., Chang, H. D., Rajewsky, N., Radbruch, A., & Mashreghi, M. F. The microRNA miR-182 is induced by IL-2 and promotes clonal expansion of activated helper T lymphocytes. Nat.Immunol. 11[11], 1057-1062. 2010.

Surdziel, E., Cabanski, M., Dallmann, I., Lyszkiewicz, M., Krueger, A., Ganser, A., Scherr, M., & Eder, M. Enforced expression of miR-125b affects myelopoiesis by targeting multiple signaling pathways. Blood 117[16], 4338-4348. 4-21-2011.

Taganov, K. D., Boldin, M. P., Chang, K. J., & Baltimore, D. NF-kappaB-dependent induction of microRNA miR-146, an inhibitor targeted to signaling proteins of innate immune responses. Proc.Natl.Acad.Sci.U.S.A 103[33], 12481-12486. 8-15-2006.

Tan, L. P., Wang, M., Robertus, J. L., Schakel, R. N., Gibcus, J. H., Diepstra, A., Harms, G., Peh, S. C., Reijmers, R. M., Pals, S. T., Kroesen, B. J., Kluin, P. M., Poppema, S., &

van den, Berg A. miRNA profiling of B-cell subsets: specific miRNA profile for germinal center B cells with variation between centroblasts and centrocytes. Lab Invest 89[6], 708-716. 2009.

Tang, D., Kang, R., Zeh, H. J., III, & Lotze, M. T. High-mobility group box 1 and cancer. Biochim.Biophys.Acta 1799[1-2], 131-140. 2010.

Teichler, S., Illmer, T., Roemhild, J., Ovcharenko, D., Stiewe, T., & Neubauer, A. MicroRNA29a regulates the expression of the nuclear oncogene Ski. Blood 118[7], 1899-1902. 8-18-2011.

Thai, T. H., Calado, D. P., Casola, S., Ansel, K. M., Xiao, C., Xue, Y., Murphy, A., Frendewey, D., Valenzuela, D., Kutok, J. L., Schmidt-Supprian, M., Rajewsky, N., Yancopoulos, G., Rao, A., & Rajewsky, K. Regulation of the germinal center response by microRNA-155. Science 316[5824], 604-608. 4-27-2007.

Tili, E., Croce, C. M., & Michaille, J. J. miR-155: on the crosstalk between inflammation and cancer. Int.Rev.Immunol. 28[5], 264-284. 2009.

Tomasi, T. B., Magner, W. J., Wiesen, J. L., Oshlag, J. Z., Cao, F., Pontikos, A. N., & Gregorie, C. J. MHC class II regulation by epigenetic agents and microRNAs. Immunol.Res. 46[1-3], 45-58. 2010.

Tserel, L., Runnel, T., Kisand, K., Pihlap, M., Bakhoff, L., Kolde, R., Peterson, H., Vilo, J., Peterson, P., & Rebane, A. MicroRNA expression profiles of human blood monocyte-derived dendritic cells and macrophages reveal miR-511 as putative positive regulator of Toll-like receptor 4. J.Biol.Chem. 286[30], 26487-26495. 7-29-2011.

Turner, M. & Vigorito, E. Regulation of B- and T-cell differentiation by a single microRNA. Biochem.Soc.Trans. 36[Pt 3], 531-533. 2008.

Turner, M. L., Schnorfeil, F. M., & Brocker, T. MicroRNAs regulate dendritic cell differentiation and function. J.Immunol. 187[8], 3911-3917. 10-15-2011.

Valadi, H., Ekstrom, K., Bossios, A., Sjostrand, M., Lee, J. J., & Lotvall, J. O. Exosome-mediated transfer of mRNAs and microRNAs is a novel mechanism of genetic exchange between cells. Nat.Cell Biol. 9[6], 654-659. 2007.

van Kouwenhove M., Kedde, M., & Agami, R. MicroRNA regulation by RNA-binding proteins and its implications for cancer. Nat.Rev.Cancer 11[9], 644-656. 2011.

Velu, C. S., Baktula, A. M., & Grimes, H. L. Gfi1 regulates miR-21 and miR-196b to control myelopoiesis. Blood 113[19], 4720-4728. 5-7-2009.

Ventura, A. & Jacks, T. MicroRNAs and cancer: short RNAs go a long way. Cell 136[4], 586-591. 2-20-2009.

Ventura, A., Young, A. G., Winslow, M. M., Lintault, L., Meissner, A., Erkeland, S. J., Newman, J., Bronson, R. T., Crowley, D., Stone, J. R., Jaenisch, R., Sharp, P. A., & Jacks, T. Targeted deletion reveals essential and overlapping functions of the miR-17 through 92 family of miRNA clusters. Cell 132[5], 875-886. 3-7-2008.

Vigorito, E., Perks, K. L., breu-Goodger, C., Bunting, S., Xiang, Z., Kohlhaas, S., Das, P. P., Miska, E. A., Rodriguez, A., Bradley, A., Smith, K. G., Rada, C., Enright, A. J., Toellner, K. M., Maclennan, I. C., & Turner, M. microRNA-155 regulates the generation of immunoglobulin class-switched plasma cells. Immunity. 27[6], 847-859. 2007.

Vilar, E. & Gruber, S. B. Microsatellite instability in colorectal cancer-the stable evidence. Nat.Rev.Clin.Oncol. 7[3], 153-162. 2010.

Wang, F., Wang, X. S., Yang, G. H., Zhai, P. F., Xiao, Z., Xia, L. Y., Chen, L. R., Wang, Y., Wang, X. Z., Bi, L. X., Liu, N., Yu, Y., Gao, D., Huang, B. T., Wang, J., Zhou, D. B., Gong, J. N., Zhao, H. L., Bi, X. H., Yu, J., & Zhang, J. W. miR-29a and miR-142-3p downregulation and diagnostic implication in human acute myeloid leukemia. Mol.Biol.Rep. 6-16-2011a.

Wang, P., Hou, J., Lin, L., Wang, C., Liu, X., Li, D., Ma, F., Wang, Z., & Cao, X. Inducible microRNA-155 feedback promotes type I IFN signaling in antiviral innate immunity by targeting suppressor of cytokine signaling 1. J.Immunol. 185[10], 6226-6233. 11-15-2010.

Wang, W., Corrigan-Cummins, M., Hudson, J., Maric, I., Simakova, O., Neelapu, S. S., Kwak, L. W., Janik, J. E., Gause, B., Jaffe, E. S., & Calvo, K. R. MicroRNA profiling of follicular lymphoma identifies microRNAs related to cell proliferation and tumor response. Haematologica . 11-18-2011b.

Wasiuk, A., de, Vries, V, Hartmann, K., Roers, A., & Noelle, R. J. Mast cells as regulators of adaptive immunity to tumours. Clin.Exp.Immunol. 155[2], 140-146. 2009.

Wieser, R., Scheideler, M., Hackl, H., Engelmann, M., Schneckenleithner, C., Hiden, K., Papak, C., Trajanoski, Z., Sill, H., & Fonatsch, C. microRNAs in acute myeloid leukemia: expression patterns, correlations with genetic and clinical parameters, and prognostic significance. Genes Chromosomes.Cancer 49[3], 193-203. 2010.

Williams, M. E., Connors, J. M., Dreyling, M. H., Gascoyne, R. D., Kahl, B. S., Leonard, J. P., Press, O. W., & Wilson, W. H. Mantle cell lymphoma: report of the 2010 Mantle Cell Lymphoma Consortium Workshop. Leuk.Lymphoma 52[1], 24-33. 2011.

Wistuba, I. I. & Gazdar, A. F. Lung cancer preneoplasia. Annu.Rev.Pathol. 1, 331-348. 2006.

Wu, H., Neilson, J. R., Kumar, P., Manocha, M., Shankar, P., Sharp, P. A., & Manjunath, N. miRNA profiling of naive, effector and memory CD8 T cells. PLoS.ONE. 2[10], e1020. 2007.

Xiao, C., Calado, D. P., Galler, G., Thai, T. H., Patterson, H. C., Wang, J., Rajewsky, N., Bender, T. P., & Rajewsky, K. MiR-150 controls B cell differentiation by targeting the transcription factor c-Myb. Cell 131[1], 146-159. 10-5-2007.

Xiao, C. & Rajewsky, K. MicroRNA control in the immune system: basic principles. Cell 136[1], 26-36. 1-9-2009.

Xiong, Y., Li, Z., Ji, M., Tan, A. C., Bemis, J., Tse, J. V., Huang, G., Park, J., Ji, C., Chen, J., Bemis, L. T., Bunting, K. D., & Tse, W. MIR29B regulates expression of MLLT11 (AF1Q), an MLL fusion partner, and low MIR29B expression associates with adverse cytogenetics and poor overall survival in AML. Br.J.Haematol. 153[6], 753-757. 2011.

Yamamichi, N., Shimomura, R., Inada, K., Sakurai, K., Haraguchi, T., Ozaki, Y., Fujita, S., Mizutani, T., Furukawa, C., Fujishiro, M., Ichinose, M., Shiogama, K., Tsutsumi, Y., Omata, M., & Iba, H. Locked nucleic acid in situ hybridization analysis of miR-21 expression during colorectal cancer development. Clin.Cancer Res. 15[12], 4009-4016. 6-15-2009.

Yu, P. & Fu, Y. X. Tumor-infiltrating T lymphocytes: friends or foes? Lab Invest 86[3], 231-245. 2006.

Yu, S. L., Chen, H. Y., Chang, G. C., Chen, C. Y., Chen, H. W., Singh, S., Cheng, C. L., Yu, C. J., Lee, Y. C., Chen, H. S., Su, T. J., Chiang, C. C., Li, H. N., Hong, Q. S., Su, H. Y., Chen, C. C., Chen, W. J., Liu, C. C., Chan, W. K., Chen, W. J., Li, K. C., Chen, J. J., &

Yang, P. C. MicroRNA signature predicts survival and relapse in lung cancer. Cancer Cell 13[1], 48-57. 2008.

Zauli, G., Voltan, R., di Iasio, M. G., Bosco, R., Melloni, E., Sana, M. E., & Secchiero, P. miR-34a induces the downregulation of both E2F1 and B-Myb oncogenes in leukemic cells. Clin.Cancer Res. 17[9], 2712-2724. 5-1-2011.

Zhang, M., Liu, Q., Mi, S., Liang, X., Zhang, Z., Su, X., Liu, J., Chen, Y., Wang, M., Zhang, Y., Guo, F., Zhang, Z., & Yang, R. Both miR-17-5p and miR-20a alleviate suppressive potential of myeloid-derived suppressor cells by modulating STAT3 expression. J.Immunol. 186[8], 4716-4724. 4-15-2011.

Zhang, N. & Bevan, M. J. Dicer controls CD8+ T-cell activation, migration, and survival. Proc.Natl.Acad.Sci.U.S.A 107[50], 21629-21634. 12-14-2010.

Zhao, J. J., Lin, J., Lwin, T., Yang, H., Guo, J., Kong, W., Dessureault, S., Moscinski, L. C., Rezania, D., Dalton, W. S., Sotomayor, E., Tao, J., & Cheng, J. Q. microRNA expression profile and identification of miR-29 as a prognostic marker and pathogenetic factor by targeting CDK6 in mantle cell lymphoma. Blood 115[13], 2630-2639. 4-1-2010.

Zhao, J. L., Rao, D. S., Boldin, M. P., Taganov, K. D., O'Connell, R. M., & Baltimore, D. NF-kappaB dysregulation in microRNA-146a-deficient mice drives the development of myeloid malignancies. Proc.Natl.Acad.Sci.U.S.A 108[22], 9184-9189. 5-31-2011.

Zhou, L., Seo, K. H., He, H. Z., Pacholczyk, R., Meng, D. M., Li, C. G., Xu, J., She, J. X., Dong, Z., & Mi, Q. S. Tie2cre-induced inactivation of the miRNA-processing enzyme Dicer disrupts invariant NKT cell development. Proc.Natl.Acad.Sci.U.S.A 106[25], 10266-10271. 6-23-2009.

Zhou, X., Jeker, L. T., Fife, B. T., Zhu, S., Anderson, M. S., McManus, M. T., & Bluestone, J. A. Selective miRNA disruption in T reg cells leads to uncontrolled autoimmunity. J.Exp.Med. 205[9], 1983-1991. 9-1-2008.

Zhu, D. X., Miao, K. R., Fang, C., Fan, L., Zhu, W., Zhu, H. Y., Zhuang, Y., Hong, M., Liu, P., Xu, W., & Li, J. Y. Aberrant microRNA expression in Chinese patients with chronic lymphocytic leukemia. Leuk.Res. 35[6], 730-734. 2011.

Zitvogel, L., Tesniere, A., & Kroemer, G. Cancer despite immunosurveillance: immunoselection and immunosubversion. Nat.Rev.Immunol. 6[10], 715-727. 2006.

Zou, W. Immunosuppressive networks in the tumour environment and their therapeutic relevance. Nat.Rev.Cancer 5[4], 263-274. 2005.

12

The Role of Mesenchymal Stem Cells in the Tumor Microenvironment

Aline M. Betancourt and Ruth S. Waterman
Tulane University School of Medicine and Ochsner Clinic Foundation, New Orleans, Louisiana, USA

1. Introduction

Currently, there are many promising clinical trials using mesenchymal stem cells (MSCs) in cell-based therapies of diseases ranging widely from graft-versus-host to joint and cartilage disorders (Salem and Thiemermann 2010; Tolar, Le Blanc et al.). Increasingly, however, there is a concern over the clinical use of MSCs because they are also known to home to tumors and once resident in the tumor microenvironment (TME) to support tumor growth and spread (Karnoub, Dash et al. 2007; Kidd, Spaeth et al. 2008; Coffelt, Marini et al. 2009; Klopp, Gupta et al. 2010; Klopp, Gupta et al. 2011). Conversely, other studies have reported that MSCs found in the TME diminish tumor growth, which has further generated some controversy in this field (reviewed in (Klopp, Gupta et al. 2010; Klopp, Gupta et al. 2011). Either way as a result of the MSC propensity for the TME, genetically modified MSCs that can act as "Trojan horses" and deliver anti-cancer therapeutics into the tumor stroma are being evaluated as a promising new specific cell-based therapy for cancer.

Our group established that MSCs in the ovarian tumor microenvironment promoted tumor growth and favored angiogenesis (Zwezdaryk, Coffelt et al. 2007; Coffelt and Scandurro 2008; Coffelt, Marini et al. 2009). We also developed new methodology to induce the conventional mixed pool of MSCs into two uniform but distinct phenotypes, *MSC1* and *MSC2* (Waterman, Tomchuck et al. 2010). We based their classification on several parallel observations reported within the monocyte literature. Like MSCs, heterogeneous bone marrow-derived monocytes respond to stress or "danger" inflammatory signals and home to tissue injury. Monocyte polarization into pro-inflammatory macrophages (M1) occurs early on in tissue repair whereas, monocyte polarization into anti-inflammatory macrophages (M2) follows later to help in tissue injury resolution (Mantovani, Sozzani et al. 2002; Martinez, Gordon et al. 2006). Although, this is a much simplified view of what occurs in the complex process of wound healing and repair, it provides a convenient paradigm to begin to dissect critical components within this biological process (Mantovani, Sica et al. 2007; Mosser and Edwards 2008; Mosser and Zhang 2008). Likewise, we believe that pro-inflammatory *MSC1* and anti-inflammatory *MSC2* provide convenient tools with which to begin to interrogate the role of MSCs in the tumor microenvironment.

In recent studies we found that *MSC2* supported ovarian cancer growth and spread while surprisingly *MSC1* had an opposite anti-tumor effect (Waterman 2011). We suggest that by more closely studying the distinct tumor effects observed for these MSC phenotypes we may figure out why in the studies mentioned above MSCs favor tumor growth while in others MSCs attenuate tumors. In other words, induction into each discrete but uniform phenotype may help resolve some of the controversies surrounding the use of MSCs in cell based-therapies.

It is known that MSCs resident in the TME contribute mitogens, extracellular matrix proteins, angiogenic, and inflammatory factors. These contributions are not trivial to tumor growth and spread and serve to recruit specific subsets of leukocytes and endothelia to the TME that profoundly influence tumors. *MSC1* in the TME are expected to attenuate tumor growth by secretion of anti-tumor factors and recruitment of anti-tumor immunity. *MSC2* found in TME should promote tumor growth and spread by secretion of mitogens and supressing anti-tumor immune responses. We expect that by identifying the differences between these two phenotypes we will shed some light on the growing controversy on the role of MSCs in tumors, and provide a means to safely deliver MSCs in cell-based therapies. We have attempted to provide all relevant information that is available concerning these issues in the sections included in this chapter.

2. Current understanding of MSCs function in the TME

Mesenchymal stem cells (MSCs) are a group of heterogeneous multipotent cells that can be easily isolated from many tissues throughout the body. Though initially isolated from the bone marrow, they are now recognized to be mostly in perivascular regions throughout the body (Feng, Mantesso et al. ; Zwezdaryk, Coffelt et al. 2007; da Silva Meirelles, Caplan et al. 2008). The discovery of these cells dates back to the 1960s (Friedenstein, Piatetzky et al. 1966). In recent years, MSCs have been widely studied due to their ability to be expanded in culture and stored without losing their capacity to differentiate into many different cells of mesodermal origin such as osteoblasts, chondrocytes, and adipocytes (Bruder, Jaiswal et al. 1997; Jaiswal, Haynesworth et al. 1997; Digirolamo, Stokes et al. 1999; Phinney, Kopen et al. 1999; Pittenger, Mackay et al. 1999). MSCs can also transdifferentiate into cells of ectodermal (Kopen, Prockop et al. 1999) and endodermal (Sun, Chen et al. 2007; Ju, Teng et al. 2010) origins. As a result, many preclinical studies have focused on evaluating the capacity of MSCs to repair and replace injured or diseased tissues of all origins.

Despite these research efforts however, there is growing evidence that the clinical benefit of MSCs in cell-based therapies is not the replacement of the injured tissue, but rather their efficiency in modulating aberrant host immune responses (Pittenger, Mackay et al. 1999; Prockop 2003; Prockop 2009). Following the remarkable clinical observations by the Le Blanc group who used the successful delivery of MSCs as a last resort to stave off graft-versus-host disease in a young boy, the immune modulating capability of MSCs is now more widely recognized (Le Blanc, Rasmusson et al. 2004). Further evidence indicating that immunomodulation is the primary activity of MSCs can be gleaned from the observation in many studies that although infused MSCs home to sites of injury and provide treatment benefit in widely ranging diseases, they can rarely be detected within the repaired tissue. Subsequent research efforts are beginning to identify the myriad ways that MSCs affect host immune responses. These appear to be mediated both by direct cell-to-cell contact and indirectly by the secretion of inflammatory factors (further discussed below) (Aggarwal and Pittenger 2005; Abdi, Fiorina et al. 2008; Uccelli, Moretta et al. 2008; Nemeth, Mayer et al. 2009; Bunnell, Betancourt et al. 2010; Singer and Caplan 2011).

Thus far, the immune modulating effects of MSCs include inhibition of the proliferation of activated CD8+ and CD4+ T lymphocytes and natural killer (NK) cells, recruitment and support of regulatory T cells, suppression of Th17 lymphocytes and immunoglobulin production by plasma cells, inhibition of maturation of dendritic cells (DCs), as well as attenuation of mast cells (Aggarwal and Pittenger 2005; Abdi, Fiorina et al. 2008; Uccelli, Moretta et al. 2008; Nemeth, Mayer et al. 2009; Nemeth, Keane-Myers et al. 2010). MSCs secrete various inflammatory factors including TNF-α-induced protein 6 (TNAIP6 or TSG-6), prostaglandin E2 (PGE2), human leukocyte antigen G5 (HLA-G5), hepatocyte growth factor (HGF), inducible nitric oxide synthase (iNOS), indoleamine-2,3-dioxygenase (IDO), transforming growth factor β (TGF-β), leukemia-inhibitory factor (LIF), and interleukin (IL)-10 (Krampera, Pasini et al. 2006; Gur-Wahnon, Borovsky et al. 2009; Bunnell, Betancourt et al. 2010; Singer and Caplan 2011).

MSCs express low levels of human leukocyte antigen (HLA) major histocompatibility complex (MHC) class I, do not express co-stimulatory molecules (B7-1/CD80 and -2/CD86, CD40, or CD40L), and must be induced to express MHC class II and Fas ligand that likely allows the safe delivery of these cells in non-self (allogeneic) hosts (Aggarwal and Pittenger 2005; Bunnell, Betancourt et al. 2010). Indeed, MSCs stand alone among the other types of stem cells such as embryonic or induced pluripotent (iPS) cells being considered in regenerative medicine for their safe, non-immune provoking, allogeneic host delivery capability. This has prompted many new and established businesses to amass expanded stockpiles of MSCs ready for use in the treatment of many human diseases including cancer (Salem and Thiemermann 2010).

Given the ability to deliver expanded, stockpiled clinical grade MSCs, knowing that they specifically home to the TME, and that they secrete mitogens, extracellular matrix proteins, angiogenic and inflammatory factors, it is not hard to conceive that MSCs might on the one hand influence tumors, and on the other hand, be used as vehicles to deliver anti-cancer agents. At issue is that despite intense study over the past few years, the effect of MSCs on tumors or their function in the TME is far from clear. Some studies report that MSCs promote tumor growth and spread while others report that MSCs attenuate tumor growth (Table 1). The distinct effects by MSCs on tumors has recently been attributed to differences in the experimental cancer model, the heterogeneity of MSC preparations, the dose or timing of the delivered MSCs, the animal host, or some as yet unknown factor (Klopp, Gupta et al. 2010; Klopp, Gupta et al. 2011). Also at play may be that the primary immunomodulatory function of MSCs is not realized in the context of most of these studies, which rely on immune compromised animal models. It is clear however, that with all of their unique properties MSCs make attractive candidates in cell therapies of cancer. In fact, a few promising pre-clinical reports have shown the delivery by MSCs of several anti-cancer therapeutics such as interferon (IFN)-β, cytosine deaminase, tumor necrosis factor-related apoptosis-inducing ligand (TRAIL), and oncolytic viruses to tumors (Pittenger, Mackay et al. 1999; Studeny, Marini et al. 2002; Prockop 2003; Studeny, Marini et al. 2004; Nakamizo, Marini et al. 2005; Ren, Li et al. 2007; Kim, Lim et al. 2008; Ren, Kumar et al. 2008; Ren, Kumar et al. 2008; Mader, Maeyama et al. 2009; Prockop 2009). Though it would seem from these reports that any pro-tumor MSC effect is outweighed by the anti-cancer strategy, it is important to fully understand all of the contributions that MSCs have in the TME of immune competent tumors to safely use them in cell-based therapies of human disease.

It is appreciated that MSCs contribute in a number of ways within the TME. As mentioned above, it has long been documented that MSCs elaborate a number of factors directly, after stimulation, or after contact with adjacent cells. These include mitogens, extracellular matrix (ECM) proteins, angiogenic factors, and inflammatory factors, all of which could potentially influence tumor growth and spread. These are summarized below along with some of the pro-tumorigenic and anti-tumorigenic evidence for MSCs.

2.1 Pro-tumorigenic evidence

There are a growing number of studies implicating a role for MSCs derived from various tissues in tumor growth and spread. Upon review of these studies and the anti-tumorigenic

Study	MSC Source	MSC:Tumor Ratio	Immune Status of animal model	Tumor Model	MSC Effect
(Muehlberg, Song et al. 2009)	Hu, Mu ASCs	10:1	-	Br	Larger tumor, increased SDF-1
(Karnoub, Dash et al. 2007)	Hu BMSCs	3:1	-	Br	Larger tumor, increased spread, CCL5-mediated
(Galie, Konstantinidou et al. 2008)	Mu ASCs	1:1	+	Br	Larger tumors, pro-angiogenesis
(Yu, Ren et al. 2008)	Hu ASCs	1:1, 1:2, 1:10	-	Lu, Glioma	Larger tumor, anti-apoptosis
(Djouad, Plence et al. 2003; Djouad, Fritz et al. 2005)	Mu BMSCs	1:1	+	Melanoma	Larger tumors, inflammation
(Kucerova, Matuskova et al.)	Hu ASCs	1:5-1:10	-	Melanoma Glioblastoma	Larger tumors, VEGF and SDF1-CXCR4
(Coffelt, Marini et al. 2009)	Hu BMSCs	1:10	-	Ova	Larger tumors, pro-angiogenesis
(Lin, Yang et al. 2010)	Hu ASCs	1:2	-	Pr	Larger tumors, pro-angiogenesis and CXCR4
(Prantl, Muehlberg et al.)	Hu ASCs	1:10	-	Pr	Larger tumors, pro-angiogenesis
(Zhu, Xu et al. 2006)	Hu BMSCs	10:1, 1:1	-	Co	Larger tumors, pro-angiogenesis
(Shinagawa, Kitadai et al.)	Hu BMSCs	1:2	-	Co	Larger tumors, anti-apoptosis

Abbreviations: Hu- human, Mu- murine, ASC- adipose-derived MSCs, BMSCs- bone marrow-derived MSCs, Immune Status of animal model- - immune compromised +- immune competent, Br- breast, Lu- lung, Ov- ovarian, Pr- prostate, and Co- colon cancer cell lines.

Table 1. Pro-tumorigenic evidence for MSCs in the TME.

ones below it is tempting to speculate that cancers of endo- and ectodermal tissue origin are likely supported by MSCs whereas cancers of mesodermal tissue origin are likely inhibited by MSCs. However, as stated above, the fact that most of the studies are for technical reasons conducted in immune compromised animals greatly limits these conclusions and our understanding of the final outcome of MSCs in cancer. Evidence that MSCs promote tumor growth and their stated mechanism(s) is given by the studies summarized in Table 1. MSCs supported growth of breast, brain, lung, ovary, prostate, and colon, as well as lymphoma and melanoma (Kucerova, Matuskova et al. ; Shinagawa, Kitadai et al. ; Djouad, Plence et al. 2003; Djouad, Fritz et al. 2005; Zhu, Xu et al. 2006; Karnoub, Dash et al. 2007; Galie, Konstantinidou et al. 2008; Yu, Ren et al. 2008; Coffelt, Marini et al. 2009; Muehlberg, Song et al. 2009; Lin, Yang et al. 2010). The MSCs delivered at high ratios to the experimental tumor cell lines most commonly promoted tumor growth and metastasis. Most studies reported an increase in angiogenesis as a result of increased VEGF production by the MSCs in the TME. Some studies reported attenuation of tumor apoptosis. Chemokines such as Chemokine Ligand-5 (CCL5 or RANTES) and stromal-derived factor-1 (SDF-1)-C-X-C chemokine receptor-4 (CXCR4) axis effects by the MSCs were associated with elevated tumor migration and spread.

The secretion of pro-angiogenic molecules by the MSCs likely assist the tumors in capturing essential nutrients—perhaps also explaining the anti-apoptosis effects-- and in gaining the ability to spread to remote tissues—explaining the role of the chemokines. MSCs are known to secrete pro-angiogenic factors such as VEGF and possibly erythropoietin (Epo) thus this chief effect is not unexpected (Zwezdaryk, Coffelt et al. 2007; Singer and Caplan 2011). More studies are needed that focus on whether MSC conditioned medium is sufficient to elicit these responses and to test whether cell-to-cell contact by the MSCs, leukocytes, and/or cancer cells is required for the promotion of tumor growth and spread by MSCs.

2.2 Anti-tumorigenic evidence

While the pro-tumorigenic activity of MSCs is largely characterized by the secretion of pro-angiogenic molecules, the anti-tumorigenic activity of these cells is exemplified by modulation of members of the Wnt-signaling family (Table 2). MSCs inhibited the growth of tumors in several different models (Maestroni, Hertens et al. 1999; Ohlsson, Varas et al. 2003; Khakoo, Pati et al. 2006; Lu, Yuan et al. 2008; Qiao, Xu et al. 2008; Qiao, Xu et al. 2008; Cousin, Ravet et al. 2009; Otsu, Das et al. 2009; Zhu, Sun et al. 2009; Dasari, Kaur et al. ; Dasari, Velpula et al. ; Secchiero, Zorzet et al.). For instance, in studies that used fetal tissue derived MSCs, their secretion of the Wnt-signalling inhibitor Dickkopf-related protein-1 (DKK-1) inhibited breast and liver cancer cell lines (Qiao, Xu et al. 2008; Qiao, Xu et al. 2008). When the researchers used a neutralizing antibody or small interfering RNA to block DKK-1 within MSCs, the inhibitory tumor effects were attenuated. In the DKK-1 associated inhibition of primary leukemia by adipose-derived MSCs (ASCs), the stem cell transcription factor NANOG was also implicated (Zhu, Sun et al. 2009).

Interestingly, in an immune competent model, MSCs typically believed to be immune suppressive, recruited leukocytes and appeared to favor pro-inflammatory monocyte/granulocyte infiltration, which promoted rat colon carcinoma growth (Ohlsson, Varas et al. 2003). In the other immune competent model studies, one reported lack of immune suppression or attenuation of T-cell activation by the admixed MSCs but did not report the changes in any other pro-inflammatory leukocytes, and the other study was focused more on the effect on angiogenesis by the MSCs rather than on inflammatory cells (Lu, Yuan et al. 2008; Otsu, Das et al. 2009).

Study	MSC Source	MSC:Tumor Ratio	Immune Status of animal model	Tumor Model	MSC Effect
(Khakoo, Pati et al. 2006)	Hu BMSCs	1:1, 2:1	-	Kaposi's Sarcoma	Smaller tumors, E-cadherin dependent AKT-inhibition
(Secchiero, Zorzet et al.)	Hu BMSCs	1:2, 1:10	-	NH-Lymphoma	Smaller tumors, increased animal survival
(Lu, Yuan et al. 2008)	Mu BMSCs	2-4:1	+	Insulinoma Li	Decreased ascites, pro-apoptosis
(Zhu, Sun et al. 2009)	Hu ASCs	1:10	-	Leukemia	DKK-1 mediated anti-proliferation
(Cousin, Ravet et al. 2009)	Hu ASCs	10^3 ASCs/mm^3 tumor	-	Pan	Smaller tumors
(Otsu, Das et al. 2009)	Mu BMSCs	10^6 MSCs/700mm^3 tumor	+	Melanoma	Smaller tumors, anti-angiogenesis
(Maestroni, Hertens et al. 1999)	Hu BMSCs	1:1	-	Melanoma, Lu	Smaller tumors and mets with GM-CSF tx MSCs
(Dasari, Kaur et al. ; Dasari, Velpula et al.)	Hu UCSCs	1:4	-	Glioma	Smaller tumors, ↑PTEN, ↓PI3K,AKT
(Qiao, Xu et al. 2008)	Hu MSCs-TERT tx	1:100	-	Br	Smaller tumors, less mets, DKK-1 mediated Wnt1 inhibition
(Qiao, Xu et al. 2008)	Hu MSCs-TERT tx	1:1	-	Li	Smaller tumors, less mets, DKK-1 mediated Wnt1 inhibition
(Ohlsson, Varas et al. 2003)	Mu BpMSCs-*c-myc*	1:1-10	+	Co	Smaller tumors, ↑inflammation

Abbreviations: Hu- human, Mu- murine, ASC- adipose-derived MSCs, BMSCs- bone marrow-derived MSCs, UCSCs- umbilical cord-derived MSCs, MSCs-TERT tx –MSC cell line immortalized with telomerase vectors, BpMSCs-*c-myc*-bone marrow-derived MSC progenitor cells immortalized with *c-myc*, Immune Status of animal model- - immune compromised +- immune competent, Br- breast, Co-colon, Li- liver, Lu- lung, NH- Non-Hodgkin's lymphoma, and Pan- pancreas cancer cell lines. DKK-1-dickkopf-related protein 1, GM-CSF-granulocyte/monocyte-colony stimulating factor, PTEN-phosphatase and tensin homolog 10, PI3K-phosphoinositol-3-kinase.

Table 2. Anti-tumorigenic evidence for MSCs in the TME.

2.3 Controversies

Greater than a 100 clinical trials are underway or completed that investigate MSC-based therapy of human disease, and thus far the reports of adverse effects related to the therapy have been unremarkable (Salem and Thiemermann 2010; Tolar, Le Blanc et al. 2010; Singer and Caplan 2011). Therapy-related tumorigenicity has not been found, yet the preclinical studies presented above argue that we should carefully study this MSC potential. The question is why did MSCs promote cancer growth and spread in some studies, while in others MSCs diminished growth and spread? To begin to address this question there are a few important issues that have to be considered. First is the fact that surprisingly the chief effect of MSC-based therapies on disease is the modulation of the inflammatory host responses and not the replacement of injured tissue. Secondly, this observed therapeutic benefit is carried out by a few lingering MSCs that survive the relatively quick clearance of the cell bolus from the circulation—given that very small numbers of MSCs are ever detected at the sites of injury (Prockop 2009). Thirdly, it is known that both the adaptive and innate immune response arms profoundly influence tumor growth and spread by a complex interplay between inflammation and immunosurveillance (Frese and Tuveson 2007; Cheng, Ramesh et al. 2010). To resolve some of this controversy and to better understand the complex nature of the MSC-tumor interaction these issues need to be taken into account in future studies.

It is difficult to accurately model tumorigenesis with human tumor xenograft models in immunodeficient mice to finally resolve the effect that MSC-based therapy will have on cancer (Frese and Tuveson 2007; Cheng, Ramesh et al. 2010). Moreover, the number of MSCs interacting with the tumor must reflect more closely what is observed by the clinical experience. To more precisely model tumorigenicity attempts have been made at humanizing the murine immune system by eliminating the endogenous immune system followed by engraftment of human bone marrow or immune cells (Frese and Tuveson 2007). The problem with this approach has been that species-specific differences in both arms of the immune system confound interpretations. Immunocompetent autochthonous mouse models of human cancer provide a valuable tool that better addresses some of these issues. Though far from perfect, these models more closely parallel human carcinogenesis by allowing intrinsic tumor formation with immune surveillance and offer a better alternative system to study MSC-tumor interactions.

Apart from the limitations of current cancer models there are many other reasons that have been suggested to explain the divergent effects of MSCs in tumors (Klopp, Gupta et al. 2010; Klopp, Gupta et al. 2011). These include the heterogeneity of cells present in current MSC preparation protocols. Convention dictates that more homogeneous preparations of MSCs will also yield more consistent therapeutic outcomes with these cells. However, provided that we can overcome this hurdle and deliver more uniform cells, we may never get away from the variability that comes from the human donors. The age, gender, weight, and disease status of the donor may always affect efficacy outcomes and needs to be investigated more closely. Differences in the tissue source of the MSCs, whether bone marrow, adipose, umbilical cord, or other, also appear to affect a number of MSC functions (Sakaguchi, Sekiya et al. 2005; Hass, Kasper et al. 2011). Further complicating matters in all MSC-based therapy is the cell number and dosing frequency used to achieve a particular therapeutic efficacy. Cancer is a complex disease and to fully understand the contribution of MSCs, which are also intricate, more careful consideration of all these issues needs to be given. Despite these hurdles, MSCs remain an intriguing vehicle that can specifically target tumors.

3. Contributions by MSCs to tumors

In spite of all the limitations described, there is agreement about certain factors that MSCs elaborate that are important to tumorigenesis. It has long been know that MSCs synthesize a broad spectrum of growth factors, extracellular matrix proteins (ECM), cytokines, chemokines, and angiogenic molecules that have effects on cells in their vicinity. The effects of the bioactive molecules that MSCs secrete can be either direct, indirect, or even both: direct by causing intracellular signaling or indirect by causing another cell in the vicinity to secrete a bioactive factor. The indirect activity is typically termed "trophic", based on the original use of this word in neurobiology to distinguish neurotransmitters from other bioactive molecules released from nerve terminals (Caplan and Dennis 2006; Meirelles Lda, Fontes et al. 2009; Singer and Caplan 2011).

Typically, the bioactive molecules that are released from MSCs are reported to be relatively constant between different donors, regardless of age or health status of the donor. However, there can be some donor-specific differences in the levels of the secreted molecules-- that can be as high as a ten-fold difference. Moreover, the specific bioactive agents secreted by individual MSCs are also controlled by their functional status, level of differentiation, and the influence of their local microenvironments (Phinney, Kopen et al. 1999; Djouad, Fritz et al. 2005; Caplan and Dennis 2006; Krampera, Pasini et al. 2006; Tomchuck, Zwezdaryk et al. 2008; Nemeth, Mayer et al. 2009; Prasanna, Gopalakrishnan et al. ; Singer and Caplan 2011). It is expected that MSCs, as multipotent stem cells, will elaborate different levels and arrays of bioactive molecules as they differentiate into defined lineages. Additionally, the pattern and quantity of these secreted factors is well known to feed back on the MSC itself and change both its functional status and physiology.

These MSC paracrine and autocrine factors can have profound effects on local cellular dynamics. For instance, the marrow stroma derived from MSCs not only provides the matrix that supports cell anchorage, but also helps to maintain nearby endothelia and hematopoietic cells. In stroma poor niches within the marrow the hematopoetic stem cells (HSCs) will begin distinct programs of differentiation. The interdependence of MSCs and HSCs in the marrow is governed by the secretion of bioactive molecules such as the stromal-derived factor-1 (SDF1) to C-X-C chemokine receptor-4 (CXCR4) axis that helps support full hematopoietic lineage progression (Lopez Ponte, Marais et al. 2007).

3.1 Soluble, Extracellular Matrix (ECM), and angiogenic factors

The secretion of these broad range bioactive molecules is now believed to be the main mechanism by which MSCs achieve their therapeutic effect and that likely most affect the tumor microenvironment. These are typically divided by the processes they affect, such as mitogenic, angiogenic, apoptotic, or inflammatory/immune modulating (Table 3). We have added exosomes as a new category to these bioactive factors. Exosomes appear to be a previously unrecognized secretory vesicle that can affect neighboring cells. We include mitogens, Extracellular Matrix (ECM) proteins, and angiogens, exosomes and inflammatory/immune modulating bioactive factors as molecules potentially contributed by MSCs but caution that this is not an exhaustive list of all MSC products. Some of the molecules overlap in function, some of the molecules play greater roles in one species versus another (e.g.-mouse vs. human), and some of the molecules are released only following specific stimulation or activation (Tomchuck, Zwezdaryk et al. 2008; Klopp, Gupta et al. 2010; Waterman, Tomchuck et al. 2010; Klopp, Gupta et al. 2011). These have been recently reviewed (da Silva Meirelles, Caplan et al. 2008; Klopp, Gupta et al. 2010; Klopp, Gupta et al. 2011; Singer and Caplan 2011).

Molecule Types	Molecules	Study
Mitogens	bFGF, G-CSF, GM-CSF, HGF, IGF-I, IL6, Leptin, LIF, SCF, SDF-1, stanniocalcin-1, TGFβ, VEGF	(Zwezdaryk, Coffelt et al. 2007; Block, Ohkouchi et al. 2009; Meirelles Lda, Fontes et al. 2009[Tomchuck, 2008 #621; Klopp, Gupta et al. 2010; Waterman, Tomchuck et al. 2010; Klopp, Gupta et al. 2011)
Extracellular Matrix Proteins	Collagens, Fibronectin, Laminin	(Zuckerman and Wicha 1983; Hashimoto, Kariya et al. 2006; Zwezdaryk, Coffelt et al. 2007; Tomchuck, Zwezdaryk et al. 2008; Meirelles Lda, Fontes et al. 2009; Waterman, Tomchuck et al. 2010)
Angiogens	Angiopoetin-1, bFGF, IL6, IL8, Leptin, stanniocalcin-1, VEGF	(Zwezdaryk, Coffelt et al. 2007; Tomchuck, Zwezdaryk et al. 2008; Meirelles Lda, Fontes et al. 2009; Waterman, Tomchuck et al. 2010)
Exosomes	Pro-inflammatory molecules, miRNAs	(Anand 2010; Chen, Lai et al. 2010; Lai, Arslan et al. 2010)
Inflammatory/ Immune Modulating	galectin-3, galectin-1, HGF, HLA-G, IDO, IL1β, IL1RA, IL6, IL8, IL12, iNOS, IP-10, LIF, MCP-1, MIP-1, PGE2, semaphorin-3A, RANTES, SDF-1, stanniocalcin-1, TGFβ, TSG-6	(Zwezdaryk, Coffelt et al. 2007; Tomchuck, Zwezdaryk et al. 2008; Block, Ohkouchi et al. 2009; Meirelles Lda, Fontes et al. 2009; Bartosh, Ylostalo et al. 2010; Bunnell, Betancourt et al. 2010; Klopp, Gupta et al. 2010; Waterman, Tomchuck et al. 2010; Danchuk, Ylostalo et al. 2011; Klopp, Gupta et al. 2011)

Abbreviations: bFGF- basic fibroblast growth factor, CCL- C-C motif chemokine ligand, CXC- C-X-C-motif chemokine, CXCL-CXC-ligand, G-CSF-granulocyte-colony stimulating factor, GM-CSF-granulocyte-macrophage-colony stimulating factor, HGF-hepatocyte growth factor (scatter factor), HLA-G- human leukocyte antigen-G, IDO- indoleamine 2,3-dioxygenase, IGF-I-insulin-like growth factor-1, IL-interleukin, IL-1RA- interleukin-receptor 1 antagonist, iNOS-inducible nitric oxide synthase, IP-10-interferon-gamma-inducible protein 10 (CXCL10), LIF-leukemia inhibitory factor, MCP-1-monocyte chemoatractant protein-1 (CCL2), MIP1-macrophage inflammatory protein-1 (CCL3), PGE2-prostaglandin-E2, PlGF-placental-derived growth factor, RANTES- regulated upon activation normal T cell expressed and secreted (CCL5), SCF-stem cell factor, SDF-1-stromal-derived factor-1, TGFβ–transforming growth factor–β, TSG-6- TNF-alpha stimulated gene/protein 6, VEGF-vascular-derived endothelial growth factor (vascular permeability factor, VPF).

Table 3. Molecules Contributed by MSCs.

3.2 Exosomes

A recently described form of intercellular communication that may also be important in MSC-tumor exchanges is exosomes. These are endosome-derived vesicles of about 40–100 nm that are formed by the involution of endosome membranes resulting in the formation of multi-vesicular bodies (MVBs). Following certain physiological conditions, the MVBs fuse with the plasma membrane and release the exosomes into the circulation or tissue microenvironment. Exosomes have a "saucer-shaped" morphology as determined from electron microscopy analyses. Various methods have been developed to enrich for exosomes derived from a number of cell types including antigen-presenting cells (APCs), monocytes, T-lymphocytes, reticulocytes, mast cells, platelets, fibroblasts, tumor cells, and MSCs (Anand 2010; Lai, Arslan et al. 2010; Tan, De La Pena et al. 2010).

Investigators studying the cardioprotective effect of human embryonic stem cell-derived MSC-conditioned medium (CM) on myocardial ischemia/reperfusion injury reasoned based on proteomic analyses that exosomes were responsible for the beneficial effect (Sze, de Kleijn et al. 2007; Lai, Arslan et al. 2010). Their unbiased proteomic profiling of proteins secreted by MSCs revealed an abundance of membrane and cytosolic proteins. This suggested to them that the trophic effects of MSCs were not mediated by soluble growth factors and cytokines alone. Sze *et al.* proceeded to enrich for particles by size-exclusion fractionation on HPLC. Based on the size and the composition of the particles they figured exosomes were present in the condition medium of MSCs. Moreover they demonstrated that the enriched fraction of exosomes reduced infarct size in a mouse model of myocardial ischemia/reperfusion injury.

The particles could be visualized by electron microscopy and were shown to be phospholipid vesicles consisting of cholesterol, sphingomyelin, and phosphatidylcholine. Moreover, they were composed of known exosome-associated proteins-- CD81, CD9, and Alix. Exosomes are known to have a specific protein composition, including CD9, CD81, Alix, TSP-1, SOD-1, and pyruvate kinase. CD9 and CD81 are tetrapannin membrane proteins that are also localized in the membrane of exosomes. Consistent with the presence of exosomes in the CM of the MSCs this study further demonstrated that CD9 in the CM was a membrane-bound protein while SOD-1 was localized within a lipid vesicle. They eliminated the possibility of immune cells or platelets as sources of exosomes with an *ex vivo* mouse model of myocardial ischemia/reperfusion injury.

Similarly in human ESC-derived MSC conditioned medium other investigators found exosomes that contained small RNAs (less than 300 nt) encapsulated in cholesterol-rich phospholipid vesicles. The small RNAs were identified by a number of biochemical and genetic criteria to be microRNAs (miRNAs). Of interest the *Let-7* family of miRNAs figured prominently in these studies (Chen, Lai et al. 2010; Koh, Sheng et al. 2010). It is becoming increasingly clear that miRNAs are potent global gene regulators of many diverse cell functions including adaptation to mitogens, low oxygen (hypoxia), and inflammation. Perhaps this might explain why exosomes are potent immune modulators (Anand 2010). Apart from the molecules present inside the lumen of exosomes, it has been suggested that certain exosomal membrane molecules can interact with their surface receptors on the target cells thereby inducing an immunomodulatory response or activating the immune system. Consistent with this notion, exosome release is enhanced following pathologies where immune activation is required. It has been suggested that immunogenic molecules on the exosomal membrane can activate leukocytes. In support of this idea is the fact that exosomes are analogous to inverted endosomes and thus display inflammatory intracellular factors present normally within plasma membrane. Taking advantage of this inflammatory nature of exosomes, clinicians are developing cancer vaccines based on loading dendritic cells (DCs) with tumor antigens, expanding the DCs *ex vivo*, and subsequently isolating their enriched exosomes (Tan, De La Pena et al. 2010). The tumor antigen loaded exosomes are then reintroduced into patients to elicit tumor specific anti-tumor immunity.

Lastly, highlighting the interactions of tumors and MSCs, exosomes derived from tumors appear to drive adipose-derived MSC differentiation toward tumor associated myofibroblasts that can then contribute to tumor growth and spread (Webber, Steadman et al. 2010; Cho, Park et al. 2011; Cho, Park et al. 2011). Interestingly and perhaps providing a mechanism for the Wnt-signaling mediated anti-tumor effect of MSCs mentioned above, β-catenin was found to be contained within exosomes (Chairoungdua, Smith et al. 2010). Furthermore, exosomal release of β-catenin antagonized Wnt-signaling in the recipient cell. These studies emphasize the need for more intense investigations that clarify the role of both tumor- and MSC-derived exosomes in tumorigenesis. Besides identifying new components of tumor biology such studies may identify new therapeutic interventional agents.

3.3 Immune modulation

Apart from the ability of MSCs to contribute mitogens, ECM proteins, pro-angiogenic molecules, inflammatory agents, and exosomes to the TME, their most significant contribution may be modulating specific subsets of immune cells (Table 4)(Fibbe, Nauta et al. 2007; Nauta and Fibbe 2007; Bunnell, Betancourt et al. 2010; Roddy, Oh et al. 2011; Singer and Caplan 2011; Weiss, Bertoncello et al. 2011). The specific mechanism for this MSC role is not completely understood and may involve direct immune cell-MSC cell contact or indirect effects such as by the contribution of the factors just described or both. However, knowing the importance of immune and inflammatory cells in cancer growth and metastasis, the manner that MSCs in the TME might influence this process deserves closer attention and study.

Though initially described as an *ex vivo* phenomena requiring the stimulation of the MSCs to lead to suppression of T-lymphocyte activation or proliferation, many clinical trials have asserted immune modulation to be a primary effect of MSC-based therapies (Di Nicola, Carlo-Stella et al. 2002; Krampera, Glennie et al. 2003; Le Blanc, Rasmusson et al. 2004; Aggarwal and Pittenger 2005). In addition, these early observations prompted a number of studies to explore the distinct immune modulatory effects of MSCs derived from a variety of sources and species. Of note, although MSCs influence many immune cells, part of what makes them attractive candidates in cell-based therapies is their muted host immune responses even when delivered into a non-self (allogeneic) host. This is partly due to the fact that MSCs express low levels of human leukocyte antigen (HLA) major histocompatibility complex (MHC) class I, do not express co-stimulatory molecules (B7-1/CD80 and B7-2/CD86, CD40, or CD40L), and express MHC class II and Fas ligand only after specific stimulation.

MSCs are now known to inhibit dendritic cell maturation, B and T cell proliferation and differentiation, attenuate natural killer cell and mast cell activity, as well as support the production of suppressive T regulatory cells (Tregs) while attenuating pro-inflammatory Th17 cells (Table 4) (Najar, Raicevic et al. ; Di Nicola, Carlo-Stella et al. 2002; Krampera, Glennie et al. 2003; Aggarwal and Pittenger 2005; Beyth, Borovsky et al. 2005; Ramasamy, Fazekasova et al. 2007; Ren, Zhang et al. 2008; Uccelli, Moretta et al. 2008; Gur-Wahnon, Borovsky et al. 2009; Meirelles Lda, Fontes et al. 2009; Nemeth, Mayer et al. 2009; Bunnell, Betancourt et al. 2010; Salem and Thiemermann 2010; Tolar, Le Blanc et al. 2010; Brown, Nemeth et al. 2011; Singer and Caplan 2011).

Immune Response Arm	Cells	MSC effects
Innate	Dendritic Cells (APC)	Inhibition of maturation (CD80/86 expression) by STAT3 and IL10 (Beyth, Borovsky et al. 2005; Gur-Wahnon, Borovsky et al. 2009; Mezey, Mayer et al. 2009; Nemeth, Leelahavanichkul et al. 2009)
	Monocyte/Macrophages (APC)	PGE2 mediated increased IL10 secretion and attenuation of maturation (Beyth, Borovsky et al. 2005; Gur-Wahnon, Borovsky et al. 2009; Mezey, Mayer et al. 2009; Nemeth, Leelahavanichkul et al. 2009)
	Natural Killer Cells	Inhibition of proliferation and cytolytic activity (Giuliani, Oudrhiri et al. 2011)
	Mast Cells	COX-2 mediated suppression (Brown, Nemeth et al. 2011)
Adaptive	Th1	Inhibition of proliferation/activation (class switching) by HLA-G5, HGF, iNOS, COX2, IDO, PGE2, TGFβ and indirectly through support of immature APCs reviewed in (Singer and Caplan 2011)
	Th2	Inhibition of proliferation/activation (class switching) by HLA-G5, HGF, iNOS, COX2, IDO, PGE2, TGFβ and indirectly through support of immature APCs reviewed in (Singer and Caplan 2011)
	Tregs	Recruitent and support (class switching) IL10, TGFβ, LIF
	Th17	Inhibition of proliferation/activation (class switching) by COX-2 and PGE2 (Duffy, Pindjakova et al. 2011; Duffy, Ritter et al. 2011)
	B lymphocyte	Suppression of terminal differentiation to plasma cell (Asari, Itakura et al. 2009)

Abbreviations: COX-2- cyclooxygenase-2, HGF-hepatocyte growth factor (scatter factor), HLA-G-human leukocyte antigen-G, IDO- indoleamine 2,3-dioxygenase, iNOS-inducible nitric oxide synthase, IL10-interleukin-10, LIF-leukemia inhibitory factor, PGE2- prostaglandin-E2, STAT3- signal transducer and activator of transcription-3, TGFβ–transforming growth factor–β.

Table 4. Immune cells modulated by MSCs.

3.3.1 MSCs and myelomonocytic cells

Although the details of the interactions of MSCs with T lymphocytes, B lymphocytes, natural killer cells, and dendritic cells have been investigated in some detail, the effects of MSCs on cells of myelomonocytic lineages (MMCs) observed early on by the Rachmilewitz group remained under investigated until recently (Figure 1. Beyth, Borovsky et al. 2005). The growing clinical evidence for MSCs as major regulators of immune and inflammatory processes and the central role played by MMCs (including monocytes and granulocytes) within them has sparked new interest in studies on the interplay between MSCs and MMCs. Kim and Hematti (2009) reported that human macrophages generated *in vitro* after co-culture with MSCs assume an immunophenotype defined as IL-10–high, IL-12–low, IL-6–high, and

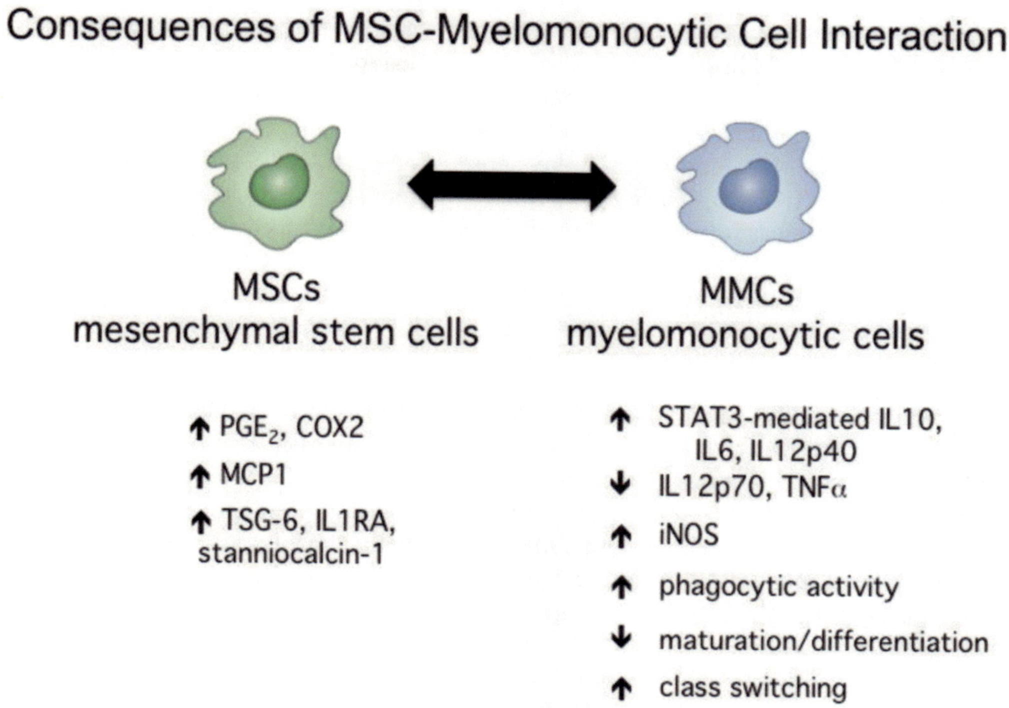

Abbreviations: COX-2- cyclooxygenase-2, IL-interleukin, IL-1RA- interleukin-receptor 1 antagonist, iNOS-inducible nitric oxide synthase, MCP-1-monocyte chemoatractant protein-1 (CCL2), PGE2-prostaglandin-E2, STAT3- signal transducer and activator of transcription-3, TSG-6- TNF-alpha stimulated gene/protein.

Fig. 1. The Consequences of the Interaction Between MSCs and Myelomonocytic Cells. Though still in their infancy the studies that have begun to identify the effect of the interactions between MSCs and MMCs whether cell-cell contact dependent or not have so far described those included in the figure. Please refer to the text for details.

TNF-a–low secreting cells (Kim and Hematti 2009). They proposed that these MSC-educated monocytes represent a unique and novel type of alternatively activated macrophage with a potentially significant role in tissue repair. Initially, Beyth *et al.* reported that human MSCs affect monocytes or dendritic antigen-presenting cell (APC) maturation in a contact-dependent manner (Beyth, Borovsky et al. 2005). Later, it was reported that the MSCs co-cultured with the APCs induced the expression of the anti-inflammatory IL10 and that activation of the signal transducer and activator of transcription 3 (STAT3) within APCs is linked to abnormal APC differentiation and function by a new contact-dependent mechanism, that plays a critical role in mediating the immunomodulatory effects of MSCs (Gur-Wahnon, Borovsky et al. 2007; Gur-Wahnon, Borovsky et al. 2009). In order to understand this process better, they further extended their studies to tumor cells since tumors secrete a variety of bioactive factors that activate STAT3 within infiltrating APCs. Their studies demonstrated that in at least certain cellular microenvironments, cell-to-cell dependent interactions represent a novel way to activate STAT3 signaling different from the activation of STAT3 seen with soluble bioactive factors. As such this observation suggests an uncoupling of APC activation events and that may consequently independently regulate immunity and tolerance. In agreement with these studies, the Mezey group identified other pathways involved in MSC-murine macrophage interactions (Nemeth, Leelahavanichkul et al. 2009). They also showed that LPS-stimulated macrophages produced more IL-10 when cultured with MSCs, but this effect was eliminated if the MSCs lacked the genes encoding TLR4, myeloid differentiation primary response gene-88 (MyD88), TNF-receptor-1α or cyclooxygenase-2 (COX-2). Their observations demonstrated that MSCs reprogram macrophages by releasing PGE2 that then acts on the macrophages through the prostaglandin EP2 and EP4 receptors. A unique population of MSCs isolated from human gingiva (GMSCs) with similar stem cell-like properties, immunosuppressive, and anti-inflammatory functions as bone marrow-derived MSCs were also studied in this context with similar effects (Zhang, Su et al. 2010).

When co-cultured with GMSCs, macrophages acquired an anti-inflammatory M2 phenotype similarly characterized by an increased expression of IL10 and IL6, mannose receptor (MR; CD206), a suppressed production of TNFα, and also decreased the ability to induce Th-17 cell expansion. Interesting to the discussion on tumors and their microenvironments, they demonstrated that systemically infused GMSCs could home to wounds-- specifically to sites where host macrophages were found-- promoted M2 polarization of the co-localized monocytes, significantly enhanced wound repair, and thus presumably could promote tumor growth by similar mechanisms. In addition, they noted that GMSC treatment suppressed local inflammation by reducing the infiltration of inflammatory cells and the production of IL6 and TNFα, and by increased expression of IL10. Another complementary study used muine macrophages stimulated with LPS and co-cultured with MSCs and found the suppression of TNFα, IL6, IL12p70 and interferonγ but increased levels of secreted IL10 and IL12p40. They noted that the murine MSC effect could be reproduced with MSC conditioned medium suggesting that bioactive factors constitutively released by the murine MSCs may be sufficient for the monocyte effect in this animal species (Maggini, Mirkin et al. 2010). They also found in cell-based therapy of mouse models that MSCs supported macrophages that showed a low expression of CD86 and MHC class II, and with a high ability to secrete IL10 and IL12p40, but not IL12 p70. They suggested in agreement with the other studies, that MSCs switch monocytes into a regulatory profile characterized by enhanced IL10 secretion, reduced inflammatory cytokine elaboration and enhanced phagocytic activity. Apart from elevated IL10 and related signaling mechanisms, other new players in the effects observed for MSCs on monocytes were recently advanced (Block, Ohkouchi et al. 2008; Block, Ohkouchi et al. 2009; Danchuk, Ylostalo et al. 2011; Prockop and Youn Oh 2011)]. Anti-inflammatory effects supported by MSC-monocyte interactions were suggested to also be partly mediated by elevated IL1 receptor antagonist (IL1RA) and by a negative feedback loop in which TNFα and other pro-inflammatory cytokines from resident macrophages activate MSCs to secrete the anti-inflammatory protein TNFα stimulated gene/protein 6 (TSG-6). These reports demonstrate that MSC derived TSG-6 acts to repress NF-κB signaling in the resident macrophages causing attenuation of pro-inflammatory cytokine synthesis. The investigators of these studies also proposed that MSC secreted PGE2 promotes monocytes toward an IL10 secreting phenotype as well as, that anti-inflammatory effects may also be mediated by stanniocalcin-1.

Finally, in another recent report using pre-clinical murine models it was shown that MCP1 secreted by activated MSCs contributes to the bone marrow egress, trafficking, and recruitment of monocytes towards remote sites (Shi, Jia et al. 2011). This elegant study demonstrated the intimate and complex cooperation that exists between MSCs and myelomonocytic cells that occurs not only in peripheral tissues or tumors but also in their originating bone marrow niche. It is widely recognized that tumor infiltrating cells can include macrophages, myeloid-derived suppressor cells (MDSCs), MSCs, and TIE2-expressing monocytes that are all mostly derived from the bone marrow. MDSCs represent a heterogeneous population of cells of myeloid origin that are expanded and activated in response to growth factors and cytokines released by tumors much like MSCs. The details of the effects of MDSCs on tumors are better understood. It is known that once MDSCs are activated, they accumulate in lymphoid organs and tumors where they exert specific T cell mediated immune suppression. However, not much is known about whether MDSCs and MSCs cooperate at tumor sites or the nature of that interaction. It is tempting to suggest that MSC-myelomononocytic cell interactions including MSC-MDSC ones represent an intriguing new target for cancer therapies that would break the anti-inflammatory tumor tolerance mechanisms established by these two cell types however, there is still much left to learn before this can come to fruition. Furthermore, while the vast majority of these reports demonstrate the ability of MSCs to suppress immune responses or act in an anti-inflammatory manner, there is emerging evidence that supports their contrasting ability to elicit pro-inflammatory responses-- which may also be mediated by their interaction with myelomonocytic cells. Both anti-inflammatory and pro-inflammatory effects will be important to know in dissecting their specific roles in tumors. This information will ultimately help in the design of more effective and targeted cancer therapeutics.

3.3.2 Immune suppressive or anti-inflammatory responses

The expression of IDO and iNOS by MSCs has been associated with its immune suppression of T-cell proliferation. Recently, secretion of IDO by MSCs therapeutically delivered in an experimental autoimmune myasthenia gravis model inhibited the proliferation of acetylcholine receptor-specific T cells and B cells and normalized the distribution of Th1, Th2, Th17 and Treg cells (Kong, Sun et al. 2009). IDO catalyzes the conversion of tryptophan, an essential amino acid for T-cell proliferation, into kynurenine. Immune suppression by IDO results from the local accumulation of tryptophan metabolites, rather than through tryptophan depletion (Ryan, Barry et al. 2007). Expression of IDO by MSCs was thought to be IFN-γ dependent (Krampera, Cosmi et al. 2006; Ryan, Barry et al. 2007; Bunnell, Betancourt et al. 2010). However, Opitz and colleagues recently demonstrated that IDO expression in MSCs can also be induced by activation of Toll-like receptor 3 (TLR3) and TLR4 via induction of an autocrine IFN-β signaling loop involving protein kinase R and independent of IFN-γ (Opitz, Litzenburger et al. 2009). Interestingly, when MSCs were treated with IFN-γ *in vitro*, they expressed extremely high levels of IDO and very low levels of iNOS, whereas mouse MSCs expressed abundant iNOS and very little IDO. These data suggest there is species variation in the mechanisms of MSC immunosuppression (Opitz, Litzenburger et al. 2009).

Prostaglandin E2 (PGE2) is emerging as a central mediator of many of the anti-inflammatory properties of MSCs (Nauta and Fibbe 2007; Uccelli, Moretta et al. 2008). PGE-2 is synthesized from arachidonic acid by cyclooxygenase (COX) enzymes COX-1 and COX-2.

COX-1 is constitutively expressed in MSCs and COX-2 expression can be induced by inflammatory cytokines such as IL-1β, IL-6, IFN-γ, and TNF-α (Chen, Wang et al. 2010). Inhibitors of PGE2 synthesis attenuated MSC suppression of T cells and natural killer cells (Sotiropoulou, Perez et al. 2006; Chen, Wang et al. 2010). PGE2 is associated also with the MSC-mediated inhibition of dendritic cell maturation. Nemeth *et al.* reported that activated MSCs released PGE2 causing increased production of IL10 by macrophages, and decreased production of the pro-inflammatory cytokines TNF-α and IL-6 in a murine sepsis model (Sotiropoulou, Perez et al. 2006). Maggini *et al.* similarly reported macrophage alterations by PGE2 (Maggini, Mirkin et al. 2010).

Mezey's group demonstrated that COX-2 is also involved in MSCs ability to suppress mast cell activation (Brown, Nemeth et al. 2011). Mast cells (MCs) have a key role in the induction of allergic inflammation and contribute to the severity of certain autoimmune diseases. An increasing body of literature also implicates MCs in the TME to affect tumor inflammation, angiogenesis, and growth (Ribatti, Nico et al. 2011). To date, few studies have investigated the potential of mast cell-MSC interactions. Since MCs are critical effector cells in allergic inflammation and they represent an important cell type to therapeutically target using the immune modulatory properties of MSCs, Mezey's group set out to study murine MC-MSCs effects. They reported that MSCs effectively suppressed specific MC functions *in vitro* and in animal models. MCs co-cultured with MSCs in direct contact, had dampened MC degranulation, pro-inflammatory cytokine production, chemokinesis, and chemotaxis. They also found that MC degranulation within mouse skin or the peritoneal cavity was suppressed following delivery of MSCs. Lastly, they discovered that these inhibitory effects were dependent on COX2 in MSCs (Brown, Nemeth et al. 2011).

Transforming growth factor-β (TGFβ) is an anti-inflammatory cytokine that is constitutively expressed by MSCs. The immune modulatory function of MSCs on T cells and natural killer cells can be impaired by treatment with neutralizing antibodies to TGFβ (Di Nicola, Carlo-Stella et al. 2002; Sotiropoulou, Perez et al. 2006). In contrast, several studies have also established that TGFβ had no effect on the immunosuppressive properties of MSCs (Tse, Pendleton et al. 2003; Xu, Zhang et al. 2007). These discrepancies are likely explained by differences in species or experimental conditions. The importance of TGFβ in MSC therapy was recently established in a mouse model of ragweed-induced asthma. Mezey's group again demonstrated this assertion with neutralizing antibodies and the use of MSCs derived from TGFβ knockout mice (Nemeth, Keane-Myers et al. 2010). Notably, the number of Tregs in this model was elevated by the MSC-therapy. However, the role of TGFβ in this process was not directly studied, as was done by Patel *et al.* who showed that in co-cultures of peripheral blood mononuclear cells (PBMCs) with MSCs, TGFβ produced by MSCs resulted in increased numbers of Tregs (Patel, Meyer et al. 2010).

Several other factors are associated with the potential anti-inflammatory properties of MSCs including HLA-G, hepatocyte growth factor (HGF), leukemia inhibitory factor (LIF), IL1 receptor antagonist (IL1RA), CCL2, galectin-3, galectin-1 and semaphorin-3A, most of which attenuate T lymphocyte activation and are highly expressed by MSCs (Di Nicola, Carlo-Stella et al. 2002; Ortiz, Dutreil et al. 2007; Di Ianni, Del Papa et al. 2008; Kang, Kang et al. 2008; Nasef, Ashammakhi et al. 2008; Rafei, Hsieh et al. 2008; Lepelletier, Lecourt et al. 2009; Selmani, Naji et al. 2009; Sioud, Mobergslien et al. 2010; Volarevic, Al-Qahtani et al. 2010). A recently advanced culprit is TNF-α-induced protein 6 TNAIP6 or TSG-6 (Lee, Pulin et al.

2009; Prockop and Youn Oh 2011). TSG-6 secretion is known to suppress inflammation through the inhibition of the inflammatory network of proteases primarily by increasing the inhibitory activity of inter-α-inhibitor, sequestration of hyaluronan fragments, and decreasing neutrophil infiltration into sites of inflammation. In a model of acute inflammation induced by myocardial infarction, TSG-6 knockdown in MSCs significantly reduced their anti-inflammatory therapeutic effect. The administration of recombinant TSG-6 protein largely duplicated the therapeutic effects of the delivered MSCs on inflammatory responses and infarct size (Getting, Mahoney et al. 2002; Wisniewski and Vilcek 2004; Milner, Higman et al. 2006; Forteza, Casalino-Matsuda et al. 2007; Lee, Pulin et al. 2009). Together these results make TSG-6 an interesting new factor in the anti-inflammatory effects of MSCs.

3.3.3 Pro-inflammatory MSC responses

Though we are beginning to better understand the many complex mechanisms associated with the secretion by MSCs of immune suppressive mediators like TSG-6, so far only a few reports have described a contrasting pro-inflammatory activity of MSCs that could be important in understanding the distinct role of MSCs in tumors. Indeed, the observation of this distinct MSCs immune effect came from studies primarily focused on the downstream consequences of TLR stimulation within these cells. TLRs are a conserved family of receptors that recognize pathogen- associated molecular patterns (PAMPs) and promote the activation of immune cells (Wright 1999-76; Triantafilou, Triantafilou et al. 2001; Sabroe, Read et al. 2003; Anders, Banas et al. 2004; Miggin and O'Neill 2006; West, Koblansky et al. 2006; Bunnell, Betancourt et al. 2010). Many TLRs (TLR1 to TLR13) have been identified and characterized in a variety of immune cell types and species. Agonists for TLRs include exogenous microbial components, such as LPS (TLR2 and 4), lipoproteins and peptidoglycans (TLR1, 2, 6), viral RNA (TLR3), bacterial and viral unmethylated CpG-DNA (TLR9), and endogenous molecules shed following cell injury, including heat shock proteins and extracellular matrix molecules (Wright 1999-77; Triantafilou, Triantafilou et al. 2001; Sabroe, Read et al. 2003; Anders, Banas et al. 2004; Miggin and O'Neill 2006; West, Koblansky et al. 2006; Bunnell, Betancourt et al. 2010). Specific agonist engagement of TLRs leads to the expression of inflammatory cytokines or co-stimulatory molecules by a MyD88 (a TLR adapter protein)-dependent or MyD88-independent signaling pathways and can promote chemotaxis of the stimulated cell. TLRs are differentially expressed on leukocyte subsets and non-immune cells and may regulate important aspects of innate and adaptive immune responses (Mempel, Voelcker et al. 2003; Hwa Cho, Bae et al. 2006; Nagai, Garrett et al. 2006; Pevsner-Fischer, Morad et al. 2006; West, Koblansky et al. 2006; Tomchuck, Zwezdaryk et al. 2008).

MSCs are among the cells that express an array of TLRs, including TLR2, 3, 4, 5, 6 and 9 (Hwa Cho, Bae et al. 2006; Pevsner-Fischer, Morad et al. 2006; Tomchuck, Zwezdaryk et al. 2008). Furthermore, studies by our group established that the stimulation of MSCs with TLR agonists led to the activation of downstream signaling pathways, including NF-kB, AKT, and mitogen-activated protein kinase (MAPK). Consequently, activation of these pathways triggers the previously unreported induction and secretion of pro-inflammatory cytokines, chemokines, and related TLR gene products. Interestingly, the unique patterns of affected genes, cytokines, and chemokines measured identified the TLRs as potential players in the established MSC immune modulatory properties, as well as their ability to migrate towards injured tissues. Surprisingly, we noted that TLR4 stimulation with LPS led to the secretion of primarily pro-inflammatory mediators, such as IL-1β and IL6 (Tomchuck, Zwezdaryk et al. 2008). Though unexpected, previous observations reported by Beyth *et al.* recognized that LPS priming affected co-cultures of leukocytes with human MSCs and attenuated the expected human MSC- mediated inhibition of T-lymphocyte activation as well as affected their capacity to secrete interferon (Beyth, Borovsky et al. 2005). More recently, Romieu-Mourez *et al.* showed that TLR stimulation in murine MSCs similarly resulted in the production of inflammatory mediators, such as IL-1, IL-6, IL-8, and CCL5 (Romieu-Mourez, Francois et al. 2009). Furthermore, they demonstrated that TLR and IFN activated murine MSCs injected within Matrigel matrices into mice resulted in the formation of an inflammatory site attracting innate immune cells and resulting in a dramatic recruitment of neutrophils. Raicevic *et al.*, studying the effect of TLR activation within MSCs in an inflammatory milieu, observed that this environment shifted the cytokine profile to a pro-inflammatory one rather than the expected immunosuppressive one (Raicevic, Rouas et al. 2010). They similarly observed an increase in IL-1β, IL-6, and IL-12 after TLR activation in this inflammatory context.

Though somewhat confounding, this recent body of work on the downstream consequences of TLRs provides emerging evidence for a new pro-inflammatory immune modulating role for MSCs. The identification of the molecular details for this new pro-inflammatory MSC role, and whether it is innate or just an *in vitro* artifact, awaits further investigation. However, this novel observation is important to consider given the accelerated use of MSCs in anti-inflammatory cell-based therapies. Additionally, as Raicevic *et al.* suggest targeting of TLRs in MSCs, may avoid deleterious consequences in their use as anti-inflammatory therapies (Raicevic, Rouas et al. 2010). By contrast, TLR-activated pro-inflammatory MSCs could prove useful in breaking tolerance in the therapy of immune evasive diseases, such as cancer.

4. New MSC paradigm: Pro-inflammatory *MSC1* and anti-inflammatory *MSC2*

Our recent studies are partly an attempt to resolve some of the controversy surrounding the potential of MSCs to be anti-inflammatory in some cases and pro-inflammatory in others or to be pro-tumor in some cancers and anti-tumor in others, as described above. These studies led us to propose a new paradigm for MSCs based on the premise that these heterogeneous cells can be induced to polarize into two distinct but homogeneously acting phenotypes-- that we modeled after monocytes, the other heterogeneous bone marrow-derived cells (Figure 2. Verreck, de Boer et al. 2006).

It is established that stimulation of monocytes with known cytokines or agonists to their TLRs, including IFN-γ and endotoxin (LPS, TLR4-agonist), polarizes them into a classical M1 phenotype that participates in early pro-inflammatory responses. IL-4 treatment of monocytes yields the alternative M2 phenotype that is associated with anti-inflammatory resolution responses (Verreck, de Boer et al. 2006). We proposed that MSCs, like monocytes, are polarized by downstream TLR signaling into two homogenously acting phenotypes, classified as *MSC1* and *MSC2*, following the monocyte nomenclature. We reported that TLR4 agonists polarized MSCs toward a pro-inflammatory *MSC1* phenotype while the downstream consequences of TLR3 stimulation of MSCs was a skewing toward an anti-inflammatory *MSC2* phenotype. This novel MSC polarization paradigm is based on the consistent but novel outcomes observed for *MSC1* when compared with *MSC2* for several parameters, including dissimilar patterns of secretion of cytokines and chemokines and differences in differentiation capabilities, extracellular matrix deposition, TGF-β signaling pathways, and Jagged, IDO and PGE-2 expression (Waterman, Tomchuck et al. 2010). The most compelling outcome was opposite effects of each cell type on T-lymphocyte activation (Waterman, Tomchuck et al. 2010).

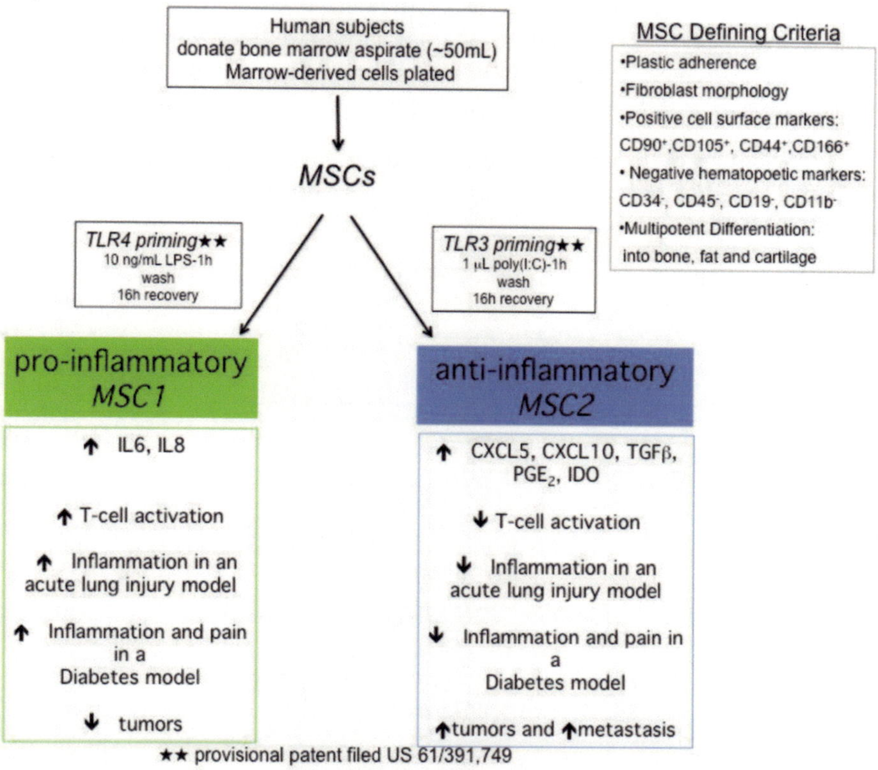

Fig. 2. Characteristics of the MSC1 and MSC2 Phenotypes. Short-term and low-level priming of TLR4 (left side) and TLR3 (right side) leads to the induction of heterogeneous hMSC preparations into a pro-inflammatory *MSC1* phenotype or an anti-inflammatory *MSC2* phenotype. (adapted from (Tomchuck, Zwezdaryk et al. 2008; Waterman, Tomchuck et al. 2010)).

4.1 Evidence for *MSC1* and *MSC2*

Our previous work, as well as that of others, established that MSCs reside in TMEs or tumor stroma, provide structural support for the malignant cells, modulate the tumor microenvironment, and consequently promote tumor growth and spread. Therefore, gene-modified MSCs that can act as "Trojan horses" and deliver anti-cancer therapeutics into the tumor stroma are being evaluated as a promising new specific cell-based therapy for cancer. We also previously established that MSCs recruited to ovarian tumors by elevated secretion of LL-37 play a supportive role in ovarian tumor stroma. We found that specific induction of MSCs into *MSC1* causes the secretion of pro-inflammatory mediators rather than anti-inflammatory ones, as well as promotes collagen rather than fibronectin deposition into the extracellular matrix (Figure 1)(Waterman, Tomchuck et al. 2010). Our preliminary studies support the notion that *MSC1* may be effective in new cell-based treatment of cancers. Indeed, ovarian cancer cell lines co-cultured with *MSC1* formed smaller tumor spheroids and had markedly reduced tumor colony forming potential; whereas, co-cultures with *MSC2* phenotype had the expected pro-tumor effect. Moreover, *MSC1*-treated ovarian cancer cells were less invasive than *MSC2*-treated ones in matrigel coated transwell migration assays. Pilot tests in murine ovarian cancer models were consistent with these findings. *MSC1* delivered in mice with established tumors had attenuated growth and spread. Mice treated with *MSC2* had larger and more metastatic tumors.

MSC1 and MSC2 therapy has been successfully tested in several animal disease models and has resulted in predictable inflammatory responses and distinct effects on tumor growth and spread (Table 5).

Animal Disease Model	MSC-based Therapy	MSC Dose (cells)	Treatment Frequency (Time of treatment)	Disease Impact	Length of study	Adverse Effects
1. LPS-induced Acute Lung Injury (ALI) (BalbC and C57BL/6J, *n*=12)	MSCs	$0.5X10^6$	1X (24hrs post-disease onset)	Mostly anti-inflammatory	1 week post-treatment	**NONE**
	MSC1	$0.5X10^6$	1X (24hrs post-disease onset)	Pro-inflammatory	1 week post-treatment	**NONE**
	MSC2	$0.5X10^6$	1X (24hrs post-disease onset)	Anti-inflammatory	1 week post-treatment	**NONE**
2. Streptozotocin-Induced Diabetes and neuropathic pain (C57BL/6J, *n*=30)	MSCs	$1\text{-}3X10^6$	3X (given in 10-day intervals post-disease onset)	Mostly anti-inflammatory	70 days post-treatment	**NONE**
	MSC1	$1\text{-}3X10^6$	3X (given in 10-day intervals post-disease onset)	Pro-inflammatory	70 days post-treatment	**NONE**
	MSC2	$1\text{-}3X10^6$	3X (given in 10-day intervals post-disease onset)	Anti-inflammatory	70 days post-treatment	**NONE**
3. Immune-incompetent human tumor xenografts (Balb *scid* and *nude* *n*=60)	MSCs	$0.5X10^6$	3X (given weekly post-disease onset)	Mostly anti-inflammatory	>120 days post-treatment	**NONE**
	MSC1	$0.5X10^6$	3X (given weekly post-disease onset)	Pro-inflammatory	>120 days post-treatment	**NONE**
	MSC2	$0.5X10^6$	3X (given weekly post-disease onset)	Anti-inflammatory	>120 days post-treatment	**NONE**
4. Immune-competent MOSEC (C57/BL6J *n*=20)	MSCs	$0.5X10^6$	3X (given weekly post-disease onset)	Mostly anti-inflammatory	>70 days post-treatment	**NONE**
	MSC1	$0.5X10^6$	3X (given weekly post-disease onset)	Pro-inflammatory	>70 days post-treatment	**NONE**

Table 5. Human MSC-based therapy of murine disease models.

Please NOTE that for all of the data presented MSCs represent conventionally prepared human MSCs, *MSC1* are defined as the hMSCs incubated for 1hr with 10 ng/mL LPS and washed prior to delivery. *MSC2* are defined as the hMSCs incubated for 1hr with 1 mg/mL poly(I:C) and washed prior to delivery (provisional patent filed US 61/391,749).

Cancer models: Pilot studies with the mouse ovarian cancer model (MOSEC) and with a xenograft model demonstrate our assertions. A single delivery of *MSC1*-based therapy resulted in slower growing tumors, whereas comparable therapy with MSCs or *MSC2* resulted in larger tumors and metastasis at the end of the study (day 65, Figure 3).

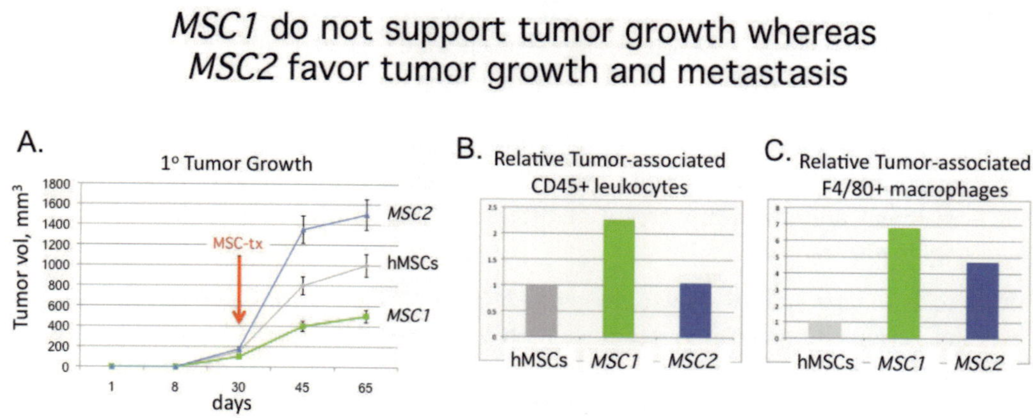

Fig. 3. MSC1 do not support tumor growth whereas MSC2 favor tumor growth and metastasis. The data show differences in tumor volume, CD45+leukocyte, and F4/80+ macrophage recruitment after the treatment of mice with established ovarian tumors, with human *MSC1*- and *MSC2*-based therapies. Methods The established syngeneic mouse model for epithelial ovarian cancer used is based upon a spontaneously transformed mouse ovarian surface epithelial cell (MOSEC) line ID8 that has been previously described (Roby, Taylor et al. 2000). 4-6 week-old female mice (n>10 mice/MSC-treatment) were injected subcutaneously (s.c.) in the right hind leg with 1 X10^7 MOSEC cells. At approximately 4 weeks a single dose of labeled human MSCs (hMSCs), *MSC1*, or *MSC2* (1X10^6/per mouse) were injected intraperitonealy (IP) as indicated by red arrow ↓. (A.) Tumor growth was measured with callipers as standard at weekly intervals until day of mouse sacrifice (Day 65). Harvested tumors and metastasis were weighed, counted and processed for flow cytometry and immunohistochemical analysis (IHC, Coffelt et al., 2009). Metastasis was found only in *MSC2*-treated mice (data not shown). MSCs were detected by flow cytometry and IHC. All MSC-treated samples had similar detectable MSCs within the tumor tissue-trending towards more *MSC1* and *MSC2* measured than hMSCs: approximately 15-25 cells counted per 200X field after 24hr of MSC-treatment and 2-5 cells at time of tissue harvest (day 65, data not shown). Sectioned tumor sample slides were stained with murine CD45 (B.) or F4/80 (C.) antibodies and the number of positively stained immune cells per 200X field were scored as described previously (Coffelt et al., 2009). Data are expressed as average cells counted in 4 fields/slide relative to hMSC sample. Data indicate in vivo stability and predictably distinct effects by the *MSC1* and *MSC2*.

ALI model: In an established endotoxin-induced acute lung injury (ALI) mouse model, LPS, or endotoxin (0.1 mg/kg) was instilled intratracheally into adult Balb/C mice. After 24 hrs, mice were each treated with 0.5x10^6 MSCs, *MSC1, MSC2,* or HBSS vehicle. To characterize inflammation, the lungs of the animals were lavaged and bronchioalveolar lavage fluid (BALF) was analyzed after 24 hr for changes in neutrophil/monocyte recruitment (myeloperoxidase activity), total cell content by flow cytometry, and lung integrity by total protein leaked into the BALF *(n=12)*. *MSC1*-therapy aggravated the disease and resulted in increased neutrophil recruitment and more compromised lungs than the conventional MSC or *MSC2* therapy.

Diabetes Model: Streptozotocin (STZ)-induced diabetic mice were procured from Jackson Laboratory (Bar Harbor, Maine). Blood glucose levels and animal weights were measured by standard methods. A month post STZ-injection, mice received intraperitonealy (IP) $0.5x10^6$ cells of MSCs, *MSC1, MSC2,* or HBSS vehicle for a total of 3 times in 10-day intervals. Established behavioral assays to evaluate hyperalgesia and allodynia were conducted one day prior to each MSC therapy, as well as prior to sacrifice. Inflammatory factors and immune cell changes were measured as before to characterize the treatment effects on inflammation *(n=30).* Again, all indicators were consistent with enhanced inflammation by *MSC1*-treatment and an improvement of disease by the *MSC2*- or MSC-treated animals. *Manuscript in preparation.*

Additionally *in vitro* studies show divergent effects of *MSC1* and *MSC2* on cancer cells. Co-culture of various human cancer cell lines with *MSC1* and *MSC2* in Colony Forming Units (CFU) assays and 3-D tumor spheroid assays agree with the *in vivo* tumor models with different *MSC1* and *MSC2* treatment effects (Figure 4).

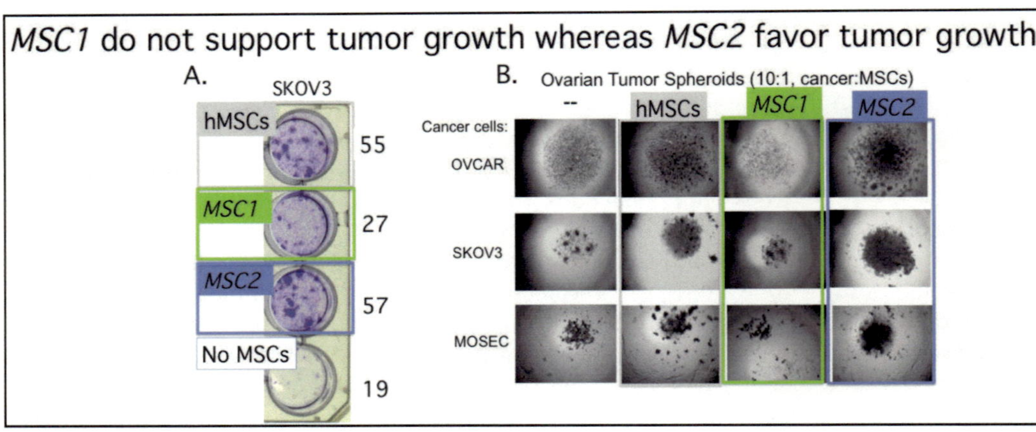

Fig. 4. MSC1 do not support tumor growth whereas MSC2 favor tumor growth: A. Data demonstrates that there are distinct effects on colony forming units (CFU) after coculture of different human cancer cell lines with untreated MSCs (hMSCs), MSC1, or MSC2. Methods: CFU assay was performed by culturing human tumor cells (200 cells/well) mixed with hMSCs, MSC1, or MSC2 (2 cells/well) at a ratio of 10 cancer cells per 1 MSC and plated in 24-well plates in growth medium supplemented with 10% FBS as indicated in figure. Cultures were grown for 14 days at 37°C in a humidified atmosphere of 5% carbon dioxide balance air. Growth medium was changed every 3-4 days. Colonies were visualized by staining with a crystal violet solution (0.5% crystal violet/10% ethanol). The resulting colonies were enumerated by the colony counting macro in ImageJ software, SKOV3-ovarian cancer cell lines. Micrographs of the stained plates are shown. Colony counts are at right.(n=8) B. Data demonstrates that there are distinct effects on tumor spheroids after coculture of different cancer cell lines with unprimed MSCs, MSC1, or MSC2. Methods: Tumor spheroids were formed by culturing tumor cells (2000 cells/well) mixed without any other cells (--) or with hMSCs, MSC1, or MSC2 (20 cells/well) at a ratio of 10 cancer cells per

1 MSC and plated over 1.5% agarose in 96-well plates in growth medium supplemented with 10% FBS as indicated in figure. Cultures were grown for 14 days at 37°C in a humidified atmosphere of 5% carbon dioxide balance air. Growth medium was changed every 3-4 days. Micrographs shown represent 20X magnified field of the 96-well plate. Cancer cell lines used are: OVCAR-human ovarian cancer, SKOV3-human ovarian cancer cell lines, and MOSEC-murine ovarian surface epithelium carcinoma cells. Data indicate distinct effects by MSC1 and MSC2 on cancer cell growth and spread.

5. Conclusion

The unique pathology of individual tumors presents a huge problem for conventional mono-specific therapies. New approaches aiming at developing effective treatments against cancer include the use of MSC-based therapies. There are many features that make this new strategy attractive and feasible. First, MSC-based therapies are already in clinical use and thus far have not been associated with adverse effects. Second, MSCs can be easily expanded and stored without any impact to their capabilities—a phenomenom that has triggered the creation of many new biotech start-ups. Third, once delivered, MSCs preferentially home to tumors and affect tumor growth and spread. Fourth, MSCs from non-self (allogeneic) or autologous (self) hosts can be safely delivered since they do not elicit immunity. Lastly, pre-clinical studies have demonstrated efficacy with genetically-engineered MSCs that carry anti-cancer therapeutics that reached the tumors and prevented their growth.

MSCs targeted to cancers are expected to contribute many soluble factors such as mitogens, extracellular matrix proteins, angiogenic and inflammatory factors, as well as exosomes with as yet poorly defined potentials, once resident in the TME. MSCs are also expected to affect tumor-associated leukocytes either directly by cell-cell contact or indirectly by the secretion of trophic factors. MSCs are known to affect the proliferation and differentiation of dendritic cells, monocytes/macrophages, B and T cells, NK cells, and even mast cells. There has been a great deal of debate in the field in trying to assert whether MSCs resident in the TME contribute to tumor growth and spread or prevent it, and if so, by what mechanisms. Many reasons have been advanced to explain the contradictory MSC role in cancer including the heterogeneity of MSC preparations, the age or health of the MSC donor, and the experimental model or condition, to name a few. Our group has suggested a new paradigm for MSCs that we believe will help resolve some of the conflicting issues. The induction of MSCs into uniform and consistently acting pro-inflammatory *MSC1* or anti-inflammatory *MSC2* phenotypes should provide convenient experimental tools that dissect the potential pro- and anti-tumor contributions of MSCs. MSC-based therapies stand to revolutionize medicine with the myriad ways that they can be manipulated and guided to reach pathologic tissue sites such as tumors. The continued investigation of these cells will ensure safe and effective therapy of human disease.

6. Acknowledgment

This work was supported by the National Institutes of Health grant 1P20RR20152-01, Department of Defense OC073102 Concept Award and research support from the Tulane Cancer Center and the Center for Stem Cell Research and Regenerative Medicine.

7. References

Abdi, R., P. Fiorina, et al. (2008). "Immunomodulation by mesenchymal stem cells: a potential therapeutic strategy for type 1 diabetes." *Diabetes* 57(7): 1759-67.

Aggarwal, S. and M. F. Pittenger (2005). "Human mesenchymal stem cells modulate allogeneic immune cell responses." *Blood* 105(4): 1815-22.

Anand, P. K. (2010). "Exosomal membrane molecules are potent immune response modulators." *Commun Integr Biol* 3(5): 405-8.

Anders, H. J., B. Banas, et al. (2004). "Signaling danger: toll-like receptors and their potential roles in kidney disease." *J Am Soc Nephrol* 15(4): 854-67.

Asari, S., S. Itakura, et al. (2009). "Mesenchymal stem cells suppress B-cell terminal differentiation." *Exp Hematol* 37(5): 604-15.

Bartosh, T. J., J. H. Ylostalo, et al. (2010). "Aggregation of human mesenchymal stromal cells (MSCs) into 3D spheroids enhances their antiinflammatory properties." *Proc Natl Acad Sci U S A* 107(31): 13724-9.

Beyth, S., Z. Borovsky, et al. (2005). "Human mesenchymal stem cells alter antigen-presenting cell maturation and induce T-cell unresponsiveness." *Blood* 105(5): 2214-9.

Block, G. J., S. Ohkouchi, et al. (2008). "Multipotent Stromal Cells (MSCs) are Activated to Reduce Apoptosis in Part by Upregulation and Secretion of Stanniocalcin-1 (STC-1)." *Stem Cells*.

Block, G. J., S. Ohkouchi, et al. (2009). "Multipotent stromal cells are activated to reduce apoptosis in part by upregulation and secretion of stanniocalcin-1." *Stem Cells* 27(3): 670-81.

Brown, J. M., K. Nemeth, et al. (2011). "Bone marrow stromal cells inhibit mast cell function via a COX2-dependent mechanism." *Clin Exp Allergy* 41(4): 526-34.

Bruder, S. P., N. Jaiswal, et al. (1997). "Growth kinetics, self-renewal, and the osteogenic potential of purified human mesenchymal stem cells during extensive subcultivation and following cryopreservation." *J Cell Biochem* 64(2): 278-94.

Bunnell, B. A., A. M. Betancourt, et al. (2010). "New concepts on the immune modulation mediated by mesenchymal stem cells." *Stem Cell Res Ther* 1(5): 34.

Caplan, A. I. and J. E. Dennis (2006). "Mesenchymal stem cells as trophic mediators." *J Cell Biochem*.

Chairoungdua, A., D. L. Smith, et al. (2010). "Exosome release of beta-catenin: a novel mechanism that antagonizes Wnt signaling." *J Cell Biol* 190(6): 1079-91.

Chen, K., D. Wang, et al. (2010). "Human umbilical cord mesenchymal stem cells hUC-MSCs exert immunosuppressive activities through a PGE2-dependent mechanism." *Clin Immunol* 135(3): 448-58.

Chen, T. S., R. C. Lai, et al. (2010). "Mesenchymal stem cell secretes microparticles enriched in pre-microRNAs." *Nucleic Acids Res* 38(1): 215-24.

Cheng, L., A. V. Ramesh, et al. (2010). "Mouse models for cancer stem cell research." *Toxicol Pathol* 38(1): 62-71.

Cho, J. A., H. Park, et al. (2011). "Exosomes from ovarian cancer cells induce adipose tissue-derived mesenchymal stem cells to acquire the physical and functional characteristics of tumor-supporting myofibroblasts." *Gynecol Oncol*.

Cho, J. A., H. Park, et al. (2011). "Exosomes from breast cancer cells can convert adipose tissue-derived mesenchymal stem cells into myofibroblast-like cells." *Int J Oncol*.

Coffelt, S. B., F. C. Marini, et al. (2009). "The pro-inflammatory peptide LL-37 promotes ovarian tumor progression through recruitment of multipotent mesenchymal stromal cells." *Proc Natl Acad Sci U S A* 106(10): 3806-11.

Coffelt, S. B. and A. B. Scandurro (2008). "Tumors sound the alarmin(s)." *Cancer Res* 68(16): 6482-5.

Cousin, B., E. Ravet, et al. (2009). "Adult stromal cells derived from human adipose tissue provoke pancreatic cancer cell death both in vitro and in vivo." *PLoS One* 4(7): e6278.

da Silva Meirelles, L., A. I. Caplan, et al. (2008). "In search of the in vivo identity of mesenchymal stem cells." *Stem Cells* 26(9): 2287-99.

Danchuk, S., J. H. Ylostalo, et al. (2011). "Human multipotent stromal cells attenuate lipopolysaccharide-induced acute lung injury in mice via secretion of tumor necrosis factor-alpha-induced protein 6." *Stem Cell Res Ther* 2(3): 27.

Dasari, V. R., K. Kaur, et al. (2010). "Upregulation of PTEN in glioma cells by cord blood mesenchymal stem cells inhibits migration via downregulation of the PI3K/Akt pathway." *PLoS One* 5(4): e10350.

Dasari, V. R., K. K. Velpula, et al. (2010). "Cord blood stem cell-mediated induction of apoptosis in glioma downregulates X-linked inhibitor of apoptosis protein (XIAP)." *PLoS One* 5(7): e11813.

Di Ianni, M., B. Del Papa, et al. (2008). "Mesenchymal cells recruit and regulate T regulatory cells." *Exp Hematol* 36(3): 309-18.

Di Nicola, M., C. Carlo-Stella, et al. (2002). "Human bone marrow stromal cells suppress T-lymphocyte proliferation induced by cellular or nonspecific mitogenic stimuli." *Blood* 99(10): 3838-43.

Digirolamo, C. M., D. Stokes, et al. (1999). "Propagation and senescence of human marrow stromal cells in culture: a simple colony-forming assay identifies samples with the greatest potential to propagate and differentiate." *Br J Haematol* 107(2): 275-81.

Djouad, F., V. Fritz, et al. (2005). "Reversal of the immunosuppressive properties of mesenchymal stem cells by tumor necrosis factor alpha in collagen-induced arthritis." *Arthritis Rheum* 52(5): 1595-603.

Djouad, F., P. Plence, et al. (2003). "Immunosuppressive effect of mesenchymal stem cells favors tumor growth in allogeneic animals." *Blood* 102(10): 3837-44.

Duffy, M. M., J. Pindjakova, et al. (2011). "Mesenchymal stem cell inhibition of T-helper 17 differentiation is triggered by cell-cell contact and mediated by prostaglandin E2 via the EP4 receptor." *Eur J Immunol.*

Duffy, M. M., T. Ritter, et al. (2011). "Mesenchymal stem cell effects on T-cell effector pathways." *Stem Cell Res Ther* 2(4): 34.

Feng, J., A. Mantesso, et al. "Dual origin of mesenchymal stem cells contributing to organ growth and repair." *Proc Natl Acad Sci U S A* 108(16): 6503-8.

Fibbe, W. E., A. J. Nauta, et al. (2007). "Modulation of immune responses by mesenchymal stem cells." *Ann N Y Acad Sci* 1106: 272-8.

Forteza, R., S. M. Casalino-Matsuda, et al. (2007). "TSG-6 potentiates the antitissue kallikrein activity of inter-alpha-inhibitor through bikunin release." *Am J Respir Cell Mol Biol* 36(1): 20-31.

Frese, K. K. and D. A. Tuveson (2007). "Maximizing mouse cancer models." *Nat Rev Cancer* 7(9): 645-58.

Friedenstein, A. J., S. Piatetzky, II, et al. (1966). "Osteogenesis in transplants of bone marrow cells." *J Embryol Exp Morphol* 16(3): 381-90.

Galie, M., G. Konstantinidou, et al. (2008). "Mesenchymal stem cells share molecular signature with mesenchymal tumor cells and favor early tumor growth in syngeneic mice." *Oncogene* 27(18): 2542-51.

Getting, S. J., D. J. Mahoney, et al. (2002). "The link module from human TSG-6 inhibits neutrophil migration in a hyaluronan- and inter-alpha -inhibitor-independent manner." *J Biol Chem* 277(52): 51068-76.

Giuliani, M., N. Oudrhiri, et al. (2011). "Human mesenchymal stem cells derived from induced pluripotent stem cells downregulate NK cell cytolytic machinery." *Blood.*

Gur-Wahnon, D., Z. Borovsky, et al. (2007). "Contact-dependent induction of regulatory antigen-presenting cells by human mesenchymal stem cells is mediated via STAT3 signaling." *Exp Hematol* 35(3): 426-33.

Gur-Wahnon, D., Z. Borovsky, et al. (2009). "The induction of APC with a distinct tolerogenic phenotype via contact-dependent STAT3 activation." *PLoS One* 4(8): e6846.

Hashimoto, J., Y. Kariya, et al. (2006). "Regulation of proliferation and chondrogenic differentiation of human mesenchymal stem cells by laminin-5 (laminin-332)." *Stem Cells* 24(11): 2346-54.

Hass, R., C. Kasper, et al. (2011). "Different populations and sources of human mesenchymal stem cells (MSC): A comparison of adult and neonatal tissue-derived MSC." *Cell Commun Signal* 9: 12.

Hwa Cho, H., Y. C. Bae, et al. (2006). "Role of Toll-Like Receptors on Human Adipose-Derived Stromal Cells." *Stem Cells %R 10.1634/stemcells.2006-0189* 24(12): 2744-2752.

Jaiswal, N., S. E. Haynesworth, et al. (1997). "Osteogenic differentiation of purified, culture-expanded human mesenchymal stem cells in vitro." *J Cell Biochem* 64(2): 295-312.

Ju, S., G. J. Teng, et al. (2010). "In vivo differentiation of magnetically labeled mesenchymal stem cells into hepatocytes for cell therapy to repair damaged liver." *Invest Radiol* 45(10): 625-33.

Kang, J. W., K. S. Kang, et al. (2008). "Soluble factors-mediated immunomodulatory effects of canine adipose tissue-derived mesenchymal stem cells." *Stem Cells Dev* 17(4): 681-93.

Karnoub, A. E., A. B. Dash, et al. (2007). "Mesenchymal stem cells within tumour stroma promote breast cancer metastasis." *Nature* 449(7162): 557-63.

Khakoo, A. Y., S. Pati, et al. (2006). "Human mesenchymal stem cells exert potent antitumorigenic effects in a model of Kaposi's sarcoma." *J Exp Med* 203(5): 1235-47.

Kidd, S., E. Spaeth, et al. (2008). "The (in) auspicious role of mesenchymal stromal cells in cancer: be it friend or foe." *Cytotherapy* 10(7): 657-67.

Kim, J. and P. Hematti (2009). "Mesenchymal stem cell-educated macrophages: a novel type of alternatively activated macrophages." *Exp Hematol* 37(12): 1445-53.

Kim, S. M., J. Y. Lim, et al. (2008). "Gene therapy using TRAIL-secreting human umbilical cord blood-derived mesenchymal stem cells against intracranial glioma." *Cancer Res* 68(23): 9614-23.

Klopp, A. H., A. Gupta, et al. (2010). "Dissecting a Discrepancy in the Literature: Do Mesenchymal Stem Cells Support or Suppress Tumor Growth?" *Stem Cells.*

Klopp, A. H., A. Gupta, et al. (2011). "Concise review: Dissecting a discrepancy in the literature: do mesenchymal stem cells support or suppress tumor growth?" *Stem Cells* 29(1): 11-9.

Koh, W., C. T. Sheng, et al. (2010). "Analysis of deep sequencing microRNA expression profile from human embryonic stem cells derived mesenchymal stem cells reveals possible role of let-7 microRNA family in downstream targeting of hepatic nuclear factor 4 alpha." *BMC Genomics* 11 Suppl 1: S6.

Kong, Q. F., B. Sun, et al. (2009). "BM stromal cells ameliorate experimental autoimmune myasthenia gravis by altering the balance of Th cells through the secretion of IDO." *Eur J Immunol* 39(3): 800-9.

Kopen, G. C., D. J. Prockop, et al. (1999). "Marrow stromal cells migrate throughout forebrain and cerebellum, and they differentiate into astrocytes after injection into neonatal mouse brains." *Proc Natl Acad Sci U S A* 96(19): 10711-6.

Krampera, M., L. Cosmi, et al. (2006). "Role for interferon-gamma in the immunomodulatory activity of human bone marrow mesenchymal stem cells." *Stem Cells* 24(2): 386-98.

Krampera, M., S. Glennie, et al. (2003). "Bone marrow mesenchymal stem cells inhibit the response of naive and memory antigen-specific T cells to their cognate peptide." *Blood* 101(9): 3722-9.

Krampera, M., A. Pasini, et al. (2006). "Regenerative and immunomodulatory potential of mesenchymal stem cells." *Curr Opin Pharmacol* 6(4): 435-41.

Kucerova, L., M. Matuskova, et al. "Tumor cell behaviour modulation by mesenchymal stromal cells." *Mol Cancer* 9: 129.

Lai, R. C., F. Arslan, et al. (2010). "Exosome secreted by MSC reduces myocardial ischemia/reperfusion injury." *Stem Cell Res* 4(3): 214-22.

Le Blanc, K., I. Rasmusson, et al. (2004). "Treatment of severe acute graft-versus-host disease with third party haploidentical mesenchymal stem cells." *Lancet* 363(9419): 1439-41.

Lee, R. H., A. A. Pulin, et al. (2009). "Intravenous hMSCs improve myocardial infarction in mice because cells embolized in lung are activated to secrete the anti-inflammatory protein TSG-6." *Cell Stem Cell* 5(1): 54-63.

Lepelletier, Y., S. Lecourt, et al. (2009). "Galectin-1 and semaphorin-3A are two soluble factors conferring T-cell immunosuppression to bone marrow mesenchymal stem cell." *Stem Cells Dev* 19(7): 1075-9.

Lin, G., R. Yang, et al. (2010). "Effects of transplantation of adipose tissue-derived stem cells on prostate tumor." *Prostate* 70(10): 1066-73.

Lopez Ponte, A., E. Marais, et al. (2007). "The in vitro migration capacity of human bone marrow mesenchymal stem cells: Comparison of chemokine and growth factor chemotactic activities." *Stem Cells.*

Lu, Y. R., Y. Yuan, et al. (2008). "The growth inhibitory effect of mesenchymal stem cells on tumor cells in vitro and in vivo." *Cancer Biol Ther* 7(2): 245-51.

Mader, E. K., Y. Maeyama, et al. (2009). "Mesenchymal stem cell carriers protect oncolytic measles viruses from antibody neutralization in an orthotopic ovarian cancer therapy model." *Clin Cancer Res* 15(23): 7246-55.

Maestroni, G. J., E. Hertens, et al. (1999). "Factor(s) from nonmacrophage bone marrow stromal cells inhibit Lewis lung carcinoma and B16 melanoma growth in mice." *Cell Mol Life Sci* 55(4): 663-7.

Maggini, J., G. Mirkin, et al. (2010). "Mouse bone marrow-derived mesenchymal stromal cells turn activated macrophages into a regulatory-like profile." *PLoS One* 5(2): e9252.

Mantovani, A., A. Sica, et al. (2007). "New vistas on macrophage differentiation and activation." *Eur J Immunol* 37(1): 14-6.

Mantovani, A., S. Sozzani, et al. (2002). "Macrophage polarization: tumor-associated macrophages as a paradigm for polarized M2 mononuclear phagocytes." *Trends Immunol* 23(11): 549-55.

Martinez, F. O., S. Gordon, et al. (2006). "Transcriptional profiling of the human monocyte-to-macrophage differentiation and polarization: new molecules and patterns of gene expression." *J Immunol* 177(10): 7303-11.

Meirelles Lda, S., A. M. Fontes, et al. (2009). "Mechanisms involved in the therapeutic properties of mesenchymal stem cells." *Cytokine Growth Factor Rev* 20(5-6): 419-27.

Mempel, M., V. Voelcker, et al. (2003). "Toll-like receptor expression in human keratinocytes: nuclear factor kappaB controlled gene activation by Staphylococcus aureus is toll-like receptor 2 but not toll-like receptor 4 or platelet activating factor receptor dependent." *J Invest Dermatol* 121(6): 1389-96.

Mezey, E., B. Mayer, et al. (2009). "Unexpected roles for bone marrow stromal cells (or MSCs): a real promise for cellular, but not replacement, therapy." *Oral Dis.*

Miggin, S. M. and L. A. O'Neill (2006). "New insights into the regulation of TLR signaling." *J Leukoc Biol* 80(2): 220-6.

Milner, C. M., V. A. Higman, et al. (2006). "TSG-6: a pluripotent inflammatory mediator?" *Biochem Soc Trans* 34(Pt 3): 446-50.

Mosser, D. M. and J. P. Edwards (2008). "Exploring the full spectrum of macrophage activation." *Nat Rev Immunol* 8(12): 958-69.

Mosser, D. M. and X. Zhang (2008). "Activation of murine macrophages." *Curr Protoc Immunol* Chapter 14: Unit 14 2.

Muehlberg, F. L., Y. H. Song, et al. (2009). "Tissue-resident stem cells promote breast cancer growth and metastasis." *Carcinogenesis* 30(4): 589-97.

Nagai, Y., K. P. Garrett, et al. (2006). "Toll-like receptors on hematopoietic progenitor cells stimulate innate immune system replenishment." *Immunity* 24(6): 801-12.

Najar, M., G. Raicevic, et al. "Mesenchymal stromal cells use PGE2 to modulate activation and proliferation of lymphocyte subsets: Combined comparison of adipose tissue, Wharton's Jelly and bone marrow sources." *Cell Immunol* 264(2): 171-9.

Nakamizo, A., F. Marini, et al. (2005). "Human bone marrow-derived mesenchymal stem cells in the treatment of gliomas." *Cancer Res* 65(8): 3307-18.

Nasef, A., N. Ashammakhi, et al. (2008). "Immunomodulatory effect of mesenchymal stromal cells: possible mechanisms." *Regen Med* 3(4): 531-46.

Nauta, A. J. and W. E. Fibbe (2007). "Immunomodulatory properties of mesenchymal stromal cells." *Blood* 110(10): 3499-506.

Nemeth, K., A. Keane-Myers, et al. (2010). "Bone marrow stromal cells use TGF-beta to suppress allergic responses in a mouse model of ragweed-induced asthma." *Proc Natl Acad Sci U S A* 107(12): 5652-7.

Nemeth, K., A. Leelahavanichkul, et al. (2009). "Bone marrow stromal cells attenuate sepsis via prostaglandin E(2)-dependent reprogramming of host macrophages to increase their interleukin-10 production." *Nat Med* 15(1): 42-9.

Nemeth, K., B. Mayer, et al. (2009). "Modulation of bone marrow stromal cell functions in infectious diseases by toll-like receptor ligands." *J Mol Med.*

Ohlsson, L. B., L. Varas, et al. (2003). "Mesenchymal progenitor cell-mediated inhibition of tumor growth in vivo and in vitro in gelatin matrix." *Exp Mol Pathol* 75(3): 248-55.

Opitz, C. A., U. M. Litzenburger, et al. (2009). "Toll-like receptor engagement enhances the immunosuppressive properties of human bone marrow-derived mesenchymal stem cells by inducing indoleamine-2,3-dioxygenase-1 via interferon-beta and protein kinase R." *Stem Cells* 27(4): 909-19.

Ortiz, L. A., M. Dutreil, et al. (2007). "Interleukin 1 receptor antagonist mediates the antiinflammatory and antifibrotic effect of mesenchymal stem cells during lung injury." *Proc Natl Acad Sci U S A* 104(26): 11002-7.

Otsu, K., S. Das, et al. (2009). "Concentration-dependent inhibition of angiogenesis by mesenchymal stem cells." *Blood* 113(18): 4197-205.

Patel, S. A., J. R. Meyer, et al. (2010). "Mesenchymal stem cells protect breast cancer cells through regulatory T cells: role of mesenchymal stem cell-derived TGF-beta." *J Immunol* 184(10): 5885-94.

Pevsner-Fischer, M., V. Morad, et al. (2006). "Toll-like receptors and their ligands control mesenchymal stem cell functions." *Blood %R 10.1182/blood-2006-06-028704*: blood-2006-06-028704.

Phinney, D. G., G. Kopen, et al. (1999). "Plastic adherent stromal cells from the bone marrow of commonly used strains of inbred mice: variations in yield, growth, and differentiation." *J Cell Biochem* 72(4): 570-85.

Phinney, D. G., G. Kopen, et al. (1999). "Donor variation in the growth properties and osteogenic potential of human marrow stromal cells." *J Cell Biochem* 75(3): 424-36.

Pittenger, M. F., A. M. Mackay, et al. (1999). "Multilineage potential of adult human mesenchymal stem cells." *Science* 284(5411): 143-7.

Prantl, L., F. Muehlberg, et al. "Adipose tissue-derived stem cells promote prostate tumor growth." *Prostate* 70(15): 1709-15.

Prasanna, S. J., D. Gopalakrishnan, et al. (2010). "Pro-inflammatory cytokines, IFNgamma and TNFalpha, influence immune properties of human bone marrow and Wharton jelly mesenchymal stem cells differentially." *PLoS One* 5(2): e9016.

Prockop, D. J. (2003). "Further proof of the plasticity of adult stem cells and their role in tissue repair." *J Cell Biol* 160(6): 807-9.

Prockop, D. J. (2009). "Repair of tissues by adult stem/progenitor cells (MSCs): controversies, myths, and changing paradigms." *Mol Ther* 17(6): 939-46.

Prockop, D. J. and J. Youn Oh (2011). "Mesenchymal Stem/Stromal Cells (MSCs): Role as Guardians of Inflammation." *Mol Ther.*

Qiao, L., Z. Xu, et al. (2008). "Suppression of tumorigenesis by human mesenchymal stem cells in a hepatoma model." *Cell Res* 18(4): 500-7.

Qiao, L., Z. L. Xu, et al. (2008). "Dkk-1 secreted by mesenchymal stem cells inhibits growth of breast cancer cells via depression of Wnt signalling." *Cancer Lett* 269(1): 67-77.

Rafei, M., J. Hsieh, et al. (2008). "Mesenchymal stromal cell-derived CCL2 suppresses plasma cell immunoglobulin production via STAT3 inactivation and PAX5 induction." *Blood* 112(13): 4991-8.

Raicevic, G., R. Rouas, et al. (2010). "Inflammation modifies the pattern and the function of Toll-like receptors expressed by human mesenchymal stromal cells." *Hum Immunol* 71(3): 235-44.

Ramasamy, R., H. Fazekasova, et al. (2007). "Mesenchymal stem cells inhibit dendritic cell differentiation and function by preventing entry into the cell cycle." *Transplantation* 83(1): 71-6.

Ren, C., S. Kumar, et al. (2008). "Therapeutic potential of mesenchymal stem cells producing interferon-alpha in a mouse melanoma lung metastasis model." *Stem Cells* 26(9): 2332-8.

Ren, C., S. Kumar, et al. (2008). "Cancer gene therapy using mesenchymal stem cells expressing interferon-beta in a mouse prostate cancer lung metastasis model." *Gene Ther* 15(21): 1446-53.

Ren, G., T. Li, et al. (2007). "Lentiviral RNAi-induced downregulation of adenosine kinase in human mesenchymal stem cell grafts: a novel perspective for seizure control." *Exp Neurol* 208(1): 26-37.

Ren, G., L. Zhang, et al. (2008). "Mesenchymal stem cell-mediated immunosuppression occurs via concerted action of chemokines and nitric oxide." *Cell Stem Cell* 2(2): 141-50.

Ribatti, D., B. Nico, et al. (2011). "Tryptase-positive mast cells and CD8-positive T cells in human endometrial cancer." *Pathol Int* 61(7): 442-4.

Roby, K. F., C. C. Taylor, et al. (2000). "Development of a syngeneic mouse model for events related to ovarian cancer." *Carcinogenesis* 21(4): 585-91.

Roddy, G. W., J. Y. Oh, et al. (2011). "Action at a Distance: Systemically Administered Adult Stem/Progenitor Cells (MSCs) Reduce Inflammatory Damage to the Cornea Without Engraftment and Primarily by Secretion of TSG-6." *Stem Cells*.

Romieu-Mourez, R., M. Francois, et al. (2009). "Cytokine modulation of TLR expression and activation in mesenchymal stromal cells leads to a proinflammatory phenotype." *J Immunol* 182(12): 7963-73.

Ryan, J. M., F. Barry, et al. (2007). "Interferon-gamma does not break, but promotes the immunosuppressive capacity of adult human mesenchymal stem cells." *Clin Exp Immunol* 149(2): 353-63.

Sabroe, I., R. C. Read, et al. (2003). "Toll-like receptors in health and disease: complex questions remain." *J Immunol* 171(4): 1630-5.

Sakaguchi, Y., I. Sekiya, et al. (2005). "Comparison of human stem cells derived from various mesenchymal tissues: superiority of synovium as a cell source." *Arthritis Rheum* 52(8): 2521-9.

Salem, H. K. and C. Thiemermann (2010). "Mesenchymal stromal cells: current understanding and clinical status." *Stem Cells* 28(3): 585-96.

Secchiero, P., S. Zorzet, et al. (2010). "Human bone marrow mesenchymal stem cells display anti-cancer activity in SCID mice bearing disseminated non-Hodgkin's lymphoma xenografts." *PLoS One* 5(6): e11140.

Selmani, Z., A. Naji, et al. (2009). "HLA-G is a crucial immunosuppressive molecule secreted by adult human mesenchymal stem cells." *Transplantation* 87(9 Suppl): S62-6.

Shi, C., T. Jia, et al. (2011). "Bone marrow mesenchymal stem and progenitor cells induce monocyte emigration in response to circulating toll-like receptor ligands." *Immunity* 34(4): 590-601.

Shinagawa, K., Y. Kitadai, et al. "Mesenchymal stem cells enhance growth and metastasis of colon cancer." *Int J Cancer* 127(10): 2323-33.

Singer, N. G. and A. I. Caplan (2011). "Mesenchymal stem cells: mechanisms of inflammation." *Annu Rev Pathol* 6: 457-78.

Sioud, M., A. Mobergslien, et al. (2010). "Evidence for the involvement of galectin-3 in mesenchymal stem cell suppression of allogeneic T-cell proliferation." *Scand J Immunol* 71(4): 267-74.

Sotiropoulou, P. A., S. A. Perez, et al. (2006). "Interactions between human mesenchymal stem cells and natural killer cells." *Stem Cells* 24(1): 74-85.

Studeny, M., F. C. Marini, et al. (2002). "Bone marrow-derived mesenchymal stem cells as vehicles for interferon-beta delivery into tumors." *Cancer Res* 62(13): 3603-8.

Studeny, M., F. C. Marini, et al. (2004). "Mesenchymal stem cells: potential precursors for tumor stroma and targeted-delivery vehicles for anticancer agents." *J Natl Cancer Inst* 96(21): 1593-603.

Sun, Y., L. Chen, et al. (2007). "Differentiation of bone marrow-derived mesenchymal stem cells from diabetic patients into insulin-producing cells in vitro." *Chin Med J (Engl)* 120(9): 771-6.

Sze, S. K., D. P. de Kleijn, et al. (2007). "Elucidating the secretion proteome of human embryonic stem cell-derived mesenchymal stem cells." *Mol Cell Proteomics* 6(10): 1680-9.

Tan, A., H. De La Pena, et al. (2010). "The application of exosomes as a nanoscale cancer vaccine." *Int J Nanomedicine* 5: 889-900.

Tolar, J., K. Le Blanc, et al. (2010). "Concise review: hitting the right spot with mesenchymal stromal cells." *Stem Cells* 28(8): 1446-55.

Tomchuck, S. L., K. J. Zwezdaryk, et al. (2008). "Toll-like receptors on human mesenchymal stem cells drive their migration and immunomodulating responses." *Stem Cells* 26(1): 99-107.

Triantafilou, K., M. Triantafilou, et al. (2001). "A CD14-independent LPS receptor cluster." *Nat Immunol* 2(4): 338-45.

Tse, W. T., J. D. Pendleton, et al. (2003). "Suppression of allogeneic T-cell proliferation by human marrow stromal cells: implications in transplantation." *Transplantation* 75(3): 389-97.

Uccelli, A., L. Moretta, et al. (2008). "Mesenchymal stem cells in health and disease." *Nat Rev Immunol* 8(9): 726-36.

Verreck, F. A., T. de Boer, et al. (2006). "Phenotypic and functional profiling of human proinflammatory type-1 and anti-inflammatory type-2 macrophages in response to microbial antigens and IFN-gamma- and CD40L-mediated costimulation." *J Leukoc Biol* 79(2): 285-93.

Volarevic, V., A. Al-Qahtani, et al. (2010). "Interleukin-1 receptor antagonist (IL-1Ra) and IL-1Ra producing mesenchymal stem cells as modulators of diabetogenesis." *Autoimmunity* 43(4): 255-63.

Waterman, R. S., S. L. Tomchuck, et al. (2010). "A new mesenchymal stem cell (MSC) paradigm: polarization into a pro-inflammatory MSC1 or an Immunosuppressive MSC2 phenotype." *PLoS One* 5(4): e10088.

Waterman R.S. and Betancourt A.M. (2011). "Distinct Roles for Mesenchymal Stem Cell Phenotypes: MSC1 and MSC2 in Tumors." *Cancer Research* Manuscript in Preparation.

Webber, J., R. Steadman, et al. (2010). "Cancer exosomes trigger fibroblast to myofibroblast differentiation." *Cancer Res* 70(23): 9621-30.

Weiss, D. J., I. Bertoncello, et al. (2011). "Stem cells and cell therapies in lung biology and lung diseases." *Proc Am Thorac Soc* 8(3): 223-72.

West, A. P., A. A. Koblansky, et al. (2006). "Recognition and signaling by toll-like receptors." *Annu Rev Cell Dev Biol* 22: 409-37.

Wisniewski, H. G. and J. Vilcek (2004). "Cytokine-induced gene expression at the crossroads of innate immunity, inflammation and fertility: TSG-6 and PTX3/TSG-14." *Cytokine Growth Factor Rev* 15(2-3): 129-46.

Wright, S. D. (1999). "Toll, a new piece in the puzzle of innate immunity." *J Exp Med* 189(4): 605-9.

Xu, G., L. Zhang, et al. (2007). "Immunosuppressive properties of cloned bone marrow mesenchymal stem cells." *Cell Res* 17(3): 240-8.

Yu, Y., H. Ren, et al. (2008). "[Differentiation of human umbilical cord blood-derived mesenchymal stem cells into chondroblast and osteoblasts]." *Sheng Wu Yi Xue Gong Cheng Xue Za Zhi* 25(6): 1385-9.

Zhang, Q. Z., W. R. Su, et al. (2010). "Human gingiva-derived mesenchymal stem cells elicit polarization of m2 macrophages and enhance cutaneous wound healing." *Stem Cells* 28(10): 1856-68.

Zhu, W., W. Xu, et al. (2006). "Mesenchymal stem cells derived from bone marrow favor tumor cell growth in vivo." *Exp Mol Pathol* 80(3): 267-74.

Zhu, Y., Z. Sun, et al. (2009). "Human mesenchymal stem cells inhibit cancer cell proliferation by secreting DKK-1." *Leukemia* 23(5): 925-33.

Zuckerman, K. S. and M. S. Wicha (1983). "Extracellular matrix production by the adherent cells of long-term murine bone marrow cultures." *Blood* 61(3): 540-7.

Zwezdaryk, K. J., S. B. Coffelt, et al. (2007). "Erythropoietin, a hypoxia-regulated factor, elicits a pro-angiogenic program in human mesenchymal stem cells." *Exp Hematol* 35(4): 640-52.

13

Visualisation of Myelomonocytic Cells in Tumors

Tatyana Chtanova[1,2] and Lai Guan Ng[3]
[1]*Garvan Institute of Medical Research,*
[2]*St. Vincent's Clinical School, Faculty of Medicine, University of New South Wales,*
[3]*Singapore Immunology Network (A*STAR),*
[1,2]*Australia*
[3]*Singapore*

1. Introduction

Emerging evidence suggests that inflammation is one of the major contributing factors for tumor development and progression. In this context, myelomonocytic cells, as key mediators of inflammatory responses, are essential components of the malignant microenvironment. Numerous studies have provided evidence to show that infiltrating tumor-associated macrophages (TAMs) play a critical role in promoting tumor growth. Similarly, human studies also revealed that a high frequency of infiltration by TAMs is associated with poor prognosis in many human cancers (reviewed in (Bingle et al. 2002)). There is now substantial evidence that tumor-associated neutrophils (TANs), like TAMs, have a critical role in tumor development (reviewed in (Gregory and Houghton 2011)). Despite major research efforts in this area, the role of neutrophils in cancer pathogenesis remains controversial. This is likely due to the fact that neutrophils can play a dual role in primary tumors: neutrophils can mediate tumor rejection but also promote angiogenesis and tissue remodelling which favour tumor growth. Furthermore, emerging evidence suggests that neutrophils may also have the ability to promote metastasis. Hence there is great potential for novel neutrophil-based therapies in the treatment of cancer if the contrasting roles of neutrophils in tumor growth are fully elucidated.

In this chapter, we will first briefly introduce the methodology of intravital multi-photon microscopy (MP-IVM), and then provide an overview of the application of MP-IVM for the visualisation of immune cells in tumor models. In addition, we will summarize how this technique has helped to reveal the unique interactive behavior of myelomonocytic cells, in particular neutrophils, during inflammatory responses. Our intention is to discuss the practical aspects of MP-IVM applications, with the aim of highlighting the features of MP microscopy that make it an ideal tool for investigating immune cell-tumor interactions *in vivo*.

2. Neutrophils in immunity

The immune system plays a well-established role in protecting the body from a wide variety of infectious diseases and in the elimination of endogenous tumors. In both cases, immediate but non-specific protection is mediated by the innate immune system, while the adaptive immune system provides more directed 'antigen-specific' responses and immune memory. Neutrophils, traditionally viewed as 'first wave' responders, can perform a diverse array of functions. Despite the central role of neutrophils in the acute inflammatory response, their role in immunity has only recently been "rediscovered". It is possible that neutrophils have been overlooked because they were considered to be too short-lived to play a significant role in the immune response as it evolved over time. Based on *in vitro* assays, neutrophils were thought to have a lifespan <1 day, and only 4-8 hours for activated neutrophils (Dancey et al. 1976). However, more rigorous analysis using *in vivo* deuterium-labeling has shown non-activated neutrophils to have a lifespan of 5.4 days under homeostatic conditions (Pillay et al. 2010). Although the major effector function of neutrophils is to induce rapid destruction of targets by phagocytosis and oxidative burst, emerging evidence suggests that neutrophils also play a crucial role in shaping the subsequent adaptive immune response. Neutrophils have a major effect on the recruitment and activation of additional immune cells via the release of soluble factors such as IL-8 and CXCL10. In certain circumstances, neutrophils were even shown to suppress the adaptive immune response by secreting anti-inflammatory cytokines (e.g. IL-10 and transforming growth factor-β) (reviewed in (Kasama et al. 2005)). Together, these data therefore point to a growing need to reassess the role of neutrophils in immunity.

3. Neutrophils in cancer

There is evidence to suggest that neutrophils play an important role in promoting human cancers. Clinical studies have shown that an increase in tumor-infiltrating neutrophils is correlated with a poorer outcome in bronchioalveolar carcinoma (Bellocq et al. 1998) and localized renal cell carcinomas (Jensen et al. 2009). Moreover, $CD11b^{+}$ $CD15^{+}$ neutrophils and monocytes with immunosuppressive properties were expanded in the peripheral blood of patients with malignant melanoma, and this correlated with disease stage (De Santo et al. 2010). Similarly, elevated numbers of peripheral blood neutrophils and monocytes have been associated with poor prognosis in patients with metastatic melanoma (Schmidt et al. 2005). Despite the clinical associations reported, the precise role of neutrophils in cancer remains controversial (Houghton et al. 2010; Granot et al. 2011).

There is evidence from animal studies that under some circumstances neutrophils can contribute to tumor rejection whilst under other conditions neutrophils can promote tumor growth. These two opposing phenotypes have been termed N1 and N2 by analogy to M1 and M2 polarised macrophages (Fridlender et al. 2009). Under "N1" conditions, neutrophil recruitment and activation can result in direct tumor cell killing by reactive oxygen species and further recruitment and activation of monocytes, macrophages, dendritic cells, natural killer and cytotoxic T cells (Fridlender et al. 2009). Under "N2" conditions, however, the non-specific tissue destruction and tissue remodelling induced by neutrophil-derived metalloproteases can create space, and angiogenesis induced by neutrophil-derived IL-8 and VEGF can ensure ongoing supply of oxygen and nutrients to support further tumor growth and also promote metastasis (reviewed in (Noonan et al. 2008; Gregory and Houghton 2011)). Immunosuppressive cytokines such as IL-10 and TGF-beta secreted by neutrophils can dampen anti-tumor adaptive immune responses. Furthermore, neutrophil products, such as neutrophil elastase, can directly promote tumor growth (Houghton et al. 2010).

Consistent with this, depletion of Ly6G (Gr-1) positive neutrophils was shown to inhibit tumor growth and angiogenesis in the B16-F10 mouse melanoma model (Jablonska et al. 2010). It is likely that the type of neutrophil response against a tumor is highly dependent on distinct temporal and anatomical factors. Consistent with this view, a study using melanoma cell lines transduced with the neutrophil chemoattractant IL-8 showed a biphasic dose-response curve between the number of infiltrating neutrophils and tumor growth (Schaider et al. 2003). Thus, it is possible that in the early stages of tumor development, neutrophils have an anti-tumor N1 phenotype and that later on neutrophils are conditioned to adopt a pro-tumor N2 phenotype.

Like other cells of the immune system, neutrophils appear to rely on cues from the microenvironment to regulate their functional plasticity, i.e. switching between anti-tumor and tumor-promoting functions. For instance, TGF-β can skew the population towards N2 phenotype, whilst blockade of this molecule induces an anti-tumor N1 phenotype (Fridlender et al. 2009). Inhibition of PPAR-α signals was found to switch tumor-promoting neutrophils into neutrophils with anti-tumor activities (Kaipainen et al. 2007). Delineation of neutrophil behaviour in different settings is therefore vital to our understanding of the precise role that these cells play in tumor growth and progression as well as to assess their potential as targets for therapeutic intervention.

4. Neutrophils in tumor metastasis

In addition to their role in primary tumors, neutrophils may also significantly influence tumor metastasis. Tumor metastasis is strongly associated with reduced survival of the host, making this process an important target for therapeutic intervention. Metastasis is a non-random process in which tumor cells acquire the capacity to seed particular organs, a phenomenon first observed more than 100 years ago by Stephen Paget and known as the 'seed' and 'soil' hypothesis (Paget 1889). Evidence that immunological factors (for example, cytokines, chemokines, and proteases) may direct metastasising cells to specific organs by creating permissive microenvironments for the tumor cells, led to the development of the 'pre-metastatic niche' concept (reviewed in (Kaplan et al. 2006)). Neutrophils, together with other bone marrow derived cells, have been implicated in establishing such niches (Yamamoto et al. 2008), although the precise role of neutrophils remains to be elucidated. Neutrophils may play an important role during tumor metastasis by establishing specific microenvironments that promote tumor cell 'seeding' of secondary sites. For instance, neutrophils can release tissue-remodelling factors such as matrix metalloproteases, which may assist in the establishment of a physiological niche, and also secrete chemoattractants that may recruit other cells. Interestingly a recent study by Granot et al. suggests that at least in certain conditions neutrophils 'entrained' by the tumor may actually inhibit metastasis by generating hydrogen peroxide (Granot et al. 2011). This further emphasises the potential complexity of neutrophil functions in cancer and highlights the need for further investigation.

5. Application of multi-photon microscopy in tumor-related research

Imaging has become an important tool in cancer research. Perhaps one of the biggest advancements in recent years is in the field of fluorescence-based imaging. With the availability of a wide array of fluorescent reporter mice and the rapid development of cell- and tissue-specific labeling techniques (reviewed in (Germain et al. 2006; Hickman et al.

2009)), researchers can now address important questions in cancer biology *in vivo*. One fluorescence-based imaging approach that has received a lot of attention in recent years is MP microscopy. This technique has rapidly evolved beyond merely observational to address complex biological questions at a quantitative level. It is now possible to perform dynamic, multi-dimensional imaging to simultaneously track cell populations at the single cell level in living tissues or organs (Cahalan and Parker 2008). Consequently, anatomical, cellular, and molecular information can be obtained through this approach. For more detailed technical information about the general setup of a MP microscope, please refer to these publications (Germain et al. 2006; Phan and Bullen 2010).

5.1 *In vivo* imaging of tumor development using multi-photon microscopy

Over the past few years, a number of laboratories have applied MP microscopy to investigate tumor-related biological questions. In 2001, a seminal study from Jain laboratory showed the applicability of MP imaging for studying tumor cell development *in vivo* for the first time. In this study, MP-IVM was employed to investigate cell behavior in a dorsal skin fold chamber tumor model in mice. Jain and colleagues visualized tumor cell localization, angiogenesis, as well as leukocyte-blood vessel interactions and vessel permeability with high spatial and temporal resolution (Brown et al. 2001). Since then this approach has been adopted by researchers in the field of tumor biology to study tumor cell migration and tissue invasion, as well as angiogenesis, matrix remodeling and metastasis (reviewed in (Zal and Chodaczek 2010)).

5.2 *In vivo* imaging of TAMs

Although macrophages have been implicated in many aspects of tumor development, the spatial and temporal regulation of TAMs in the context of the tumor microenvironment is still poorly understood. In 2007, the Condeelis lab provided detailed information about the localization of macrophages and tumor cells in relation to blood vessels in a three-dimensional (3D) context *in vivo*. TAMs were shown to be predominantly located in the tumor margin. In addition, Condeelis and colleagues reported the presence of a population of perivascular macrophages deep within tumors (Wyckoff et al. 2007). Importantly, this study provided evidence to support the notion that abluminally localized perivascular macrophages are important for the intravasation of tumor cells (Wyckoff et al. 2007). In another study of MP imaging of TAMs, Pittet laboratory demonstrated a novel method to specifically label M2 polarized TAMs with nanoparticles (AMTA680), thereby allowing the tracking of this subset of TAMs *in vivo* by MP-IVM (Leimgruber et al. 2009).

5.3 *In vivo* imaging of tumor killing cytotoxic cells

Arguably, the best-characterised immune imaging model during the early days of MP microscopy was that of B and T cell behaviour in lymph nodes. Most of these studies mainly focused on naïve T cells and their locomotion within the lymph node during priming (Bousso and Robey 2003; Mempel et al. 2004; Miller et al. 2002). Results from these experiments provided important framework for the subsequent studies of effector cells within target tissues. It is now well established that effector cells such as CD8 cytotoxic T cells (CTLs) and NK cells play a crucial role in host defence against malignant cells and viruses. In early MP imaging studies, three independent laboratories analysed the behaviour of infiltrating cytotoxic CD8+ T cells (CTLs) in solid tumors (Boissonnas et al. 2007; Breart et al. 2008; Mrass et al. 2006)). These studies revealed for the first time the migratory and interactive behaviour of intratumoral CTLs at different stages of tumor development, for example during progressing or regressing stages. One key observation was that CTL motility and long lasting interactions with tumor cells were dependent on the presence of cognate antigen (Boissonnas et al. 2007; Mrass et al. 2006). In addition, the Weninger lab showed that physical interaction between CTLs and tumor cells preceded the initiation of the killing of the tumor cells (Mrass et al. 2006). A study by the Bousso lab further examined the kinetics of tumor cell killing by CTLs *in vivo*. Surprisingly, this study demonstrated that it required on average 6 hours for a CTL to destroy one tumor cell, which was much longer than expected based on previous *in vitro* results (Breart et al. 2008). A subsequent study from the same lab showed that Natural Killer (NK) cell dissemination and motility within the tumor were highly dependent on the presence of its ligand, Rae-1β. Although it is known that both CTLs and NK cells mediate similar cytotoxic activity (Russell and Ley 2002), this study showed that NK cells had a distinct intratumoral behaviour compared to CTLs. Tumor infiltrating NK cells only formed transient contacts with target cells after initial interaction, whereas CTLs normally establish long lasting contacts that can last for more than 20 minutes (Deguine et al. 2011).

6. Dynamic view of neutrophil responses

As outlined in the previous section, there is now a wealth of knowledge about the behaviour of adaptive immune cells in primary tumors. Neutrophil dynamics in tumors and other inflammatory settings remain largely unexplored. However, recent studies utilizing intravital microscopy have provided some insight into the mechanisms of neutrophil adhesion and transmigration across the endothelium into the tissues, as well as the dynamics of neutrophil interstitial migration to or within their target sites (McDonald and Kubes 2011). Specifically intravital imaging studies including infection models in the skin, lymph nodes, and lungs have provided us with the first clues as to how neutrophil interstitial migration is regulated *in vivo* (Chtanova et al. 2008; Kreisel et al. 2010; Peters et al. 2008; Zinselmeyer et al. 2008). A seminal study by Sacks and colleagues provided the first *in vivo* observations of neutrophil recruitment from the blood vessels into the skin in response to *Leishmania Major* transmitted by sand bite (Peters et al. 2008). Interestingly, neutrophils readily internalised the parasites but failed to destroy them, thus aiding parasite dissemination by acting as Trojan horses.

Another important step in characterising neutrophil function *in vivo* came from a study of the immune response to *Toxoplasma gondii* infection in mice. Analysis of neutrophil behaviour in toxoplasma-infected lymph nodes revealed a strikingly coordinated pattern of migration with multiple cells simultaneously responding to an external signal to coalesce into dynamic swarms (Chtanova et al. 2008). Interestingly, neutrophil swarm formation coincided in space and time with the removal of the underlying tissue suggesting that swarm formation may present a mechanism for large scale tissue remodelling. This process could in turn provide a means for early and rapid removal of infected tissues preventing pathogen dissemination. Furthermore, these neutrophils also destroyed infected CD169$^+$ subcapsular sinus (SCS) macrophages found in the lymph nodes. These SCS macrophages play a key role in sampling antigen from the periphery drained by the lymph, and are responsible for antigen presentation to B cells (Phan et al. 2007), CD8$^+$ T cells (Chtanova et al. 2009) and NK T cells (Barral et al. 2010). Thus, the results of this study imply that not only can neutrophils clear infected cells but may also indiscriminately destroy cells that are important for the initiation of anti-pathogen immune responses. Dynamic clustering (or swarming) of neutrophils was also observed in lung tissues in response to bacterial challenge (Kreisel et al. 2010)

These findings suggest that specific molecular cues guide neutrophils through the compacted interstitial tissues towards the foci of infection/inflammation. Indeed, a recent study by Kubes lab using in vivo confocal microscopy to examine sterile liver injury has uncovered several molecular pathways involved in neutrophil sensing of injury. The authors showed that the exit of neutrophils from the circulation depended on ATP from the necrotic cells, and the Nlrp3 inflammasome, whereas migration towards the site of injury required a chemokine gradient and formyl-peptide signals as guidance cues (McDonald et al. 2011).

Using MP-IVM, we have recently characterised the cascade of events and molecular cues that guide neutrophils through the extravascular space within skin (Figure 1). In this study, we demonstrated that following confined physical injury, neutrophil accumulation at the injury site takes place in three distinct sequential steps (Ng et al. 2011). Initially, rare scouting neutrophils migrate in a directional manner towards the injury site. This is followed by the amplified attraction of additional waves of neutrophils in a highly

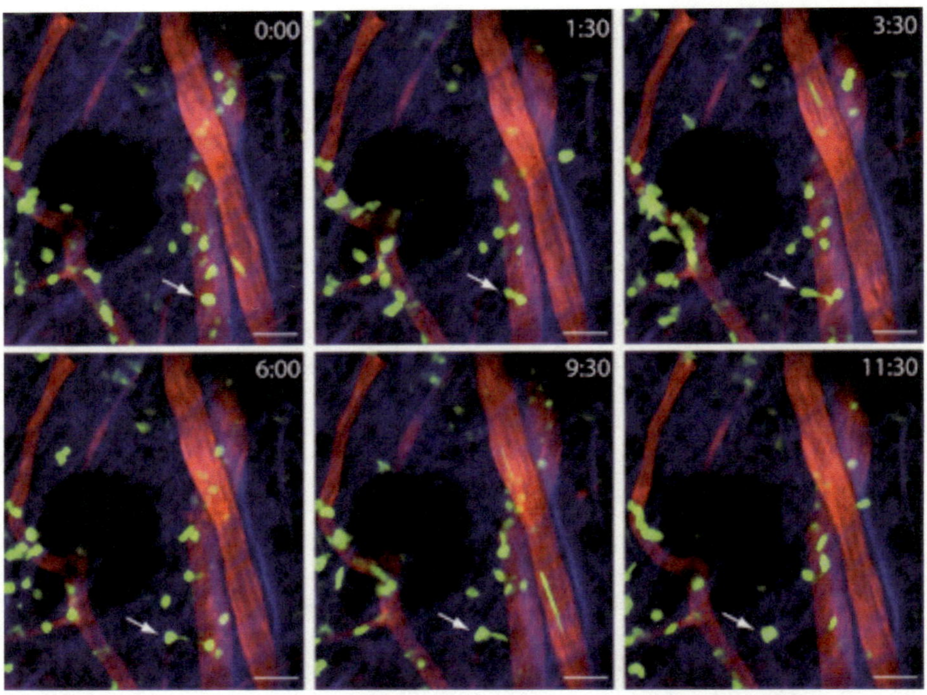

Fig. 1. Multiphoton imaging of neutrophil responses in Lysozyme-GFP mice

Time-lapse images showing the applicability of Lysozyme-GFP mice for studying neutrophil dynamic *in vivo* (skin), allowing co-visualization of neutrophils (green, tagged by green fluorescent protein), blood vessels (red, highlighted by Evans blue injection) and dermal collagen fibers (blue, detected through second harmonic generation signals). White arrows indicate the migratory path of an extravasating neutrophil over time. Time: min:sec. Scale bar: 30 μm.

synchronized manner, and finally there is a stabilisation of the neutrophil cluster around the injury. Interestingly, while neutrophil migration during steady-state conditions and during the scouting phase depended on G protein-coupled receptor signaling, the amplification phase was sensitive to interference with the cyclic adenosine diphosphate ribose pathway (Ng et al. 2011).

Together, these studies show that neutrophil responses to pathogen or injury are regulated by complex mechanisms. These observations also clearly demonstrate that neutrophil responses are highly dependent on the nature of the initial stimuli, injury versus pathogenic. Understanding the molecular cues governing the distinct neutrophil behaviour in response to different stimuli may lead to new knowledge about neutrophil function.

7. Mouse models and experimental considerations

As outlined above are heavily involved in immune responses to pathogens and injury, and that their recruitment and behaviour are intricately controlled. Although neutrophil dynamics in the context of tumors remain to be visualised, it is likely that a similarly complex picture will emerge for neutrophils inside primary tumors and at potential sites of metastasis. Here we will provide information about the tools available for *in vivo* microscopic examination of neutrophil-tumor interactions. In addition, we will also several experimental considerations in applying MP microscopy to visualise intratumoral cellular activities.

7.1 Visualizing neutrophils, blood vessels and extracellular matrix structures in tumors

Currently, there is a wide array of fluorescent transgenic mice suitable for MP microscopy. Lysozyme-GFP (Faust et al. 2000) and MacGreen-GFP mice (MacDonald et al. 2005) are the most widely used mice for direct visualisation of neutrophils *in vivo*. Although all myeloid cells in these mice express GFP, neutrophils express the highest amount of the fluorescent protein (Ng et al. 2011), which makes them distinguishable from monocytes or macrophages based on the fluorescent intensity and cell morphology. To visualize blood vessels, quantum dots, fluorescent dextrans and lectins or Evans blue dye can be injected intravenously (Ng et al. 2011; Hickman et al. 2009; Germain et al. 2006; Li et al. 2012). Furthermore, changes in the extracellular matrix within tumors can be monitored by second and third harmonic generation signals (Friedl et al. 2007). Alternatively cells of implanted tumors can be labeled by genetically expressing a fluorescent protein of choice (Mrass et al. 2006; Wyckoff et al. 2007).

7.2 *In vivo* versus explanted tumor imaging

Most tumor imaging studies have been performed *in vivo*, either through skin flaps or the skin window chamber approach (Wyckoff et al. 2007; Boissonnas et al. 2007). Although these approaches are useful, they only allow a limited field of view of the tumor cells due to physical constraints. Furthermore, some tumors are inaccessible. These limitations can be circumvented by using tumor explant models (Mrass et al. 2008; Mrass et al. 2006), which allow imaging of multiple fields of view per explanted tumor. The ability to image multiple regions is important, as tumor tissues are highly heterogeneous in composition in terms of tumor cell density, extracellular matrix remodeling and angiogenesis, as well as cellular infiltration. However, important drawbacks of this approach include lack of blood circulation and lymphatic flow, as well as innervations.

7.3 Choice of tumor models

When selecting an appropriate tumor model for MP imaging in addition to the biological question being asked, it is important to review several technical considerations. For instance, we have observed that pigmented tissues and cells are highly sensitive to MP illumination due to their high MP absorption, and contribute to the generation of non-specific high intensity signals ("speckling") (Ng et al. 2011; Li et al. 2012). This speckling not only compromises the image quality, but also induces heat injury that can trigger an inflammatory response and severely damage the tissue. We therefore recommend the use of non-pigmented tumor models in order to minimise artifacts caused by photodamage during imaging.

8. Neutrophil dynamics in tumors – A prospective

Great strides have been made in understanding the function of different immune cell subsets in cancer. Intravital MP imaging has played an important role in this process, and has allowed us to view CD8 T cells and NK cells killing tumor cells, and TAMs aiding tumor intravasation in vivo. However, many more questions remain unanswered. This is particularly true with regard to neutrophils. Recent technological advances in MP microscopy together with an ever-growing array of biological tools now make it possible to unravel the role that neutrophils may play in tumor growth and metastasis by directing visualising their activities within their native environment.

Intravital imaging experiments have already demonstrated neutrophil recruitment and subsequent swarming in inflamed tissues during immune responses to injury and infection. We anticipate that a similarly complex picture will emerge for neutrophils inside primary tumors and also at potential sites of metastasis. We expect that N1 and N2 neutrophils might exhibit different patterns of behaviour. For instance, neutrophils of the anti-tumor phenotype might function as they do in infection, that is, by initiating cell recruitment followed by a coordinated response to external signals with formation of dynamic swarms, which remodel underlying tissue. On the other hand a change in neutrophil behaviour might reflect a conversion to a pro-tumor phenotype. Pro-tumor neutrophils maybe less motile reflecting their angiogenesis-promoting role. Thus, by directly observing the behaviour of these cells in tumors, we will be able to gain unique insight into their role in tumor growth.

9. Conclusion

In conclusion, although neutrophils are frequently dismissed as short-lived 'foot-soldiers' of immunity, recent studies point to an important contribution of these cells to cancer. Furthermore, the apparent functional plasticity of neutrophils makes them a great target for therapeutic intervention and further highlights the need to unravel the role of neutrophils in cancer pathogenesis. We envision that MP imaging will not only contribute to the basic knowledge related to tumor development, but also will gradually become an important tool for preclinical studies for assessing drug delivery to tumor cells as well as the effects of therapeutic agents on immune and tumor cells.

10. Acknowledgement

We would like to thank Dr. Jo Keeble for critical comments on the manuscript. Lysozyme-GFP mice were kindly provided by Dr. Thomas Graf and neutrophil images were provided by Dr. Yilin Wang.

11. References

Barral P, Polzella P, Bruckbauer A, van Rooijen N, Besra GS, Cerundolo V, Batista FD (2010) CD169(+) macrophages present lipid antigens to mediate early activation of iNKT cells in lymph nodes. *Nat Immunol* 11 (4):pp. 303-312

Bellocq A, Antoine M, Flahault A, Philippe C, Crestani B, Bernaudin JF, Mayaud C, Milleron B, Baud L, Cadranel J (1998) Neutrophil alveolitis in bronchioloalveolar carcinoma: induction by tumor-derived interleukin-8 and relation to clinical outcome. *Am J Pathol* 152 (1):pp. 83-92

Bingle L, Brown NJ, Lewis CE (2002) The role of tumor-associated macrophages in tumor progression: implications for new anticancer therapies. *J Pathol* 196 (3):pp. 254-265

Boissonnas A, Fetler L, Zeelenberg IS, Hugues S, Amigorena S (2007) In vivo imaging of cytotoxic T cell infiltration and elimination of a solid tumor. *J Exp Med* 204 (2):pp. 345-356

Bousso P, Robey E (2003) Dynamics of CD8+ T cell priming by dendritic cells in intact lymph nodes. *Nat Immunol* 4 (6):pp. 579-585

Breart B, Lemaitre F, Celli S, Bousso P (2008) Two-photon imaging of intratumoral CD8+ T cell cytotoxic activity during adoptive T cell therapy in mice. *J Clin Invest* 118 (4):pp. 1390-1397

Brown EB, Campbell RB, Tsuzuki Y, Xu L, Carmeliet P, Fukumura D, Jain RK (2001) In vivo measurement of gene expression, angiogenesis and physiological function in tumors using multiphoton laser scanning microscopy. *Nat Med* 7 (7):pp. 864-868

Cahalan MD, Parker I (2008) Choreography of cell motility and interaction dynamics imaged by two-photon microscopy in lymphoid organs. *Annu Rev Immunol* 26:pp. 585-626

Chtanova T, Han SJ, Schaeffer M, van Dooren GG, Herzmark P, Striepen B, Robey EA (2009) Dynamics of T cell, antigen-presenting cell, and pathogen interactions during recall responses in the lymph node. *Immunity* 31 (2):pp. 342-355

Chtanova T, Schaeffer M, Han SJ, van Dooren GG, Nollmann M, Herzmark P, Chan SW, Satija H, Camfield K, Aaron H, Striepen B, Robey EA (2008) Dynamics of neutrophil migration in lymph nodes during infection. *Immunity* 29 (3):pp. 487-496

Dancey GF, Levine AE, Shapiro BM (1976) The NADH dehydrogenase of the respiratory chain of Escherichia coli. I. Properties of the membrane-bound enzyme, its solubilization, and purification to near homogeneity. *J Biol Chem* 251 (19):pp. 5911-5920

De Santo C, Arscott R, Booth S, Karydis I, Jones M, Asher R, Salio M, Middleton M, Cerundolo V (2010) Invariant NKT cells modulate the suppressive activity of IL-10-secreting neutrophils differentiated with serum amyloid A. *Nat Immunol* 11 (11):pp. 1039-1046

Deguine J, Breart B, Lemaitre F, Di Santo JP, Bousso P (2011) Intravital imaging reveals distinct dynamics for natural killer and CD8(+) T cells during tumor regression. *Immunity* 33 (4):pp. 632-644

Faust N, Varas F, Kelly LM, Heck S, Graf T (2000) Insertion of enhanced green fluorescent protein into the lysozyme gene creates mice with green fluorescent granulocytes and macrophages. *Blood* 96 (2):pp. 719-726

Fridlender ZG, Sun J, Kim S, Kapoor V, Cheng G, Ling L, Worthen GS, Albelda SM (2009) Polarization of tumor-associated neutrophil phenotype by TGF-beta: "N1" versus "N2" TAN. *Cancer Cell* 16 (3):pp. 183-194

Friedl P, Wolf K, von Andrian UH, Harms G (2007) Biological second and third harmonic generation microscopy. *Curr Protoc Cell Biol* Chapter 4: Unit 4 15

Germain RN, Miller MJ, Dustin ML, Nussenzweig MC (2006) Dynamic imaging of the immune system: progress, pitfalls and promise. *Nat Rev Immunol* 6 (7):pp. 497-507

Granot Z, Henke E, Comen EA, King TA, Norton L, Benezra R (2011) Tumor entrained neutrophils inhibit seeding in the premetastatic lung. *Cancer Cell* 20 (3):pp. 300-314

Gregory AD, Houghton AM (2011) Tumor-associated neutrophils: new targets for cancer therapy. *Cancer Res* 71 (7):pp. 2411-2416

Hickman HD, Bennink JR, Yewdell JW (2009) Caught in the act: intravital multiphoton microscopy of host-pathogen interactions. *Cell Host Microbe* 5 (1):pp. 13-21

Houghton AM, Rzymkiewicz DM, Ji H, Gregory AD, Egea EE, Metz HE, Stolz DB, Land SR, Marconcini LA, Kliment CR, Jenkins KM, Beaulieu KA, Mouded M, Frank SJ, Wong KK, Shapiro SD (2010) Neutrophil elastase-mediated degradation of IRS-1 accelerates lung tumor growth. *Nat Med* 16 (2):pp. 219-223

Jablonska J, Leschner S, Westphal K, Lienenklaus S, Weiss S (2010) Neutrophils responsive to endogenous IFN-beta regulate tumor angiogenesis and growth in a mouse tumor model. *J Clin Invest* 120 (4):pp. 1151-1164

Jensen HK, Donskov F, Marcussen N, Nordsmark M, Lundbeck F, von der Maase H (2009) Presence of intratumoral neutrophils is an independent prognostic factor in localized renal cell carcinoma. *J Clin Oncol* 27 (28):pp. 4709-4717

Kaipainen A, Kieran MW, Huang S, Butterfield C, Bielenberg D, Mostoslavsky G, Mulligan R, Folkman J, Panigrahy D (2007) PPARalpha deficiency in inflammatory cells suppresses tumor growth. *PLoS ONE* 2 (2):pp. e260

Kaplan RN, Psaila B, Lyden D (2006) Bone marrow cells in the 'pre-metastatic niche': within bone and beyond. *Cancer Metastasis Rev* 25 (4):pp. 521-529

Kasama T, Miwa Y, Isozaki T, Odai T, Adachi M, Kunkel SL (2005) Neutrophil-derived cytokines: potential therapeutic targets in inflammation. *Curr Drug Targets Inflamm Allergy* 4 (3):pp. 273-279

Kreisel D, Nava RG, Li W, Zinselmeyer BH, Wang B, Lai J, Pless R, Gelman AE, Krupnick AS, Miller MJ (2010) In vivo two-photon imaging reveals monocyte-dependent neutrophil extravasation during pulmonary inflammation. *Proc Natl Acad Sci U S A* 107 (42):pp. 18073-18078

Leimgruber A, Berger C, Cortez-Retamozo V, Etzrodt M, Newton AP, Waterman P, Figueiredo JL, Kohler RH, Elpek N, Mempel TR, Swirski FK, Nahrendorf M, Weissleder R, Pittet MJ (2009) Behavior of endogenous tumor-associated macrophages assessed in vivo using a functionalized nanoparticle. *Neoplasia* 11 (5):pp. 459-468, 452 p following 468

Li JL, Goh CC, Keeble JL, Qin JS, Roediger B, Jain R, Wang Y, Chew WK, Weninger W, Ng LG (2012) Intravital multiphoton imaging of immune responses in the mouse ear skin. *Nature Protocols* 7 (2):pp.221-234

MacDonald KP, Rowe V, Bofinger HM, Thomas R, Sasmono T, Hume DA, Hill GR (2005) The colony-stimulating factor 1 receptor is expressed on dendritic cells during differentiation and regulates their expansion. *J Immunol* 175 (3):pp. 1399-1405

McDonald B, Kubes P (2011) Cellular and molecular choreography of neutrophil recruitment to sites of sterile inflammation. *J Mol Med (Berl)* 89 (11):pp. 1079-1088

McDonald B, Pittman K, Menezes GB, Hirota SA, Slaba I, Waterhouse CC, Beck PL, Muruve DA, Kubes P (2011) Intravascular danger signals guide neutrophils to sites of sterile inflammation. *Science* 330 (6002):pp. 362-366

Mempel TR, Henrickson SE, Von Andrian UH (2004) T-cell priming by dendritic cells in lymph nodes occurs in three distinct phases. *Nature* 427 (6970):pp. 154-159

Miller MJ, Wei SH, Parker I, Cahalan MD (2002) Two-photon imaging of lymphocyte motility and antigen response in intact lymph node. *Science* 296 (5574):pp. 1869-1873

Mrass P, Kinjyo I, Ng LG, Reiner SL, Pure E, Weninger W (2008) CD44 mediates successful interstitial navigation by killer T cells and enables efficient antitumor immunity. *Immunity* 29 (6):pp. 971-985

Mrass P, Takano H, Ng LG, Daxini S, Lasaro MO, Iparraguirre A, Cavanagh LL, von Andrian UH, Ertl HC, Haydon PG, Weninger W (2006) Random migration precedes stable target cell interactions of tumor-infiltrating T cells. *J Exp Med* 203 (12):pp. 2749-2761

Ng LG, Qin JS, Roediger B, Wang Y, Jain R, Cavanagh LL, Smith AL, Jones CA, de Veer M, Grimbaldeston MA, Meeusen EN, Weninger W (2011) Visualizing the neutrophil response to sterile tissue injury in mouse dermis reveals a three-phase cascade of events. *J Invest Dermatol* 131 (10):pp. 2058-2068

Noonan DM, De Lerma Barbaro A, Vannini N, Mortara L, Albini A (2008) Inflammation, inflammatory cells and angiogenesis: decisions and indecisions. *Cancer Metastasis Rev* 27 (1):pp. 31-40

Paget S (1889) The distribution of secondary growths in cancer of the breast. 1889. *Cancer Metastasis Rev* 8 (2):pp. 98-101

Peters NC, Egen JG, Secundino N, Debrabant A, Kimblin N, Kamhawi S, Lawyer P, Fay MP, Germain RN, Sacks D (2008) In vivo imaging reveals an essential role for neutrophils in leishmaniasis transmitted by sand flies. *Science* 321 (5891):pp. 970-974

Phan TG, Bullen A (2010) Practical intravital two-photon microscopy for immunological research: faster, brighter, deeper. *Immunol Cell Biol* 88 (4):pp. 438-444

Phan TG, Grigorova I, Okada T, Cyster JG (2007) Subcapsular encounter and complement-dependent transport of immune complexes by lymph node B cells. *Nat Immunol* 8 (9):pp. 992-1000

Pillay J, den Braber I, Vrisekoop N, Kwast LM, de Boer RJ, Borghans JA, Tesselaar K, Koenderman L (2010) In vivo labeling with 2H2O reveals a human neutrophil lifespan of 5.4 days. *Blood* 116 (4):pp. 625-627

Russell JH, Ley TJ (2002) Lymphocyte-mediated cytotoxicity. *Annu Rev Immunol* 20:pp. 323-370

Schaider H, Oka M, Bogenrieder T, Nesbit M, Satyamoorthy K, Berking C, Matsushima K, Herlyn M (2003) Differential response of primary and metastatic melanomas to neutrophils attracted by IL-8. *Int J Cancer* 103 (3):pp. 335-343

Schmidt H, Bastholt L, Geertsen P, Christensen IJ, Larsen S, Gehl J, von der Maase H (2005) Elevated neutrophil and monocyte counts in peripheral blood are associated with poor survival in patients with metastatic melanoma: a prognostic model. *Br J Cancer* 93 (3):pp. 273-278

Wyckoff JB, Wang Y, Lin EY, Li JF, Goswami S, Stanley ER, Segall JE, Pollard JW, Condeelis J (2007) Direct visualization of macrophage-assisted tumor cell intravasation in mammary tumors. *Cancer Res* 67 (6):pp. 2649-2656

Yamamoto M, Kikuchi H, Ohta M, Kawabata T, Hiramatsu Y, Kondo K, Baba M, Kamiya K, Tanaka T, Kitagawa M, Konno H (2008) TSU68 prevents liver metastasis of colon cancer xenografts by modulating the premetastatic niche. *Cancer Res* 68 (23):pp. 9754-9762

Zal T, Chodaczek G (2010) Intravital imaging of anti-tumor immune response and the tumor microenvironment. *Semin Immunopathol* 32 (3):pp. 305-317

Zinselmeyer BH, Lynch JN, Zhang X, Aoshi T, Miller MJ (2008) Video-rate two-photon imaging of mouse footpad - a promising model for studying leukocyte recruitment dynamics during inflammation. *Inflamm Res* 57 (3):pp. 93-96